# TOBACCO USE

## HEALTH & BEHAVIOUR

# TOBACCO USE
## HEALTH & BEHAVIOUR

**R.C. Jiloha**

*Director Professor and Head*
Department of Psychiatry
Maulana Azad Medical College
G.B. Pant Hospital
New Delhi 110002, India

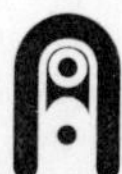

PUBLISHING FOR ONE WORLD

**NEW AGE INTERNATIONAL (P) LIMITED, PUBLISHERS**

New Delhi • Bangalore • Chennai • Cochin • Guwahati • Hyderabad
Jalandhar • Kolkata • Lucknow • Mumbai • Ranchi
Visit us at **www.newagepublishers.com**

Published by New Age International (P) Ltd., Publishers
First Edition: 2008

---



**ISBN 13: 978-81-224-2250-4**

**ISBN 10: 81-224-2250-0**

**Rs. 395.00**

**C-07-12-2150**

Printed in India at Ramprintograph, Delhi.
Typeset in-house

**PUBLISHING FOR ONE WORLD**

**NEW AGE INTERNATIONAL (P) LIMITED, PUBLISHERS**
4835/24, Ansari Road, Daryaganj, New Delhi - 110002
Visit us at **www.newagepublishers.com**

# Preface

This book gives a comprehensive account of tobacco use, particularly with respect to its addictive potential, harmful effects, treatment and control. This volume is designed as a preliminary step in the effort to acquire and disseminate more knowledge about these experiences. By allowing the experiences of the past to inform the present, and by clarifying the relationship between the two, history greatly expands our knowledge of the some of the most fundamental issues surrounding tobacco use. Tobacco use behaviour and the responses it elicits are dynamic, multifaceted phenomena which are constantly changing and which cannot be understood apart from the socio-cultural and historical context in which they unfold. This has been elaborately discussed in the book. Having placed tobacco use in its historical and current context, the book discusses cultivation and manufacture of consumable tobacco products with a detailed and reader friendly analysis, statistical information and tabulation of data. The book provides platform to discuss the pharmacological effects of nicotine present in tobacco and those external factors which influence an individual's experience with tobacco, the spread of its use, society's response and government's action. The book also helps identify which populations are most susceptible to the attraction of tobacco and under what conditions, why tobacco use is becoming more prevalent in the developing countries, and which characteristics of an individual and a society have moderated or aggravated the disruptive potential of the tobacco use behaviour. Certainly majority has abstained from the use of tobacco, but the ubiquity of its use is so striking that it must represent a basic human appetite. Nicotine in tobacco is highly addictive; it is as addictive as any hardcore dependence producing drug. There is evidence that different forms of tobacco use involve rewards derived in different degrees from social, sensory and pharmacological sources. Tobacco use in general and tobacco smoking in particular has harmful effects on the body it not only causes many diseases such as cancers and respiratory diseases, it affects the health adversely, shortens life-span and causes premature death. A series of scientific reports published by the Surgeon General of the United States of America have served, over the years, as the best source of evidence-based information on the adverse health effects of tobacco use.

The recent global surge in action against tobacco prompted me to write this book. As awareness of the dangers posed by tobacco spread, nations across the world resolved to forge a campaign strategy and frame a battle plan to overcome the tobacco threat. Close to the closure of the intergovernmental negotiations on the World Health Organization (WHO) Framework Convention on Tobacco Control (FCTC) in March 2003, came the India's anti-tobacco law in April 2003. At this point I began to contemplate to have a comprehensive source document on tobacco. This book is the effort of following four years.

This book provides a source in my effort to prevent and control tobacco use. It is also intended to inform many sections of our society who are committed to protecting the mankind from the menace of tobacco use. Since this volume is not intended exclusively for the health professionals, the attempt has been made to keep the language as free from technical jargon as possible. Most of the readers will know that tobacco is harmful but not how harmful. I believe this book will inform them. Many of our readers will want to control tobacco but not know how best to do it. I believe this book will aid them. This book will also help those physicians and students of medicine belonging to various disciplines who are interested in tobacco-cessation programmes. Finally, I believe this book will provide policy-makers the necessary impetus to initiate and implement a coordinated comprehensive strategy for tobacco control.

**R.C. JILOHA**

# Contents

# Introduction

The contemporary drug situation in the world is a unique phenomenon unlike any experienced before. Of the many ills that have plagued the human society throughout its history, abuse of drugs has remained a problem of greatest socio-medical relevance. In fact, the use of drugs or psychoactive substances is almost a universal phenomenon which has long been a complex, often highly volatile social concern. An estimated 4,000 plants yield psychoactive substances, and about 60 of these drugs have been in constant use, somewhere in the world, throughout history – with cannabis, opium, coca, tea, coffee, tobacco and alcohol predominantly. Of these, tobacco is one of the recent introductions to the list of psychoactive drugs used in the modern world as smoking and smokeless. When Christopher Columbus, a Spanish navigator and his crew discovered modern Americas in 1492, they found the natives of America smoking leaves of a plant which was later identified as tobacco. Spread of tobacco to Europe and rest of the old world was both hated and loved. On one hand it was praised to be a remedy sent by God as a panacea for all human sufferings while on the other it was feared as a plant with the powers of evil and an invention of devil. The wide-spread use of tobacco during the next four hundred years after John Rolfe and other colonists of Jamestown Virginia started cultivating tobacco for commercial purposes in 1613, indeed represents a victory for the commercial forces who have not only aggressively created a mass market, they have made many dependent on tobacco. Tobacco has become a marketed malady, a communicated disease of the consumerist modern world and its consumption an engineered addiction that has victimized members of almost all cultural and socioeconomic backgrounds. Nearly one-third of the world's adult population regularly performs this bizarre act despite of the fact that it is acknowledged, even by its adherent consumers, to be harmful to health and even repugnantly distasteful.

Tobacco is a plant product, derived from a member of *Solanaceae* family of the plant kingdom. Unlike other members of this family such as tomato and potato, which have definite nutritional role, tobacco plant carries in its leaves quantities of an alkaloid, nicotine, which gives it instead, power over man's mind. *Nicotiana tobaccum* is the species of the plant cultivated commercially to obtain tobacco all over the world; however, in some geographical areas *Nicotiana rustica* is the main source of tobacco supply.

The smoking of cigarettes (and *beedis* in Indian sub-continent) is by far the most important means of tobacco consumption, in terms of both prevalence and health consequences. From the incandescent tip of the lighted cigarette burning at a temperature of 800° C (1600-1800° F), the smoker with each puff draws along the tobacco rod and into his mouth a hot potpourri of gases and many sized particles.

About 4000 chemicals have been detected in tobacco smoke of which nicotine is the main constituent responsible for a number of patho-physiological changes in the body. This is a highly toxic and potentially lethal chemical that one-drop of the substance is sufficient to kill a dog (or a man). In an unlit cigarette the nicotine is dissolved in the moisture of tobacco leaf as water soluble salt, but in a burning cigarette nicotine volatilizes and is present in the smoke as free nicotine suspended on minute droplets of tar. Nicotine not only causes damaging effects on the body it also leads to tolerance to its own action like other dependence producing drugs.

Most of other chemicals present in tobacco smoke are also chemically active like nicotine, and trigger profound and damaging changes in the body. Carbon monoxide (CO), a highly toxic gas that combines with haemoglobin in the blood, reduces its oxygen carrying capacity and thus exposes the body to the risk of various respiratory disorders. Tar present in tobacco smoke, contains sticky, brown particles that stain teeth, fingers and lung tissue. Tar contains the carcinogen benzo(a)pyrene which triggers cancer development in various organs of the body. Nitrogen oxide another constituent of tobacco smoke, damages lung tissue and causes emphysema. Hydrogen cyanide in tobacco smoke stops the movement of cilia present in the lungs and thus impairs the foreign particle clearing capacity of the lungs and allows the poisonous tobacco smoke ingredients to accumulate in the lungs. Ammonia is a strong chemical that damages the lung tissue. Metals present in tobacco smoke such as arsenic, cadmium and lead damage the lung tissue and some of these are carcinogenic. Radioactive compounds found in tobacco smoke are also proved to be carcinogenic.

Other than nicotine, tobacco contains several other alkaloids that are structurally related to nicotine, giving rise to carcinogens N-nitrosonornicotine (NNN), 4-methyl-nitrosamino-1-butanone (NNK) and other toxic and carcinogenic nitrosamines. Tobacco-specific nitrosamines present in tobacco are formed during fermentation and curing of tobacco. Over 43 carcinogens have been found in tobacco. Tobacco smoke is rich in naphthalene and polycyclic aromatic hydrocarbons (PAH), which are known carcinogens and produce serious adverse effects on the body.

To begin with, smoking was adopted first by the men of the developed countries and then the women of the developed countries and the men of the developing countries and only recently have the *women* of the developing world taken to smoking. Reports on the ill effects of tobacco began to pour in by the beginning of the 20$^{th}$ century and most of what is known about the health effects of tobacco relates to the smoking of manufactured cigarettes, although in some parts of the world use of other forms of tobacco is also common. The most of the work on the ill effects of smoking comes from the developed countries where the prevalence of smoking is more than a century old but it is proved beyond doubt that consumption of tobacco in any form produces adverse effects on the body.

In 1937, for the first time, cancer was produced in laboratory animals by cigarette tar. Raymond Pearl of John Hopkins University, in 1938, demonstrated statistically that the non-smokers lived longer than the smokers. In 1939, the study linking lung cancer with tobacco smoking was published. Epidemiological studies in UK and the USA showed a clear statistical association between smoking and cancer. Known carcinogens were identified in the smoke and tobacco smoking is implicated in a wide range of diseases including the cancer of the oral cavity, larynx, pharynx, oesophagus, urinary bladder, coronary heart disease bronchitis and emphysema. During the 1950s and 1960s, conclusive evidence was made available that cigarette smoking was the most important cause of a wide range of diseases and death and this was the period when massive expansion of cigarette use occurred along with expansion of tobacco industry. Almost no government regulations were promulgated during this period to restrict this expansion; on the contrary, the Federal Government in the USA actively encouraged it through a variety of actions. Only since 1960s has tobacco availability been viewed as a public health issue by any major segment of the society, with many restrictions proposed and some measures instituted at all governmental levels.

US Surgeon General's Advisory Committee Report in 1964 published amid unprecedented worldwide fanfare in the mass media, convinced even most smokers that cigarette smoking shortens human life, causes lung cancer, and other forms of cancer, and exacerbates heart disease, emphysema, bronchitis and a number of other diseases — gravely increasing the risk of dying. The report provided the impetus to the renewed anti-smoking campaign when it informed people that smoking was not only harmful its control was necessary by enacting legislation. In 1965, a health warning appeared on cigarette packets. Public Health Smoking Act of 1970 was passed, essentially reflecting the position of anti-smoking interests. In 1970, radio and television advertising of cigarettes was banned throughout USA.

Per capita cigarette consumption began falling in USA annually from 1973; however, the tobacco industry continued to flourish. Despite a decline in cigarette use in Northern

Europe and USA, tobacco consumption continued to be high in other parts of the world. To some extent the smoking epidemic came under control in the developed world but this epidemic had merely shifted to the developing world where smoking continues to rise. The Asian countries have become the target of the tobacco companies as their potential customers. These companies are engaged in 'aggressive' marketing in the 'third world' countries where consumption is rising. Since the lifting of import restrictions, the Asian countries have witnessed a dramatic increase in smoking and the consequent ill effects of tobacco smoking. Smoking of tobacco became a grave concern for the governments to take remedial measures to fight this global menace that became not only a major public health threat but also a potential danger for the future world. The US Surgeon General's Advisory Committee Report, 2004 emphasizes that smoking harms almost every organ of the body, causes several diseases and reduces the health of the smoker in general.

Of all the diseases causally associated with smoking, lung cancer is the most well known, largely because in most populations, almost all lung cancer deaths are due to smoking. In 1930, lung cancer death rate for men in the USA was 4.9 per 100,000, in 1990; the rate increased to 75.6 per 100,000. Smoking is responsible for 90% of all lung cancers. However smoking causes more deaths from other diseases than lung cancer. In 1995, there were 514,000 smoking caused lung cancer deaths in developed countries, compared to 625,000 smoking attributed deaths from heart and other vascular diseases in the same year. Smoking is responsible for 75% of all cases of chronic bronchitis and emphysema. Recent epidemiological evidence suggests that cigarette smoking is also deleterious to the gastrointestinal tract. It increases the incidence and relapse rate of peptic ulcer and delays its healing process. More recent evidence points to the relationship between smoking and cancers of the stomach, liver and colon. Smokeless tobacco also poses serious health risks. The annual mortality from tobacco chewing in South Asia alone is 50,000 deaths a year.

In 1990s, about 25% of all male deaths in developing countries were due to smoking. For middle-aged women of developing countries, the percentage of all deaths caused by smoking increased more than six folds, from 2% in 1955 to 13% in 1995, and continues to increase rapidly. Cigarette kills 50% of all lifetime cigarette users and tobacco kills more than AIDS, drugs, road accidents, murder and suicide combined.

Tobacco is estimated to have caused 3 million deaths a year in early 1990s and death toll is steadily increasing and it is currently responsible for the deaths of one in 10 adult's worldwide (about five million deaths each year). If current smoking patterns continue, it will cause some ten million deaths each year by 2025. 70% of these deaths will be in the developing countries alone. Among people alive today in the world, 500 million will die prematurely due to tobacco use; most of these are children and young adults of today.

In India, cigarette smoking comprises a small part of tobacco smoking problem and a minor part of overall tobacco consumption problem. Majority of smokers in India, smoke *beedis* and large part of overall tobacco consumption is the oral use of smokeless tobacco products.

All forms of tobacco use are unsafe for human health. Mere extrapolation of results of research in the developed countries would, therefore, not provide a full picture of the dimensions of the tobacco problem in India. While much of the biological associations between tobacco and disease are applicable across the world, the varied patterns of tobacco use and the diversity of socio-cultural determinants substantially influence the profile of tobacco-related diseases. Therefore, all Indian experiences need to be carefully documented.

One aspect common to all forms of tobacco consumption across all societies is the infusion of symbolic and often moral overtones. Just as the symbolic nature of consumption is not identical among different individuals, groups or cultures, similarly the morality intrinsic to tobacco consumption varies.

The recent global surge of action against tobacco menace has proved quite favourable for the anti-tobacco movement with its special focus on the developing world. As awareness of the dangers posed by tobacco spread, nations across the world resolved to forge a campaign strategy and frame a battle plan to overcome the tobacco threat. India's anti-tobacco law emerged in May 2003, in close proximity with the closure of intergovernmental negotiations on the World Health Organization (WHO) Framework Convention on Tobacco Control (FCTC) in March 2003. Soon thereafter, the Ministry of Health and Family Welfare, Government of India, decided to commission a detailed review of status of tobacco control in India with the intention to collate the Indian experience and craft a plan for future action based on a critical appraisal of global evidence and India's specific needs.

Physicians can play a crucial role in preventing expected mortality by motivating their smoker patients to stop smoking. It is recommended that every patient approaching a physician should be enquired about his/her smoking status should be persuaded for smoking cessation and those willing should be helped to stop smoking.

While many tobacco users generally know that tobacco use is harmful, studies show that most are unaware of the true risks, even in countries in which there has been great deal of publicity about the health hazards of tobacco. According to World Bank (1999) people's knowledge of health risks of smoking appears to be partial at best, especially in low- and middle-income countries where information about these hazards is limited. Smokers tend to be even less aware of the risks of tobacco smoke to others. This book is an attempt to disseminate knowledge about tobacco. Right from the time of its discovery to its current status, every relevant aspect of tobacco is comprehensively reviewed. This book provides information not only to the general public but also serves the need of students of public health, environment, psychiatry and general medicine.

Over 500 years since its discovery, experiences with tobacco have provided enough evidence why people smoke and why they cannot easily give it up even when they clearly know that it is a preventable cause of morbidity and mortality. Nicotine dependence is a recognized psychiatric illness and has been referred to as the most prevalent, most deadly, most costly and yet most treatable of all psychiatric disorders. However, the mental health professionals often overlook it. Physician treating a patient should look into smoking status of his patients as well and persuade him for smoking cessation.

The purpose of this book is to promote a better understanding of the fluidity and mutability of understanding of our attitudes towards tobacco and of the complex process through which at any given time a society comes to differentiate acceptable from unacceptable use, or how it comes to label use as abuse.

**R. C. JILOHA**
*Director Professor and Head*
*Department of Psychiatry*
*Maulana Azad Medical College & G.B. Pant Hospital,*
*New Delhi 110002 (India)*

CHAPTER

# 1 History of Tobacco Use: New World's Revenge

*History provides a critical test for our concepts of reality and the assumptions upon which our present attitudes and policies towards drug use are based.*

— George A Austin, 1978

Introduction of tobacco from the Americas to the rest of the World some five hundred years ago generated the first great drug controversy of a global dimension. Right from the time of its introduction into Europe and other parts of the Old World, opinions regarding tobacco radically differed, in part because early reports praised its medicinal virtues but also described it as a harmful plant used in pagan religions of the natives (Wilbert, 1987). Tobacco was credited with almost miraculous healing powers and was used by the natives of America as remedy for aches, pains, snake-bite, abdominal and heart pain, chills, convulsions, epilepsy, skin disease and fatigue, among other ailments (Ashton and Stepney, 1982). While smoking for pleasure was frowned upon by many, its use as a medicine was almost universally approved with physicians leading the way in extolling the virtues of this *herbal panacea*[1], this *sanct sanctora* (holy healing herb),[2] this special remedy sent by God to man[3], this plant of "singular and divine virtues" as a panacea for all human sufferings (Dickson, 1954). On the other hand, the antagonism towards tobacco, particularly its use for pleasure or sport, was accentuated by the reports that it was employed in the magic and religion of the natives and that its use produced frenzy, stupefaction, near delirium and trance states. It, therefore, was attacked as a plant with the power of the evil and the invention of the devil[4].

---

1 Petum – The Brazilian name for tobacco – is a sort of panacea, a cure for every kind of sickness.

2 Inghi Brain, The Forbidden Game: A Serial History of Drug. Hodder and Stroughton: London, 1975.

3 Laufer Berthold, Introduction of Tobacco into Europe, Field Museum of National History, 1924.

4 Austin G.A., Perspectives of the History of Psychoactive Substance Use. NIDA: Rockville MD, 1978.

A legend among Huron natives of North America describes the origin of tobacco plant[5]:

> *"………that in ancient times, when the land was barren and the people were starving, The Great Spirit sent forth a naked woman to save humanity. As she traveled over the world, everywhere her right hand touched the soil, there grew potatoes. And everywhere her left hand touched the soil, there grew corn. And when the world was rich and fertile, she sat down and rested. When she arose, there grew tobacco……."*

Whatever the origin of tobacco plant itself, we may speculate that the peculiarly pleasurable consequences of inhaling its smoke were discovered more or less by chance during the use of various plant materials in sacred rituals involving fire and incense. Although small amounts of nicotine may be found in some Old World plants, including *Belladona* and *Nicotiana africana* and nicotine metabolites have been found in human remains and pipes in the Near East and Africa, there is no indication of habitual tobacco use in the ancient world outside of the Americas (Corti, 1996).

It is believed that the tobacco plant as we know it today began growing in Americas around 6000 BC. Tobacco seeds are discovered in archaeological excavations in Mexico and Peru, and the remains of permanent settlements built around 3500 BC show that tobacco was an important article to the inhabitants (Luthra *et al.*, 1992).

Around 1st century BC, American natives began finding ways to use tobacco, including smoking, chewing and in enemas. Experts believe that tobacco was available everywhere in Americas during 1st century AD. Pictorial record of smoking in the period from 600 AD to 1000 AD is available from Uaxactun and Guatemalan pottery. A pottery vessel found there dated before the 11th century. On it a Maya is depicted smoking a roll of tobacco leaves tied with a string. It is certain that tobacco smoking was practiced among the early Mayas (Figures 1 and 2), probably in the district of Tabasco, Mexico, as a part of their religious ceremonies. Perhaps, the word "tobacco" comes from Tobasco[6].

Over the following centuries, tobacco smoking spread in the entire Mexico region and the Antilles. It was further spread when the smoker-friendly tribes dispersed northwards by way of the Mississippi Valley and by sea to as far as Brazil.

Natives from further North made pipes, some with a bowel and mouthpiece, others shaped like a Y, with the forked extremities placed in the nostrils. They also blended their tobacco with other plants to vary its flavour or make it go deeper by enhancing the effect of tobacco with these additives[6].

In 1449, natives on Margarita Island, off the coast of Venezuela, were observed chewing a green herb that was carried in a gourd around their necks. It is assumed that the green herb was tobacco (Luthra *et al.,* 1992).

---

5 According to a mythological belief the Great Spirit *Gitche Manitou* surrendered tobacco to man.

6 Tobacco.org, tobacco news and information. The Tobacco timeline. available from URL:http://www.tobacco.org/resources/history/tobacco_history.html(accessed on 24th March 2004).

In South America, the Aztecs[7] smoked and took snuff. They also used it for certain ailments such as rumbling in the abdomen, gout and for certain recurrent illnesses[8]. Montezuma II (1446–1520), the last Aztec Emperor of Mexico, is said to have smoked a ceremonial pipe after dinner. Elsewhere in the American continent, tobacco was chewed, eaten, drunk, used as an infusion, or rubbed on the body. Certainly the use of tobacco was widespread long before the Europeans arrived to claim their 'New World'.

Inhaling of smoke was not entirely unknown in the Old World (Koskowski, 1955). Europeans inhaled smoke of unappetizing substances such as coltsfoot and dried cow dung for medicinal purposes (Corti, 1996). The use of tobacco, however, was a curious novelty - despite claims once made that a pipe still smelling of nicotine had been unearthed in the ruins of a Greek temple at Constantinople. Some historians claim that the Chinese invented the pipe and that Asians were smoking long before the Christian era, but they smoked grass and not tobacco, which has never been grown anywhere but in the Americas before Columbus.

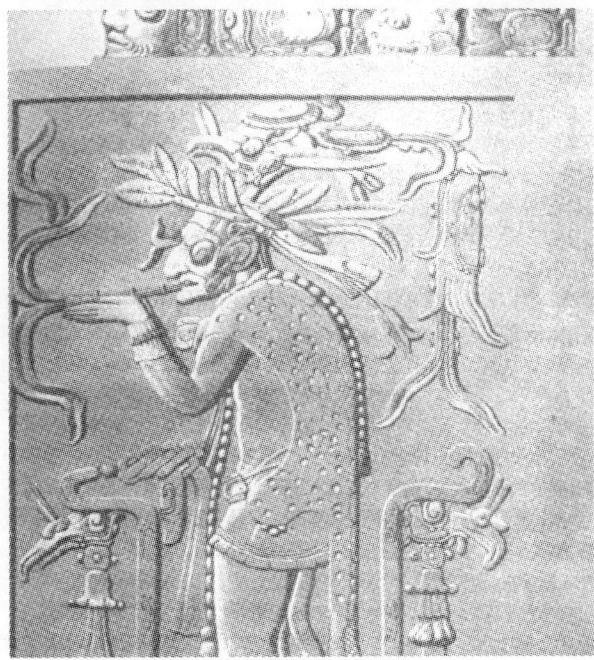

***Figure 1: A priest smoking tobacco leaves***
*Source: Corti, 1996.*

---

[7] Native Americans of Mexico.

[8] The De La Cruz – Badiano Aztec Herbal of 1555. Translated and commentary by William Gates, Publication No. 22. The Maya Society, Baltimore, 1939.

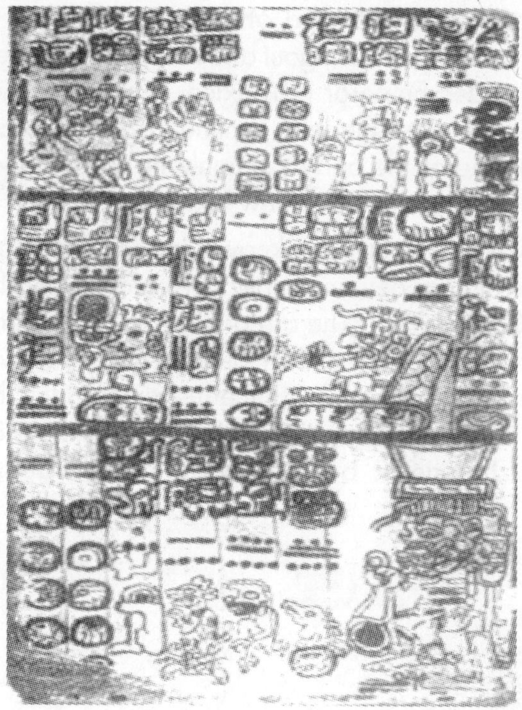

*Figure 2: A priest smoking tobacco*
*Source: Corti, 1996.*

The history of tobacco has a more clearly defined beginning after the discovery of the Americas by the European sailors. On the bright morning of 12th October 1492, Christopher Columbus, a Spanish navigator and his crewmen set foot on the New World for the first time, landing on the beach of an island in the Bahamas (called *Guanahani* by its inhabitants) that Columbus named San Salvador. The indigenous *Arawaks*, possibly thinking the strange visitors divine, offered gifts. Columbus wrote in his journal[9]:

> *"......... The natives brought fruit, wooden spears and certain dried leaves which gave of a distinct fragrance........................."*

As each item seemed much prized by the natives; Columbus accepted the gifts and ordered them brought back to the ship. The fruit was eaten; the pungent "dried leaves" were thrown away. On 15th October 1492, Columbus mentioned in his journal:

> *"We found a man in a canoe, going from Santa Maria to Fernandia. He had with him some dried leaves which are in high value among them, for a quantity of which was brought to me at San Salvador."*

---

[9] Columbus, J: Das Buch von tabak: Vienna, 1846.

The natives told Columbus of another much larger island nearby and he immediately set sail arriving off the Cuban coast on 28th October, 1492.

Not knowing what to expect, he sent two of his fellow explorers, Rodriguo de Jarez and Luis de Torres, to scout the interior and mentioned in his journal of November 1492 that these two Spanish conquistadors met a larger number of men and women in the interior:

> *"Rodriguo Jerez and Luis de Torres reported that the natives wrapped the dried tobacco leaves in palm or maize 'in the manner of musket formed of paper.' After lighting one end, they commenced "drinking" of smoke through the other."*

On the same day, Jerez took his first hesitant puff of the New World's early version of the cigarette and became the first European smoker and the first, outside the Americas. When Columbus and his crew returned home with some tobacco leaves, Rodriguo Jerez, who had taken to smoking of tobacco every day, brought the habit back to his home town but the smoke billowing from his mouth and nose so frightened his neighbors that he was imprisoned by the Holy inquisitors for 7 years. By the time he was released, smoking was a Spanish craze. Jerez thus became the first victim of anti-tobacconists. The first Old World woman to smoke was Queen Isabella of Spain, who received a cigar (made of tobacco leaves) from Columbus on his return.

Robert Romano Pane, a monk who accompanied Christopher Columbus on his second voyage in 1493, wrote the first European account on native tobacco use in 1497[10]. He reported that the natives also used tobacco by reducing it to a powder that,

> *"............................They take through a cane half a cubit long: one end of it they place in the nose, and the other upon the powder."*

However, Bartolome de las Cassas[11] provided one of the first coherent accounts of tobacco smoking in 1527:

> *"......Some dried herbs (are) put in a certain leaf, also dry, in a manner of a musket made of paper......and having lighted one part of it, by the other they suck, absorb or receive that smoke inside with breath, by which they become benumbed, almost drunk, and so it is that they do not feel fatigue. These muskets, as we will call them, they call tobacco."*
>
> *(Brooks, 1953).*

European settlers in Americas, all along the sea route, wherever they had established trading posts in Haiti and Cuba began planting of tobacco by 1531 and by 1540, they had started shipping the cultivated New World tobacco to Spain. By 1548, Portuguese were cultivating tobacco in Brazil for commercial purposes. Before the end of the 16th century Portuguese had developed small farms to a point where they could be assured of enough

---

[10] Pane Romano: *De Insularium ritibus (1497)* in: The Facts About Tobacco.

[11] Las Cassas Bartolome de: *Historie des indes 1520 – 1559.*

tobacco to meet their personal needs, for gifts and for barter. By the beginning of 17th century, these farms had, in many places, become plantations, often under native control. Andre Thevet[12] brought seeds of tobacco from Brazil and introduced in Portugal in 1558. Jean Nicot Villemain, an ambassador to the Portugese court became familiar with tobacco plant and sent it as a gift to Catherene de Medicii, the Queen mother of France to treat her son Francis II's migraine headache in 1559. Nicot and the court were the primary influence in France in the spread of knowledge about tobacco and its reputation for healing almost every complaint. It was in honour of Nicot that, in 1570, the plant was dubbed Nicotiana and its active ingredient was later called nicotine[13]. Andre Thevet also wrote the first description of tobacco in 1568 and reported that people in Brazil smoked tobacco to clean their "superfluous humor" of the brain.

The tobacco plant was introduced in Holland and Rome from France in 1560 and from the Italian posts, the information about tobacco spread to Eastern Europe. The plant was brought to Austria and Hungry, where it was cultivated as early as 1568, though chiefly in the gardens of nobility for its beauty or for its healing qualities, there being still no mention of its use for smoking.

The tobacco plant was successfully grown in Germany and Switzerland in 1560s. As a medicinal herb it intrigued the physicians everywhere since its healing powers in a variety of disorders were claimed by many. In 1571, Michael Bernhard Valentini, a German physician described several types of clysters (enemas). The tobacco clysters was said to be good for the treatment of colic, nephritis, hysteria, hernia and dysentery.

Spanish sailors visiting Americas, not only introduced tobacco to Spain they also popularized it as an aphrodisiac. Its popularity grew among physicians and lay public alike. A Seville physician named Monardes[14], - - described tobacco's craze among Spanish physicians in 1578 who considered it to be a wonder drug having miraculous effect in 36 maladies. As a result, by 1616, tobacco smoke in Spain was rampant and Spanish king Philip III established Seville as tobacco center of the world. To prevent a tobacco glut, Philip required all tobacco in the Spanish New World to be shipped to a central location, Seville, in Spain and hence Seville became the world center for the production of cigars. Spanish and Portuguese sailors spread the practice of smoking to Russia and the Levant from there.

In England, Sir John Hawkins (1532 – 1595) the first English slave-trader, who made three expeditions from Africa to Caribbean, is said to have introduced *Nicotiana rustica* from Florida in 1565, but the introduction was largely ignored initially as no use was noticed. However, in the next five years, tobacco became popular among the English aristocracy and people were intrigued to know more and more about this 'magic plant,'

---

[12] Andre Thevet: Cosmographie Universalle (1571) and *France Antarctique* (Antwerp, 1558).

[13] In 1558, Posselt and Reimanbasic isolated nicotine from tobacco leaves.

[14] Monardes Nicolo: *Herba Tobacco de' India* (Genoa, 1578).

while biologists devoted their time on the scientific inquiry of this strange member of Solaneaceae family of plant kingdom. In 1570, the first botanical book on tobacco, written in English language by Pena and Lobel[15], appeared in London markets while first attempts at tobacco cultivation in England occurred in 1571. After Sir Francis Drake[16] brought over *Nicotiana tobaccum* in 1573, the first diffusion of smoking occurred. Pipe smoking became a national recreation. Sir Walter Raleigh made the habit fashionable in the court of Elizabeth I and the polite society. Soon its use spread among all classes of Elizabethan society and among women as well as men. J.M. Barrie[17], author of "My Lady Nicotine" described in his book how tobacco turned the tide of the history:

> *"When Releigh, in honor of whom England should have changed its name, introduced tobacco, the glorious Elizabethan age began.........the men who had hitherto only concerned themselves with the narrow things of home put a pipe in their mouths and became philosophers. Poets and philosophers smoked until all ignoble ideas were driven from them, and into their place rushed such high thoughts as the world had not known before..."*

Tobacco arrived in Poland for the first time in 1580 and within few decades of its arrival its use was seen to be common and it became rampant after 1615.

In the beginning of seventeenth century smoking was an expensive fad among the court and nobility. However, by the end of Elizabeth's reign smoking was common among all classes of society; it was specially the mark of young men of fashion (Figure 3) as described by Robert Burton, in his satirical enumeration of the accomplishments necessary to be the perfect gentleman, ranked smoking with dancing, riding, hunting, and card-playing. Everybody smoked, even in theatres. However, the English physicians got upset over the indiscriminate use of tobacco by people without a doctor's prescription and complained to the King – James I in 1603. James VI, king of Scotland from 1567 and now James I of England, in 1603, started Britain's first anti-smoking campaign. The son of Mary, Queen of Scots, he ascended the throne of England on the death of Queen Elizabeth I. However, at the same time he was in need of money and discovered how easy it was to tax imported tobacco. In 1604, the king imposed a stiff duty tax on tobacco to keep the silver out of Spanish hands. He tightened his Royal monopoly by prohibiting cultivation of tobacco in and around London. The following year he extended the prohibition to the rest of England. He wrote a violent treatise against the use of tobacco but was nevertheless perceptive enough to draw attention to the fact that one of the most intriguing properties of tobacco was that it seemed capable of having contradictory effects — being used both as a sedative and as a stimulant:

---

[15] Lobel Mathia De and Petro Pena: *Nuova stripium adversaria,* Antwerp, 1576.

[16] Drake, *T.F.: The World encompassed,* London, 1628.

[17] Author of My Fair Lady Nicotine, p 106 – 107, 1890.

> *"Being taken when they go to bed, it makes one sleepe soundly, and yet being taken when a man is sleepie and drowsie, it will as they say, awaken his braine, and quicken his understanding."*
> (*James I, 1604*)

The king in his fulminations against tobacco smoking, characterized the habit as[18]

> *"A custom loathsome to the eyes, hateful to the nose, harmful to the brain, dangerous to the lungs, and in the black stinking fumes thereof, nearest resembling the horrible stygian smoke of the pit that is bottomless."*

In 1606 the king tried to impregnate the mythically rich virgin land, Virginia in the 'New World' by sending companies eager to plumb the tantalizing riches of North America. The first permanent English colony was established in 1607, when Virginia Company landed a group of adventurers in Jamestown. This colony faced a great deal of adversities — wracked by malaria epidemics, natives' attacks, intrigue, laziness, torture, starvation and ghoulish cannibalism. It was saved by Pocahontas[19] and her husband John Rolfe's cultivation of this desperate colony's only substantial resource: tobacco. Without the success of Jamestown, the dominant culture south and west of New England could well be Spanish. In 1612–1613, John Rolfe introduced the cultivation of tobacco into Jamestown, Virginia (Morrison, 1965) as a commercial crop of "tall tobacco".

The culture and export of tobacco enabled fledgling English colonies in North America to survive, and the need for a large merchant marine to transport the leaf and then for naval protection of the trade, contributed to England's supremacy at sea. This supremacy paved a path for creation of opportunities to facilitate the spread of tobacco use.

Virginia leaf found a ready market in England and it became the economic base for Britain's southern colonies in North America. Indeed, into the early 18$^{th}$ century, tobacco served as the currency of Virginia and from the colonial time onwards, tobacco regulations were devised to help further the prosperity of the industry. It began its first sale of native Virginia tobacco in England in 1614 and thus Virginia colony entered world tobacco market under the English protection. Just three years after its cultivation had begun Virginia sent 3000 lb of tobacco to London as compared with 53,000 Spanish lb to Seville. Two years later, Virginia was sending 19,000 lbs, which increased to 25,000 lbs by 1620, and the colonists had made mercantile and political allies in England. Effort was soon diverted from suppression to promotion of Virginia tobacco at the expense of the Spanish.

In 1619, the first shipment of women meant to become wives of the settlers arrived in Jamestown. A prospective husband was expected to pay for his chosen mate's passage with 120 lbs of tobacco. The same year in Jamestown, first Africans were brought to Virginia as

---

[18] James I: *Misocapnus sive de abusu Tobacci lusus regius* (London 1603) and a Counterblast to Tobacco, London, 1604.

[19] Native Chief's daughter and later John Rolfe's wife.

John Rolfe mentioned in his diary:

> *"About the last of August came in a Dutch man of Warre that sold us twenty negars. They were needed for the booming tobacco crop but had been baptized, so as Christians they could not be enslaved for life, but only indentured, just like many of the English colonists, for 5 -7 years."*

Charles I, son of James I and his successor too, shared his father's dislike of tobacco and allowed none of his courtiers to enjoy tobacco smoking in his presence. But he was also too short of money to be able to pick and choose. He realized the importance of flourishing tobacco business in European market, and therefore, strengthened the royal monopoly, restricted the foreign imports, prohibited domestic cultivation and fostered tobacco trade with colonies. In 1633, he added the licensing of retailers.

Gradually Glasgow emerged as an important port to import tobacco. By the 1720s, Glasgow was importing over half of all American tobacco brought into Britain and by 1804 the city's population had risen to 70,000, her growth founded upon a new trade — the import and re-export of tobacco from the American colonies. This dramatic growth in tobacco trade provided the impetus for developing Glasgow itself as a great port rather than relying on Port Glasgow many miles further down the Clyde. This led to the establishment of ship-building and engineering and the prosperity that followed made Glasgow the industrial center of Scotland.

Developments which occurred consequent upon introduction of tobacco in Europe reveal that the conflict about tobacco use in England was more bitter than in other Western European countries such as Spain and France, though less so than in the East. The English physicians praised tobacco's medicinal use in moderation while the aggressive fulminations by James I, the king of England, clearly express his dislike for it. Nevertheless, the events in England were typical of what occurred elsewhere: the rise of a belief in tobacco's health-giving properties, the rapidity with which it became a fad among the aristocracy and upper classes; the influence of political and social concerns, as well as health concerns, on governmental control attempts; the failure of admonitions, prohibitions, and taxes to end use; and, finally, the growth of governmental dependence on tobacco for revenue and the gradual acceptance, even encouragement, of its use.

While the reaction of Western European Governments to tobacco tended towards flexibility, at times even verging on a hypocritical opportunism and finally its acceptance, Russia and the Ottoman Turks prohibited it with the severest of punishments. Tobacco smoking was introduced into Turkey, probably in 1605 under the reign of Sultan Ahmed (1603–1617), but possibly at the end of the 16$^{th}$ century (Ortiz, 1947).

The Turkish reaction also differed from the West in the closer co-operation that developed between religious and lay opposition. From the West, tobacco spread to Turkey on mass scale and quickly became popular despite opposition from religious teachings of the Koran, in which religious taboos are placed on a number of intoxicants. One argument emphasized that Koran forbade the use of coal., and tobacco when smoked became coal. Two concerns often influenced the opposition to smoking in all countries are illustrated by the Turkish and Russian experiences: (i) the fear of fires being ignited by careless smokers, and (ii) the development of tobacco houses as centres of political and social unrest. Fear of this unexpected commercial phenomenon was partly based on the fact that the new commodity was likely to cause large and very expensive foreign imports that were not compensated for and upset the domestic economy (Austin, 1978).

The initial response to tobacco in Turkey was an excessively violent attack on the substance by secular and religious authorities that denounced tobacco as irreligious, unhealthy and a fire hazard. Sultan Murad IV[20] of Turkey ordered tobacco users executed as infidels. As many as 18 persons, using tobacco were executed every day under the law. However, despite the capital punishment, the rise in tobacco use continued and finally the authorities had to give up. In 1647, the ban was lifted and tobacco joined coffee, wine and opium as one of the four "cushions on the sofa of pleasure."

In the 17th century, Russia was in process of ending a long period of isolation from European influences. Life was harsh and characterized by extremes of drunkenness and revelry on one hand and repentance and religious prostrations on the other. The church was conservative and feared modernization and other Western influences, whereas the Czars, struggling to unify and modernize society and establish their control over it, were drawing upon western models in their efforts. It was in this period of turbulence and change that tobacco use spread into Russia, and these conditions significantly affected the subsequent Russian response. Italian, Spanish and Portuguese sailors introduced tobacco into the Eastern Europe around 1600.

The contact of various armies during the 30-year war helped in spreading the use of tobacco throughout Central and Eastern Europe. In Russia, smoking increased rapidly with people openly smoking in churches, even during services (Corti, 1996). Michael Feodorovich (1596–1645), who became the first Romanov Czar in 1613, declared tobacco use a deadly sin. In 1634, he forbade possession of tobacco for any purpose. A tobacco court was established to try people who breached the law and its usual punishments were slitting lips, or terrible and sometimes deadly — flogging. However, in spite of the terrible punishment accorded to the smokers, the habit continued (Olearius, 1696). Finally, the financial pressures let the czar to violate his own laws and establish a fiscal monopoly of the "God-hated and impious herb" (Austin, 1978). Czar Alexis (1645–1676), the second Romanov ruler also forbade tobacco smoking. Though punishments continued to be severe including death penalty, the tobacco use also continued. The Russian efforts at repression failed; these rules were finally abandoned and a trade

[20] Murad (Amurath) IV the Cruel (1623 – 1640)

monopoly was established with the English, who by this time were active purveyors of tobacco. In 1676, Russia lifted the ban on tobacco smoking.

The phenomenal spread of tobacco use was not just limited to Europe; soldiers, traders and adventurers brought the habit to the Orient, where it proved to be equally irresistible and incapable of control. Vasco da Gama, a Portuguese navigator and a contemporary of Christopher Columbus of Spain, began his voyage with a similar objective of reaching the East and basking in its tantalizing glory, but with a different sea route. He reached India in 1498, discovering the Cape route, thus, becoming the first European sailor to reach this part of the world using a sea route and introducing European usages in the Far East. This was the time that the Europeans themselves had come in contact with tobacco, for the first time, by the chance discovery of the New World. Subsequent sailors after Vasco da Gama introduced the tobacco plant in the East. There is a probability that the Chinese first received tobacco from India, where Portuguese first took the seeds of the plant in 1599.

Although, it is claimed that there were already some strains of locally grown tobacco in India, these were outclassed by the new imported varieties. Portuguese introduced tobacco in the kingdom of Adil Shah at Bijapur (presently in Karnataka) in South India. Asad Beg, ambassador of the Mughal Emperor Akbar (1556–1605) visited Bijapur in 1604–1605 and took back quantities of tobacco to the emperor's court at Agra[21].

When Portuguese ambassadors introduced tobacco in the Royal court at Agra and insisted that the emperor try smoking the leaves, he consulted his *hakeem* (the royal physician) who opined that tobacco could be safely smoked if it passed through a clay pipe immersed in water before its consumption. This way *Hookah* was invented.

Akbar's son Jahangir (1605–1627) who succeeded him as India's emperor observed that tobacco cultivation had spread to large parts of the country when he took over. Like his contemporaries, King James I of England and Shah Abas I of Persia, he believed tobacco to be a noxious drug and forbade its use (Chattopadhyay, 1995).

After his accession on 24th October 1605, Jahangir passed 12 orders amongst which one was to ban the use of intoxicants. Subsequently, Jahangir introduced taxation of tobacco products and discovered the virtues of taxing tobacco. Since then, governments all over the world have been imposing taxes on tobacco and tobacco products making it a regular source of revenue.

The Portuguese created the taste and supplied the commodity from India to Persia; besides which the Persians themselves had much interaction with India. Subsequently, the trade bloomed and tobacco quickly established itself as the most important commodity passing through Goa in the 17th century. Virtually, every household in the Portuguese

---

[21] Chattopadhyay A: Emperor Akbar as a healer and his eminent physicians. Bulletin of Indian Institute of History of Medicine, 2000.

colony took up the new fashion of smoking or chewing tobacco. Later on, the British introduced modern commercially produced cigarettes.

A Persian author documents cultivation and use of tobacco in India during seventeenth century (Gode, 1961). The report says that smoking of tobacco pervaded all ranks and classes during the reign of Shah Jahan (1628–1658) (Akbar's grandson). Tobacco was often preferred over other necessities of life. *Cheroots* were commonly smoked both by men and women in South India and *chutta* smoking was noticed on the East Coast of India in 1670 (Sanghvi, 1992).

Dutch and Portuguese trading vessels calling at ports in Nagasaki and Kagoshima introduced tobacco in Japan in 1542. It spread through the country over the ensuing decades. Japan was the first Eastern nation to practice smoking extensively both for recreation and for medicinal purposes. Corti (1996) described:

> *"In 1616 the penalties were made still more severe................But it was all of no avail: the custom spread rapidly in every direction, until, as we read in an impartial poem of the time, many smokers were to be found in the Mikado's palace. Finally even the princes who were responsible for the prohibition took to smoking, and the great landowners and the rulers of the Daimios, the military and the feudal aristocracy, who were all devoted to the habit, were glad to let the laws fall into abeyance."*

Despite a legal ban imposed on tobacco in 1620, it gradually became a socially acceptable substance in Japan. In 1667, its controlled cultivation was permitted in lands specially reclaimed for that purpose so as not to interfere with the production of rice and corn. Acceptance of tobacco grew and even the medical professionals of Japan favored smoking in moderation (Satow, 1878).

Some botanists have advanced the theory that tobacco was indigenous to China. The traveler and naturalist Pallas argued that the Chinese tobacco pre-dated the discovery of the Americas because of an almost universal prevalence of the custom among the Chinese and the Mongols — the form of their pipes and the manner in which the dried leaves were wrapped. However, most authorities agree that tobacco did not come to China until the second half of the $16^{th}$ century by way of the Portuguese and Japanese.

The Chinese must have had the habit of smoking but hardly of tobacco smoking. They might, formerly, have smoked substances other than tobacco; and the assertion, as made or understood, did not perhaps distinguish between the general habit of smoking and particular use of tobacco.

In 1567, Portuguese introduced tobacco in Southwest China and its use spread fast among the Chinese. The Chinese emperor K'ang Hsi demanded decapitation of tobacco salesmen and users after the imperial edict forbade the planting and use of tobacco in 1616. The Manchu, having conquered China, revoked all existing tobacco bans in 1644 and gradually China became the great smoking nation of Asia. Snuff, introduced by Jesuits in the mid-17th century, soon became quite popular, from the court on down, and remained so during much of the Quing Dynasty (mid 17th century to 1912). Today, over 25% of the world's smokers live in China[22].

These above mentioned experiences illustrate not only the futility of severe prohibitions on tobacco cultivation, sale and use but also the complex motivations behind such prohibitions, including fear and disdain of foreign influences, loss of valuable food crops and fires. Like Turkey and Russia, Japan and China provided examples of ineffectiveness of merciless persecution by absolutist governments against this foreign substance.

In European countries, religious and moralistic sentiments against tobacco use in any form still continued and the churches took the lead to prevent its use. In 1642, Pope Urban VIII's Bill against tobacco forbade its use in churches in Seville. Pope Innocent X forbade smoking in St Peter's basilica in Rome in 1650, under penalty of excommunication. Despite that, the practice of tobacco smoking not only continued, it became increasingly popular. During this period, the city of London witnessed an epidemic of plague in 1665–1666 claiming an estimated 70,000 lives from a population of just half a million. The victims of plague used tobacco on a large scale as a prophylactic against plague. Certainly the plague that ravaged Europe set many people smoking for what was first prescribed by doctors as a medicine or a disinfectant, and later became a habit which was continued for pleasure even after the fear of plague was gone.

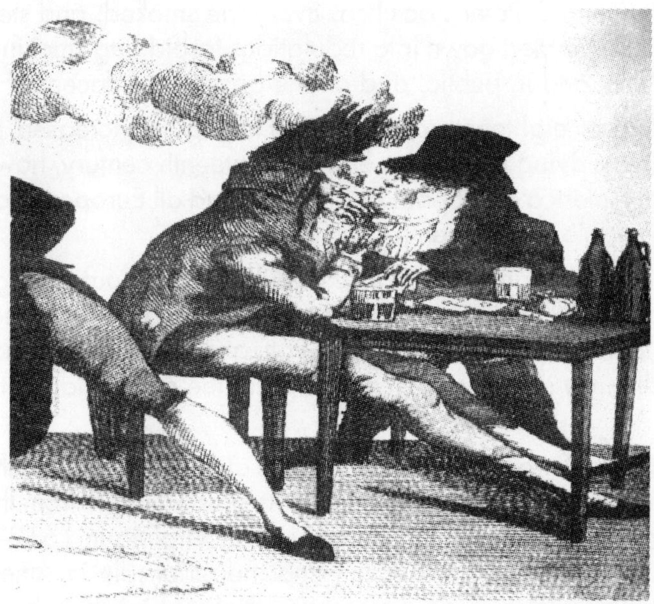

*Figure 3: Youth indulging in smoking behaviour*
*Source: Corti, 1996*

[22] World Health Organization: Tobacco Atlas, 2002.

The number of smokers grew mightily as did the glory and dignity of tobacco as expressed in the literature of the time. A growing number of writers and poets praised tobacco as a universal remedy to mankind's ills. In view of the current nearly unanimous condemnation by the medical profession, it is surprising to learn that tobacco was once much valued for its supposed medicinal properties (Brooks, 1953).

One of the most enthusiastic panegyrists of tobacco about this time was Cornelius Bontekoe, a celebrated Holland physician. In his book, *A Short Treatise on Man's Life, Health, Sickness, and Death,* he glorified tobacco and recommended it "to all who loved life and health" (Corti, 1996). Johannes Neander of Bremen in his book *Tobaccologia* lauded tobacco to the skies recommending it for all the ills to which flesh is heir.

By the beginning of eighteenth century, tobacco smoking had spread to almost the entire world and it became the passion of all people and it was believed that those who lived without tobacco had nothing to live for. A contemporary of the thirty years of war (1618–1648) pointed out its varied uses (Corti, 1996):

> *"If time hangs heavy and he has nothing else to do, a man will drink tobacco. Is he moody, angry and perplexed; he sticks his pipe between his teeth and takes a long pull at it. Should his wife begin to nag, the man will fill his mouth with smoke and puff it in her face."*

Even Peter the Great (1689–1725) advocated for tobacco smoking. By 1706 there was a decline in the prohibitions against tobacco smoking and in 1725, Pope Benedict XIII allowed snuff taking even in St Peter's basilica. Everyone smoked, and stern prohibitions of the seventeenth century dwindled down into regulations forbidding smoking at places where there was danger of fire, and in public, and on the grounds of decency.

Towards the middle of eighteenth century snuff-taking so increased that some people thought that smoking was dying out. At the end of eighteenth century, however, a new form of smoking came from America and Spain and overspread all Europe gradually culminating into cigarettes in the middle of nineteenth century.

In 1761, an English physician named John Hill published, *"Cautions Against Immoderate Use of Snuff"*—perhaps the first clinical study of tobacco effects. Hill warned snuff users that they were vulnerable to nose cancers. Dr. Percival Pott, another physician, noted the incidence of scrotal cancer in chimney smokers, hence theorizing the connection between cancer and exposure to smoke.

In colonial America, the European settlers who had already discovered the great economic power of the tobacco plant, promoted tobacco and its products right from the time when John Rolfe introduced the cultivation of tobacco in Jamestown, Virginia in 1612–1613. From then on, tobacco assumed major social., economic and industrial role in America's history and sent its ripples all over the globe. The widespread uptake of tobacco habit over these four centuries represents a victory for commercial forces, which aggressively created a mass market through engineering addiction to tobacco. All these years, a complex interplay of various socio-cultural factors in different societies influenced not only the acceptance or rejection of tobacco but also determined the patterns of its use. These four hundred years carry an ample historical evidence of tobacco's universal acceptability across socio-religious barriers.

During the American Revolution of 1776, also known as "The Tobacco War," the fledgling government used tobacco exports to build up credits abroad. When the war was over, Americans turned to tobacco taxes to help repay the revolutionary war debt. In 1794, the US Congress passed the first Federal Excise Tax on tobacco products.

Use of tobacco in the form of smoking and smokeless products spread all over the world. According to various reports of missionaries and travelers, hand-rolled cigarettes were known since the middle of the 18th century in South America, especially in Brazil where they were called *"Papelitos"*.

In 1830, the first Cuban *Segars* (as they were then known) arrived in London at the shop of Robert Lewis in St James's street. Two years later, Great Britain's first cigar divan, Simpson's-in-the-Strand opened in London.

While in Europe, from the 1830's, English and Scottish smokers were lit by the 'phosphorus' or 'Lucifer' match, followed by Vestas, Vesuvians, Flamers and Fuzees. The first commercially produced cigarettes were manufactured in France in 1843 by the state-run manufacturer *Francaise des Tabacs.* The first consignment of 20,000 cigarettes was sold at a charity bazaar organized by Queen Marie-Amelie in Paris that year. The French Emperor, Napoleon III(1808–1873) helped to popularize cigarette in France and his own consumption ran to 50 cigarettes a day. By the 1860s, the manufacturers started using better tobacco and a finer sort of paper to roll it in and cigarettes found favour throughout Europe.

The first tobacconists known to have stocked cigarettes were Messrs H. Simmons of Piccadilly and Bacon Brothers of Cambridge, who were pursuing this line of business by 1851. From 1840 to 1870, new strains of the plant and new methods of curing developed resulting into a milder and mellower form of tobacco. Don Luis Susini, who abandoned hand rolling in favor of steam-driven machines, established world's first factory for mass-production of cigarettes in Havana.

In 1854, Dr. Trall reported that the Americans had the highest per capita use of tobacco in the world (Robert 1949). During the Civil War (1861–1868) anti-tobacco movements in America practically disappeared and the habit grew appreciably. Cigarette smoking became common in the USA in 1850s when American tourists returned from Europe introduced and popularized smoking among people of every ethnic background in the USA. It is estimated that in 1850 about 19 cigarettes per capita were smoked in the USA[23]. That increased to 26 cigarettes in 1860. In 1862, the first federal excise tax on tobacco was imposed on cigarette to raise money for the Union war effort[24].

---

[23] National Commission on Marijuana and Drug-abuse Control, 1972.

[24] National Commission Report, USA, 1972.

By 1870, cigarette factories sprang up in Durham, St. Luis, Richmond and Winston and also in the Northern cities such as New York. In 1871, a Wills factory was established in Bristol and Player's factory in Nottingham in 1888. The example of cigarette production was imitated in North America where the manufacture and sale of cigarette had become one of the USA's most important industries - long after the cigarette had made a successful tour of Europe via South America. In 1874, Richard Joshua Reynolds founded his tobacco company in Winston, North Carolina. He was the first to sweeten his product with saccharine in 1891 (Tilley 1985). George Washington Hill of the American Tobacco Company later credited Reynolds for revolutionizing the tobacco industry.

Between 1876 and1888, leading cigarette manufacturers undertook a major advertising campaign and cigarette sale increased manifold. There were two critical inventions behind increased popularity and excessive consumption of cigarettes. First, Bonsack of Virginia had developed a machine by 1881 that could produce more than 200 cigarettes per minutes (Tennant, 1950). A second invention was necessary before the marketing campaign could be contemplated, however: the match, first invented in 1896 but not considered safe until 1912. Before the invention of the match, consumers would frequent the cigar-stores to light their cigarettes from a gas or oil lamp (Sobel, 1978). Match altered the way the cigarettes were smoked, encouraging their consumption during odd moments in the day; in effect, they transformed cigarette use from a thoughtful exercise into an almost unconscious habit.

The first cigarette cards appeared in America early in the 1880s and reached Britain about ten years later. The first US manufacturer was a firm called Allan and Ginter, while the first in the UK was a cigarette manufacturer with the brand name of Glove. In most cases, the card ran into sets of 50. The first brand of cigarettes to be sold in cardboard packets of the modern 'push-up' kind was Wills' Three Castles, in 1892. In May 1931, Craven A was the first brand of the cigarettes to be sold in cellophane-wrapped packets. Convenient availability of cigarettes to the public and easy lighting method contributed to a major increase in cigarette consumption from .05 billion in 1880 to 2.2 billion in 1888. Annual per capita consumption increases paralleled the total production figures.

In late 19$^{th}$ century, in India, the *beedi* industry began to grow. The oldest *beedi*-manufacturing firm was established around 1887 and by 1930 the *beedi* industry had spread across the country. The price differential from cigarettes favoured the use of *beedi* by the working classes and this domestic product soon supplanted cigarettes as the major form of tobacco consumption in Indian subcontinent[25].

In 1901, her son, Edward VII, a great smoker himself who was ticked off by his late mother when she caught him light up in Buckingham palace, succeeded Queen Victoria of England, an anti-smoking monarch.

---

25 Report on Tobacco Control in India, Ministry of Health and Family Welfare, Government of India, 2004.

Between 1895 and 1921, 14 states in USA completely banned cigarette and passed laws regulating cigarette sale. However, these prohibitions had to be lifted between 1920 and 1927, after the World War I, as cigarette smoking became rampant.

It will be reasonable to conclude from these experiences that the anti-cigarette laws and campaign in America like anywhere in the world only popularized the cigarettes and tobacco consumption in other forms. The prohibitions served as a lure. Taxation also played a part in acceptance of cigarette. Some lawmakers favored taxation as a restrictive measure. However, though smokers grumbled, they paid the taxes as they were assessed. By the time this acquiescence generally conceded, the fast growth of revenue to state and federal governments had raised cigarette taxes to a place of importance in government budgets.

In 20th century, low cost and convenience of cigarette combined with increasing prosperity, the growth of leisure and democratization of the society, provided favorable conditions for a massive growth in cigarette consumption. By 1907 in the United States, adult male per capita consumption was 86 cigarettes, and it was traditional to have a "stogy" after dinner with one or more glasses of brandy. Similar trends were evident in European countries where a significant number of adult males had adopted smoking habit. However, there was rising curiosity and fear of abuse among children and adolescents and therefore, sale of cigarettes to children below 16 years of age was declared illegal in Britain in 1908.

Cigarette smoking spread on a large scale after World War I. Cigarettes became associated with the positive values of quiet dignity, courage and dedication of the model soldier and it became an essential part of the soldier's life (Sobel, 1978). When General John J. Peshing was asked about his requirements during World War I, he stated[26]:

> *"You ask me what we need to win this war. I answer, tobacco as much as bullets. Tobacco is as much indispensable as the daily ration; we must have thousands of tons without delay."*

By 1919, during the period of rapid growth in the industry, a phenomenal 38.7% of all cigarettes manufactured in the USA were Camels. Between 1920 and 1929, an average of 80 billion cigarettes per year was produced. Increased production required increased consumption and therefore there was an increase in advertising. Tobacco industry began to advertise on a massive scale using provocative slogans appealing to youth market, women, weight-watchers and health-seekers.

European women had, in fact, developed an early taste for smoking. The French writer, George Sand, while living with Chopin in the mid-1800, loved to shock her guests by lighting up a cigar after breakfast. Some European women liked to smoke in the company of friends, however, this was not common. Cigarette smoking in women increased significantly after the First World War both in Europe and in the Americas.

In 1923, *'du Maurier'* - Britain's first filter cigarette was introduced. Introduction of filter cigarette was originally unrelated to the question of safer smoking, being initially a response to the rising importance to female smoker who was suspected to dislike conventional soggy

---

[26] Reported in Wagner, page 44, 1971.

cigarette ends. Another reason could be that the filter economized on the expansively taxed tobacco leaves preserving the cigarette length whilst avoiding wastage of tobacco in the un-smoked cigarette butt (Corina, 1975). In 1937, for the first time, cancer was produced in laboratory animals by cigarette tar. Though, case reports linking tobacco use with a specific disease – cancer – had appeared in the 19$^{th}$ century, a retrospective study of relationship between the cancer of lungs and smoking habit was carried out in Cologne in 1939. In 1938, it was statistically demonstrated that the longevity of life got reduced in tobacco smokers as compared to those who never smoked.

Following World War II, increasingly more scientific evidence gave added strength to the arguments of anti-tobacconists. During the 1950s and 1960s, conclusive evidence was made available stating that cigarette smoking was the most important cause of lung cancer as well as a major factor in coronary heart disease, chronic bronchitis, emphysema and many other diseases.

The careful epidemiological studies by Doll and Hill in the UK (Doll and Hill, 1952) and Wynder and others in the USA (Wynder *et al.*, 1956) showed a clear statistical association between smoking and cancer. Known carcinogens were identified in the smoke (Van Prosdij 1960; Wynder and Hoffman, 1967). Since then tobacco smoking has been implicated in a wide range of diseases including the cancer of the oral cavity, larynx, pharynx, oesophagus, urinary bladder, coronary heart disease etc.

In 1945, UK's Mayo Clinic issued a health warning against the use of cigarette by the patients with vascular disease or arterial injury. This warning had some effect and cigarette sale in 1950s declined for a couple of years. In 1957, the manufacturers, while pointing out shortcomings of the research said that it should stress correlation and not the causality of link between disease and smoking and cited the need for environmental studies (Fristchler 1969). Gradually the conflict grew and major cigarette manufacturers in USA formed the Tobacco Institute to counteract possible adverse political effects of the health studies (Neuhring and Markle 1974). Cigarette sale was on the rise again.

By 1960, tobacco had become a powerful force in USA. The tobacco coalition included not only the industry but also a clientele of millions whose yearly tobacco consumption exceeded billions of dollars. The recipients of this money included manufacturers, advertising agencies, mass media, farmers, shopkeepers and tax collectors. By 1962, tobacco ranked 4$^{th}$ in overall value of cash crops grown by American farmers.

The most distinctive aspect of tobacco availability concerns the massive expansion of cigarette use in the early and middle decades of the 20$^{th}$ century. Almost no government regulations were promulgated during this period to restrict this expansion; on the contrary, the Federal Government in the USA actively encouraged it through a variety of actions. Only since 1960s has tobacco availability been viewed as a public health issue by any major segment of the society, with many restrictions proposed and some measures instituted at all governmental levels.

Publication of the first report of Surgeon General's Advisory Committee in 1964 in USA provided the impetus to the renewed anti-smoking campaign, which not only attempted to inform people that smoking was dangerous — and to many morally reprehensible — and to persuade them to stop, but also sought to enact legislation to control the sale of cigarettes. In 1965, a health warning appeared on cigarette packets sold in the USA. As a result, in 1968, the use of tobacco declined. However, it increased again in 1970–1971 especially among teenagers (Brecher, 1972). Public Health Smoking Act of 1970 was passed, essentially reflecting the position of anti-smoking interests. In 1970, radio and television advertising of cigarettes was banned throughout USA.

In 1971, Federal Trade Commission (FTC) demanded larger and more prominent health warnings on packages; the tobacco industry agreed to print tar and nicotine content in all cigarette advertising. Taxes on cigarette were raised by 40% (Rublowsky, 1974). A health warning also appeared on the UK cigarette packets in 1971. In 1973, the UK government introduced 'milder' low tar brand of cigarettes that failed commercially by 1977.

Per capita cigarette consumption began falling in USA annually from 1973; however, the tobacco industry continued to flourish. Despite a decline in cigarette use in Northern Europe and USA, tobacco consumption continued to be high in other parts of the world. To some extent the smoking epidemic came under control in the developed world but this epidemic had merely shifted to the developing world where smoking continues to rise.

After the Second World War, USA had begun to export tobacco under the "Food for Peace" programme. In the first 25 years of the programme, $1 billion worth of tobacco was exported exposing developing countries to Western-style cigarettes. By the late 1960s, the leading UK companies and US were selling tobacco to dozens of countries[27]. During the 1980s, international sales rose dramatically. In 1994, 220 billion US manufactured cigarettes were shipped abroad, a 55% increase since 1989.

In the developed world, the proportion of smoking population is falling for the last few decades and the Asian countries have become the target of the US tobacco companies as their potential customers. Perhaps because of this, the tobacco companies are engaged in 'aggressive' marketing in the 'third world' countries where consumption has risen, governments are slow to action and cigarettes remain high in tar and nicotine. To encourage smoking, there has been production of less harmful cigarettes in many developing countries, leading to higher tobacco consumption (Taha and Bill, 1980). Consumption rates are rising steeply in the third world market that is supplied primarily by imports, affiliation or by licenses of the major tobacco companies (Wickstrom, 1980).

Overall cigarette consumption doubled during 1969–1986 (Chandler, 1986). During the 1980s, Japan, Taiwan, South Korea and Thailand opened their markets to American cigarette companies under US pressure. However, Thailand registered the right to ban cigarette

[27] A Deadly Business, Multi-national Monitor, July-August, 1987.

advertising under the ruling by General Agreement on Tariffs and Trade (GATT), which ruled that countries could give "priority to human health over trade liberalization."

Since the lifting of import restrictions the Asian countries have witnessed a dramatic increase in smoking. South Korea's cigarette consumption between 1980 and 1999 has increased by 30% while that in Thailand over the same period grew to the tune of 25%[28].

Scientific evidence related to the harmful effects of tobacco consumption continued to pour in clearly indicating dangerous health consequences in the affected populations.

World Health Organization (WHO), in its 39th World Health Assembly during its 14th Plenary meeting on the 15th May, 1986 urged the Member States to implement the measures to ensure that effective protection was provided to non-smokers from involuntary exposure to tobacco smoke and to protect children and young people from being addicted to the use of tobacco.

In 1988 the World Health Organization (WHO) established the first "World No Tobacco Day" set for May 31. WHO's concern intensified when lung cancer surpassed breast cancer as the number one killer in women. World No -Tobacco Day on 31st May 1989 was celebrated with the slogan: *"The female smokers at added risk."*

43rd World Health Assembly in its 14th Plenary meeting held on the 17th May, 1990 reiterated the concerns expressed in the resolution passed in 1986 and urged the Member States to consider in their tobacco control strategies for legislation and other effective measures for protecting their citizens with special attention to risk groups such as pregnant women and children from involuntary exposure to tobacco smoke, discouraging the use of tobacco and impose progressive restrictions and take concerted action to eventually eliminate all direct and indirect advertising, promotion and sponsorship concerning tobacco.

Emphasis on the ill effects of involuntary smoking and its resultant health-hazards on human body were marked by the slogan of 1991 World No Tobacco Day as *'Public Places and Transport: better be tobacco free.'* The year 1992 focused on work place. The then US president Bill Clinton banned smoking in White House in 1993, and in 1994, McDonald's banned smoking in all its 11,000 restaurants.

Anti-tobacco movement by WHO based on the massive scientific evidence that tobacco and its products were highly addictive and frequently fatal to consumers seemed quite alarming to the flourishing tobacco industry.

Therefore, cigarette manufacturers employed two complementary strategies to deal with the situation. The defensive strategy was the development of an aggressive lobbying organization, epitomized by the tobacco-Institute, and use of supporting research on health

---

[28] Projections to tobacco production, consumption and trade to the year 2010. Food and Agriculture Organization (FAO) of the United Nations.

effects through an industry controlled committee, which was founded in 1954. Research documents pointing out serious health consequences generally went unaccepted publicly by the sponsors. The tobacco industry responded to substantial evidence of harm with a variety of defensive and offensive public relation gimmicks. Finally, in 1999, Philip Morris acknowledged a scientific consensus on smoking:

> *"There is overwhelming medical and scientific consensus that cigarette smoking causes lung cancer, heart disease, emphysema and other serious diseases in smokers, there is no safe cigarette…………..cigarette smoking is addictive, as that term is most commonly used…………..."*

In May 1999, WHO's Framework Convention on Tobacco Control (FCTC) provided the basic tool for the countries to enact comprehensive tobacco control legislation and take on the powerful tobacco industry. The treaty commits nations to ban all tobacco advertising, promotion, and sponsorship (with an exception of constitutional constraints) and to require large warning labels covering at least 30% of the display area of the cigarette pack.

In May 2003, the World Health Organization (WHO) took a historic step by completing five years of work that brought scientific certainty and political will around a set of global rules for tobacco sales, promotion and consumption. The Organization's 192 Member States unanimously adopted the Framework Convention on Tobacco Control (FCTC). WHO member countries backed the resolution calling for an international attempt to regulate tobacco use; a record breaking 50 countries out of 192 pledged financial and political support. In adopting and signing the treaty, the WHO's member states have expressed their firm commitment to tackle the public health challenges posed by tobacco and have resolved to address issues such as price and tax measures, cross-border smuggling, tobacco advertising and promotion, and people's right to clean indoor air.

Indeed, this is not for the first time that law has come to secure public health gain. In its narrative, the logic of the FCTC underscores several studies and research findings that show that tobacco cultivation and consumption increases poverty, depletes national resources and causes five million preventable deaths every year. World No Tobacco Day, 2004, brings out the poverty —causing, poverty-sustaining and exploitative labour practices. This gains special significance for the next phase of FCTC as countries prepare for signature, ratification and implementation of the treaty. India is one of the participating countries in this venture. The Union Cabinet of India approved India's ratification of the Framework Convention of the Tobacco Control (FCTC)[29]. By the early August 2004, 168 WHO member countries had already signed the FCTC and 24 had ratified it[30].

Treaty became international law on 27th February 2005 on completion of 40 ratifications which was the minimum requirement for the FCTC to enter into force. FCTC is an international

[29] Economic Times: Cabinet Ratifies Global Tobacco Control Norms, December 12, 2003.

[30] Action on Smoking and Health – Fact sheet No. 21. Tobacco in the Developing World, WHO, 2004.

legal instrument designed to address the devastating health, social., environmental and economic consequences of tobacco consumption worldwide. On 26th May 2006, of the 168 signatories of FCTC, 128 countries have ratified it[31].

As stated in the Preamble of the treaty, the objective of the FCTC is "to protect present and future generations from the devastating health, social., environmental and economic consequences of tobacco consumption and exposure to tobacco smoke." The preamble also recognizes the need for countries to give priority to their right to protect public health. The FCTC requires all Parties to undertake a comprehensive ban on tobacco advertising, promotion and sponsorship within five years of ratifying the treaty.

Just a decade ago, it would have been inconceivable for an objective observer to imagine that India, in 2003, would be acclaimed as a leader in global tobacco control efforts. Given the fact that India is the second-largest tobacco producer today and had previously valued the revenue – employment generating potential of tobacco agriculture and manufacture, it would have been expected India not playing a pioneering role in tobacco control. Yet, the reality of 2003–2004 is that the Indian Parliament enacted far-reaching anti-tobacco legislation in April 2003. Smoking has been banned in public places since 2003 declaring it as a punishable offence through – the Cigarette and Other Tobacco Products Act, 2003.

This Act bans not only smoking in public places but also forbids the advertising of tobacco and tobacco products. This Act was notified and implemented on 1st May 2004.

It is sufficient time now since the Act is in force, yet the larger picture is truly alarming. India has turned into a potential market for the tobacco industry. As per estimate of National Organization for Tobacco Eradication (NOTE) about 6,000 teenagers start using tobacco products in the country every day[32] and out of 100 teenagers smoking today, 50 will eventually die of tobacco related diseases. Two-third of country's smokers begin at an early age and by the time they realize the risk, they become addicted. It is not surprising that the Indian Government is contemplating to ban smoking scenes in movies.

The World Health Organization (WHO) encourages health professionals to be proactive in minimizing the problems caused by tobacco addiction, consumption and exposure to tobacco smoke. World No Tobacco Day on 31st May 2005 dedicated to the important role of health professionals in tobacco control under the banner of *'Health Professionals against Tobacco, Action and Answers'* emphasizes the critical role of health professionals in reducing tobacco use. Brief and simple advice can substantially increase smoking cessation rates. World No Tobacco Day on 31st May 2006 encourages countries and governments to work towards stricter regulation of tobacco products. The slogan of the day is, 'Tobacco: Deadly in any form or disguise'. There is no safe tobacco product[33]. Tobacco in any form is discouraged. Year 2007 No Tobacco day stressed on keeping the environment free from tobacco-smoke.

---

[31] Tobacco free initiative. World Health Organization, 26th May, 2006.

[32] Legislation Goes up in Smoke, The Times of India, 16th May, 2005.

[33] Tobacco free initiative, World No Tobacco Day 2006, Tobacco deadly in any form or disguise, World Health Organization, 31st May, 2006.

The guidelines published by the US Public Health Service (PHS) recommend that all patients be asked about their tobacco use; those attempting to quit smoking should be prescribed at least one of the first-line pharmacotherapies in the absence of contraindications for these medications (Fiore 2000). These recommendations are especially relevant for psychiatrists as smoking is seen more commonly in patients suffering from mental disorders. All these developments point to the seriousness of the problem the world is facing today due to tobacco menace and the important role that physicians are to play in fighting this menace.

Unquestionably, tobacco was discovered by European sailors in an 'epoch propitious' toward receiving it as a panacea. The superstitious beliefs of the middle ages had not yet disappeared and the experimental curiosity had just begun making tobacco, at one and the same time, a thing of wonder and a thing of science. It became a substance that attracted interest as much by reasons of its exotic mystery and semi-fabulous origin as by strangeness of its working and unexplored field of its possible applications, all of which offered countless opportunities for experimentation. The spread of tobacco use all over Europe was facilitated by the general impression that tobacco was a medicinal plant of remarkable virtues. Though termed as an 'evil plant' by certain moralists, tobacco could not be contained in the confines of European boundaries after its introduction by the Spanish navigators, and its use spread globally despite merciless persecutions suffered by tobacco users at the hands of Turkish Murads, Russian Czars, Japanese kings and so on. Rulers came and perished but tobacco stayed. Later, governments underwent a conversion of sorts, prompted primarily by the realization that tobacco was an excellent source of revenue — derived either from customs dues or from the sale of monopolies to deal in tobacco goods. Pockets of resistance to tobacco still remained, however.

Most of the anti-tobacco crusades from the period of James I were notably for their intolerance, ignorance and more often than not their complacent stupidity. The campaign inaugurated at the end of 19$^{th}$ century and resumed prior to World War I was the most venomous and acrimonious of all. The spectacular growth of cigarette consumption immediately following the war infuriated opponents of the smoking habit and inspired them to intense effects.

Jacob Balde, a Jesuit priest, asked in an anti-tobacco tract published in Nuremberg in 1658, "What difference is there between smoking and a suicide except that one takes longer to kill him than the other?

The view that tobacco was in some way the native Americans' revenge has been expressed more than once. Fagon, the physician to the French King, Luis XIV, very poignantly addressed his fears to the Paris School of Medicine, "America triumphed over the arrogance of her conquerors by infecting them with her own vices; she hastened on the death of her new masters by giving them venereal disease — and tobacco" (Corti, 1996).

Another, more dramatic, spirit imagined meeting the 'tobacco fiend' at the court of Lucifer, said:

> *"Thus do I take revenge in full upon the Spaniardo for all their cruelty to the Indians; since by acquainting their conquerors with the use of tobacco I have done them greater injury than even the king of Spain through his agents ever did his victims; for it is more honourable and more natural to die by a pike thrust or a cannon ball than from the ignoble effects of poisonous tobacco."* (Corti, 1996)

Today, for obvious reasons, little is said in the praise of smoking or using tobacco in other forms. In the current context, smoking is clearly on the defensive and is likely to remain so. A feature of the present situation, however, is that anti-smoking sentiment is firmly anchored in widely accepted medical evidence. Surprisingly, severe and immediate punishment proved no more effective in halting smoking than current fears of long-term health consequences. However, tobacco is deeply interwoven in the world's social fabric and it is highly unlikely that the growth of tobacco, and the manufacture and sale of cigarettes and other tobacco products would stop and the consumer would voluntarily forgo smoking or tobacco use behaviour. The anti-tobacco leagues, which are to be found in one form or another all over the world have lived to see the very countries, which tried to place difficulties in the way of smoking capitulated before the spread of the custom and the opposition of the populace. At present, tobacco is a silent killer for the world and that needs to be killed.

## REFERENCES


Ashton H. and Stepney, R.: *Smoking; Psychology and Pharmacology*: Tavistock Publication London, 1982.

Austin G. A.: *Perspectives of the History of Psychoactive Substance Use*. National Institute of Drug Abuse, Rockville, Maryland, 1978.

Barrie J. M.: *My Lady Nicotine,* Hodder and Stoughton, London, 1890.

Brecher E. M.: *Licit and Illicit Drug Use,* Consumers' Union, New York, 1972.

Brooks J. E.: *The Mighty Leaf: Tobacco Through the Countries,* Alvin Redman, London. 1953.

Chandler W.: *Banishing Tobacco,* World-watch Institute, Washington DC, 1986.

Chattopadhayay A. *Jahangir's Interest in Public Health and Medicine,* Bulletin of Indian Institute of History of Medicine, 25:170–182, 1995.

Corina M.: *Trust in Tobacco: The Anglo-american Struggle for Power*, Michael Joseph, London, 1975.

Corti Count. E. C.: *A History of Smoking,* Bracken Books Random House Limited, London, 1996.

Dickson Sarah: *Panacea or Precious Bane*: *Tobacco in Sixteenth Century,* New York Public Library, New York, 1954.

Doll R. and Hill A. B.: *A Study of Etiology of Carcinoma of Lung*. British Medical Journal,2: 1271 –1286, 1952.

Fion M.: *Tobacco Use and Dependence Guideline Panel, Treating Tobacco Use and Dependence.* US Department of Health and Human Services, Public Health Service, Rockville (MD).7, 2000.

Fristchler A. Lee: *Smoking and Politics: Policy Making and the Federal Bureaucracy,* Appleton-century-crofts, New York, 1969.

Gode P.K.: *Studies in Indian Cultural History, Indological Series* 9, Institute Publication, No. 189, Vishveshvaranand Vedic Research Institute, 1:111–415, Hoshiarpur, 1961.

James I.: *A Counterblast to Tobacco*, London, 1604.

Kluger Richard: *Ashes to Ashes*, Random House of Canada Limited, 1997.

Koskowski W.: *The History of Tobacco Smoking,* Staple Press, London, 1955.

Laufer Berthold: *Introduction of Tobacco in Europe*, Field Museum of National History, Chicago, 1924.

Luthra U., Sreenvas V., Menon G., Prabhakar A.K. and Chaudhry K.: *Tobacco Control in India: Problems and Solutons,* Gupta P C, Hamner JE, Murtpr (Eds) *Control of Tobacco-related Cancer and other Diseases,* International Symposium, Oxford University Press, Bombay, 1992.

Morrison S.E.: *The Oxford History of American People*, Oxford University Press New York, 93–94, 1965.

Neahring E. and Markle G.: *Nicotine and Norms: The Re-emergence of A Deviant Behaviour, Social Problems,* 21 (4): 513–526, 1974.

Olearius Adam: Beschreibung Der Moskowitischen Und Persienisches Reise, P 100 and 140 Hamburg Edition, 1696.

Ortiz Fernando: *Cuban Counterpoint: Tobacco and Sugar*, Knopf, New York, 1947.

Robert J.: *The Story of Tobacco in America*, Knopf, New York, 1949.

Rublowsky J.: *The Stoned Age: A History of Drugs in America*, Putnam, New York, 1974.

Sanghvi L.D.: *Challenges to Tobacco Control in India: A Historical Perspective*, In: Gupta PC, Hamner JE, Murti PR (Eds) Control of Tobacco Related Cancers and other Diseases, International Symposium, 1990, Oxford University Press: Mumbai; 47–55, 1992.

Satow Ernest: *The Introduction of Tobacco Into Japan*. Translation of the Asiatic Society of Japan, 6(1): 68–86, 1878.

Sobel R: *They Satisfy: Cigarette in American Life,* Anchor Press, Garden City, New Jersey, 1978.

Taha A. and Bill K.: *Smoking and Africa: The Coming Epidemic,* British Medical Journal. 280 (6219): 991–993, 1980.

Tennant R.: *The American Cigarette Industry: A Study in Economic Analysis and Public Policy,* Yale University Press, New Haven, 1950.

Tilley, N.: *The R. J. Reynolds Tobacco Company,* University of North Carolina Press, Chapel Hill, 1985.

Van Prosidij C.: *Smoking: Its Influence on Industrial and Role in Social Medicine,* Amsterdam: Elsevier, 1960.

Wagner Susan: *Cigarette Country Tobacco in American History and Politics*, Praeger Publishers, New York, 1978.

Wickstrom B.: *Cigarette Marketing in the Third World.* in L. M. Ramstrom (Eds) The Smoking Epidemic: The Proceedings of the Fourth World Conference on Smoking and Health. Stockholm: Almqvist and Wiksell International, 1980.

Wilber Johannes: *Tobacco and Shamanism*, Yale University Press, Yale, 1987.

Wynder E. L., Bross I. J., Cornfield, J. and O' Donnell W. E.: Lung Cancer in Women. *New England Journal of Medicine.* 255 (24): 1111–1121. 1956.

Wynder E. L. and Hoffman D.: *Tobacco and Tobacco Smoke*. Academic Press, New York, 1967.

CHAPTER

# 2 Global Trends in Tobacco Use

*No doubt, tobacco use has declined in high–income countries; there have been sharp increases in tobacco use, in lower and middle income countries in recent years (especially among men). Tobacco use continues to rise in the developing countries, aided and abetted by a sophisticated, wealthy and powerful drug cartel based in New York and London.*

— Ashton and Stepneny, 1982

Within 150 years of Columbus's discovery of tobacco leaves in the New World in the last decade of fifteenth century, the use of tobacco became pervasive worldwide. Its rapid spread and widespread acceptance in both smoking and smokeless forms points to the fact that large scale tobacco consumption provided opportunities to the commercial forces to dictate massive cultivation and production to ensure its availability all over the world. In the initial years, tobacco was often chewed or smoked in various kinds of clay pipes followed by cigars and primitive cigarettes made by stuffing tobacco in a hollow cane tube, or by rolling crushed tobacco leaves in cornhusk or other vegetable materials (Luthra *et al.*, 1992). Some of these practices still persist, but they are on a decline. Mid-nineteenth century witnessed a significant development in the history of tobacco use that helped tobacco smoking to assume global proportions to the extent of its being used in all strata of human society. Cigarette appeared in mass manufactured form in the 19$^{th}$ century when the world's first factory for its mass-production was established in Havana, Cuba in 1853, and since then cigarette smoking spread worldwide on a global scale. Indeed, until about 1870 cigarettes were relatively rare in the United States from where this commodity began, and almost all tobacco consumed domestically was chewed during the mid-19$^{th}$ century (Gottsegen, 1940). Large-scale cigarette production ensured not only the easy and convenient availability it also decreased the cost to bring cigarettes within the reach of common people. Twentieth century, which brought prosperity to the world, enhanced growth of leisure and introduced democratization in the society, provided favourable conditions for a massive increase in cigarette smoking. At the dawn of this century several events occurred that contributed to increased per capita cigarette consumption. Some of these events were: (i) introduction of blend and curing process that allowed the inhalation of tobacco, (ii) improvement in mass production of cigarettes, (iii) invention of safety match which made the smoking activity easier from a planned effort to go to a cigarette store and light the cigarette to an unmindful activity; (iv) transportation that permitted widespread availability and accessibility possible even in the remotest areas and (v) use of mass media advertising to promote and popularize cigarette consumption.

Today, the smoking of cigarettes is the most important means of tobacco consumption, in terms of both prevalence and health consequences, though in some parts of the world such as India and other Asian countries, use of smokeless tobacco and other forms of tobacco smoking is also quite common. Over time, with universal spread and recognition of consequent ill effects, smoking became a major public health concern associated with a number of diseases and death[1].

## Global Tobacco Production: Changing Trends

About 100 countries around the world produce tobacco. The top ten producers, most of which are developing countries, produce 80% of the world's total tobacco. In 2003–2004, China was responsible for the production of 39.2% of all tobacco grown worldwide, with India, Brazil, and the United States, producing 25% between them. During this period, world production of un-manufactured tobacco was 5,672567 tons of which 2,224,481 tons (39.2%) were produced by China and 595,000 tons (10.5%) by India. Other top tobacco producers are Brazil, USA, Zimbabwe, Turkey, Indonesia etc. (Table 1 & 2).

***Table 1: Top ten tobacco producing countries***

| *Country* | *Tobacco Production (in million tons)* |
|---|---|
| China | 2.224 |
| India | 0.595 |
| Brazil | 0.515 |
| United States | 0.339 |
| European Union | 0.314 |
| Zimbabwe | 0.204 |
| Turkey | 0.142 |
| Indonesia | 0.135 |
| USSR(former area) | 0.116 |
| Malawi | 0.122 |
| Others | 1.187 |
| **Total World Production** | **5.667** |

***Source:*** *Higher World Tobacco Use Expected by 2010 – Growth Rate slowing down http://www.fao.org/english/newsroom/news/2003/26919-enhtml Visited on 13.6.2006*

[1] World Health Organization. Tobacco and health in the developing world. Background paper for the high level round table on Tobacco Control and Development Policy, Brussels, 2003.

For the last two decades, tobacco production is declining in the developed countries (Table 2). The share of global tobacco production by high-income countries has fallen from 30% to 15%. In 1998–1999, United States of America produced 604,131 tons of tobacco which gradually declined to 339,241 tons in 2003–2004. Similar decline is seen in the countries in Northern Europe. On the contrary, tobacco production in the developing world is consistently increasing. In the Middle East and Asia tobacco production has risen from 40 to 60% while Africa's share has increased from 4 to 6%. In 1998–1999, India was the third largest tobacco producer globally after China and USA and produced 572,200 tons (9.2% of world's share) of tobacco that year. However, in 2002–2003, India produced 592,000 tons (9.8% of world's share) of tobacco leaving USA and Brazil behind and occupied second position. Since then India is the second largest tobacco producer in the world (Table 2).[2] Lately there has been an overall decline in total world tobacco production due to various reasons including a decline in its consumption in the developed countries. Cultivation of tobacco as a cash crop is an important source of revenue for many and some countries such as Malawi and Zimbabwe depend significantly upon income generated through tobacco cultivation.

***Table 2: World unmanufactured tobacco production (in tons)***

| | *Production in tons* | | | *Share in world production (%)* | | |
|---|---|---|---|---|---|---|
| | *1998–1999* | *2002–2003* | *2003–2004* | *1998–1999* | *2002–2003* | *2003–2004* |
| China | 2,010,250 | 2,365,988 | 2,224,481 | 32.2 | 39.3 | 39.2 |
| USA | 604,131 | 358,363 | 339,241 | 9.7 | 5.9 | 5.9 |
| India | 572,200 | 592,000 | 595,000 | 9.2 | 9.8 | 10.5 |
| Brazil | 373,150 | 551,250 | 515,720 | 5.9 | 9.2 | 9.1 |
| Turkey | 217,570 | 133,812 | 142,190 | 3.5 | 2.2 | 2.5 |
| Indonesia | 123,653 | 144,700 | 135,000 | 1.9 | 2.4 | 2.4 |
| Malawi | 95,996 | 124,301 | 122,580 | 1.5 | 2.1 | 2.2 |
| Greece | 127,000 | 120,000 | 121,000 | 2.0 | 1.9 | 2.1 |
| Italy | 112,225 | 108,460 | 106,250 | 1.8 | 1.8 | 1.9 |
| Argentina | 98,100 | 106,000 | 97,700 | 1.6 | 1.8 | 1.7 |
| Pakistan | 84,636 | 84,721 | 86,389 | 1.4 | 1.4 | 1.5 |
| Others | 1,815,686 | 1,335,000 | 1,187,016 | 29.1 | 22.2 | 20.9 |
| WORLD TOTAL | 6,234,577 | 6,024,689 | 5,672,567 | 100 | 100 | 100 |

***Source:** United States Department of Agriculture (USDA) estimates for February, 2004*

2 Medium term export strategy 2002-2007 for tobacco and tobacco products. India Domain Web Service (P) Limited© 2002 Tobacco Board, Ministry of Commerce, Government of India.

## Changing Trends: Rising Cigarette Consumption in Low-income and Middle-income Countries

Annual per capita cigarette consumption in the USA was just 54 cigarettes in 1900. It increased steadily since 1930s and reached 4345 cigarettes by 1963. Consumption began to decline after that and came down to 2261 cigarettes in 1998 thanks to vigorous anti-smoking campaign and increased awareness about smoking related health risks. Declining trends are clearly witnessed since 1973. In USA, the overall cigarette smoking fell from 52.6 percent among men (peak year 1955) and 31.4 percent in women (peak year 1965) to 37.1 and 26.8 respectively in 1987. With this decline in smoking, incidence of smoking related cancers also declined and age-adjusted death rates per 100,000 persons for heart diseases decreased from 307.4 per 100,000 in 1950 to 134.6 per 100,000 in 1996. This provides a scientifically valid reason to substantiate that tobacco consumption in the form of cigarette smoking is responsible not only for causation of cancer it is responsible for significant number of deaths as well.

It is estimated that the demand of tobacco will continue to fall in these countries to 2.05 million tons in 2010 (10% lower than the 1998 figure)[3]. Decline in tobacco use is attributed to following factors:

- Scientific evidence of the relation among disease, tobacco use, and environmental exposure to tobacco—Surgeon General's Report, 1964.
- Dissemination of this information to the public.
- Surveillance and evaluation of prevention and cessation programmes.
- Campaign by advocates of non-smokers' rights.
- Restriction on cigarette advertising.
- Counter-advertising.
- Policy change (enforcement of minors' access laws, legislation restricting smoking at public places and increased taxation).
- Improvement in treatment and prevention programmes.
- Increased understanding of economic costs of tobacco.

Despite the decline in cigarette use in Northern Europe and the USA, the industry continues to flourish and the overall cigarette consumption doubled during 1969 to 1986 (Chandler, 1986). To some extent the epidemic of cigarettes is under control in USA and the UK; however, this success is not global, because the epidemic is merely transferred to other parts of the world. No doubt, tobacco use has declined in high-income countries; there have been sharp increases in tobacco use, in lower and middle income countries in recent years (especially among men). Tobacco use continues to rise in the developing countries, aided and abetted by a sophisticated, wealthy and powerful drug cartel based in New York and London.

---

[3] Cigarette Packing: The Global Survey, Published by ERC Statistical Institute, 2001.

A survey of 35 leading cigarette producing nations and cigarette markets in the world reveals that, in 1999, a total of 272 billion packs of cigarettes were consumed by these countries and the consumption increased further by 1.3% to reach 275.7 billion in 2000[4]. By contrast, tobacco consumption rates in the developing countries are expected to increase to 5.09 million tons by 2010 (1.7% increase than the 1998 figure)[5]. Currently close to 60% of total cigarettes consumed each year and 75% of total tobacco users are in developing countries alone[6].

Rising per capita consumption, a growing population, and an increasing acceptance of women smoking continue to generate new demands (Tunistra, 1998). Transnational tobacco companies have continued to identify positive aspects of market in the developing countries especially in Asia. China, despite being world's largest tobacco producer, does not export as much proportion of its tobacco as other countries do. The most populous country, China is also the world's leading tobacco consumer. Tobacco consumption is rising in the developing countries by 3.4 percent per annum.

Overall, the ratio of average cigarette consumption, per adult, between developed and developing countries have narrowed from 3.3 in the early 1970s to 1.8 in the early 1990s. Just as the gap has narrowed between developed and developing countries, it is clearly narrowing between men and women. The tobacco epidemic is being mirrored between men and women and is spreading its focus from men in higher income countries to men in developing countries and to women in both developing and developed countries. And just as the gap between men and women and developed and developing countries is narrowing, it is broadening the divide between socio-economic groups. In UK, there has been a significant decrease in smoking over time by women in upper socio-economic groups and by men in all ages and socio-economic groups (Townsend *et al.*, 1994). The governments and health agencies of the developed world have met with some limited success in the campaign to reduce the prevalence rate of smoking, but rates are rising steeply in the developing countries.

International trade agreements of liberalized global trade in many goods including cigarettes have removed trade barriers leading to greater competition, lower price, greater advertising, and other activities to stimulate demand. In four Asian economies (Japan, South Korea, Taiwan and Thailand) that opened their markets in response to the US trade pressure during the 1980s, consumption of cigarettes per person was almost 10% higher in 1991 than it would have been, if these markets had remained closed. Increased trade liberalization contributed significantly to rise in cigarette consumption, particularly in the low and middle-income countries. The entry of a multi-national tobacco company into a new market is typically accompanied by

---

4 Cigarette Packing: The Global Survey, Published by ERC Statistical Institute, 2001.

5 Cigarette Packing: The Global Survey, Published by ERC Statistical Institute, 2001.

6 Action on Smoking and Health, Fact-sheet No. 21: Tobacco in the Developing World, WHO, 2004.

sophisticated and effective advertising and promotional activities, often leading national tobacco companies to step up their marketing activities in response. As a result, overall expenditure on advertising increases with a corresponding rise in tobacco consumption. Since tobacco consumption in the high income countries is declining, it is crucial for the financial health of the tobacco companies to recruit new consumers. Tobacco industry spends billions of dollars every year around the world to advertise market and promote tobacco products. In the United States alone, tobacco companies spent more than $12.47 billion in 2002 to promote their products[7]. Asian countries in particular have been the targets of US tobacco companies.

This expanding market in the third world is supplied primarily by import, affiliation, or licensing of the major tobacco companies (Wickstrom, 1980). Nevertheless, growing tobacco itself is becoming a major part of the economy in many countries such as Malawi and India. In 2001, India exported 5.6 percent of world's tobacco export occupying 5$^{th}$ position after Brazil (17%), USA (10%), Zimbabwe (9%) and China (6%). 80% of the tobacco exported from India is in the form of un-manufactured tobacco being exported to 80 different countries of the world. From these countries, this un-manufactured tobacco is used for making manufactured goods by the tobacco companies and then re-exported with aggressive advertising.

Since the lifting of import restrictions, the Asian countries have witnessed a dramatic increase in smoking: South Korea's tobacco consumption rose from 68,000 tons in 1980–82 to 101,000 tons in 1999 while that in Thailand over the same period grew from 31,000 tons to 40,000 tons[8]. Partly because of the growth in the adult population and partly because of increased consumption in the developing countries, despite of a decline in developed countries, total number of tobacco users is on an increase globally.

In the year 2001, the annual cigarette consumption was around 1.6 trillion sticks in China, 415 billion cigarettes in the USA, 327 billion in Japan, 257 billion in Russia, 140 billion in Germany, around 100 billion in India and 97 billion in Brazil. India is the sixth largest cigarette consumer in the world, however, if *beedi* smoking is included with cigarettes, India becomes the second largest tobacco smoking country in the world.

***Table 3: Country-wise cigarette consumption, 2001***

| *Country* | *Number of cigarette sticks smoked* |
|---|---|
| China | 1.6 Trillion |
| USA | 415 Billion |
| Japan | 327 Billion |
| Russia | 257 Billion |
| Germany | 140 Billion |
| India* | 100 Billion |
| Brazil | 97 Billion |

*The Figures exclude *beedi* smoking

7 Women and Tobacco, World Health Organization, pp 63-66, 1992.

8 Mackay J and Eriksen M., The Tobacco Atlas, World Health Organization, 1992.

Today, it is estimated that there are about 1.3 billion tobacco users worldwide, approximately one billion men and more than 250 million women[9] who consume almost 6 trillion sticks of cigarettes (and *beedis)* annually or 15 billion sticks every day. If the current trends continue, it is expected that by 2025, the number of tobacco users will be 1.6 billions[10].

Globally, tobacco use is higher amongst men (47%) than it is amongst women (12%)[11]. In the developed countries, 35% of men and 22% of women smoke, while in the developing ones, figures are 50% and 9% respectively (Mackay and Eriksen, 2002). In most developing nations this is partly due to cultural tradition, although situation is changing and more women are taking up smoking in response to the marketing tactics of the tobacco industry.[12] Women in developing countries are clearly a key potential market for the tobacco industry. Britain and USA based multi-national tobacco companies are largely responsible for the rapid increase of cigarette consumption especially in the women in the developing countries.

## Global Tobacco Smoking and Gender

Cigarette smoking among women in the developed world, both in Americas and Europe, began to increase after the First World War, when targeted industry-marketing and social changes reflecting the liberalization of women's role and behaviour led to the increasing acceptability of smoking among women. Cigarette smoking was rare among women in the early 20th century; as such their smoking prevalence has always been lower than among men. However, the gender-specific difference in smoking prevalence is narrowing. Overall smoking rates are higher among men as compared to women. However, there is a considerable variation between countries, from those where the rates among men and women are nearly equal., such as in the USA and the UK, to those with rates higher among women, such as Sweden.

***Table 4: Prevalence of cigarette smoking in men & women in selected countries.***
***Smoking prevalence (%)***

| *Country* | *Males* | *Females* | *Year* |
|---|---|---|---|
| Australia | 29.0 | 21.0 | 1993 |
| Austria | 42.0 | 27.0 | 1992 |
| Bahamas | 19.3 | 3.8 | 1989 |

*Contd...*

9 Tobacco Control, Country Profile, second edition, p. 7., 2003.

10 Tobacco Control, Country Profile. WHO, second edition, p. 10., 2003.

11 Annual Survey of Industries, Central Statistical Organization, New Delhi, 1997-98.

12 World No Tobacco Day 2004, Tobacco Control and Poverty, WHO, 2004.

| Country | Males | Females | Year |
|---|---|---|---|
| Belgium | 31.0 | 19.0 | 1993 |
| Canada | 31.0 | 29.0 | 1991 |
| China | 56.0 | 6.0 | 1991 |
| Cyprus | 42.5 | 7.2 | 1990 |
| Denmark | 37.0 | 37.0 | 1993 |
| Finland | 27.0 | 19.0 | 1994 |
| France | 40.0 | 27.0 | 1993 |
| Germany | 36.8 | 21.5 | 1992 |
| Iceland | 31.0 | 28.0 | 1994 |
| Ireland | 29.0 | 28.0 | 1993 |
| Israel | 45.0 | 30.0 | 1989 |
| Italy | 38.0 | 26.0 | 1994 |
| Japan | 59.0 | 14.8 | 1994 |
| Korea | 68.0 | 6.7 | 1989 |
| Kuwait | 52.0 | 12.0 | 1991 |
| Luxembourg | 32.0 | 26.0 | 1993 |
| Netherlands | 36.0 | 29.0 | 1994 |
| New Zealand | 24.0 | 22.0 | 1992 |
| Norway | 36.4 | 35.5 | 1994 |
| Portugal | 38.0 | 15.0 | 1994 |
| Singapore | 32.0 | 3.0 | 1995 |
| Spain | 48.0 | 25.0 | 1993 |
| Sweden | 22.0 | 24.0 | 1994 |
| Switzerland | 36.0 | 26.0 | 1992 |
| United Kingdom | 28.0 | 26.0 | 1994 |
| USA | 37.7 | 22.5 | 1993 |

**Source:** *Ranson K; Jha P; Chaloupka F; Yurekli A (2000) Effectiveness and cost effectiveness of price increases and other tobacco control policy interventions. In: Jha P and Chaloupka F (eds) Tobacco Control Policies in Developing Countries, Oxford University Press, New York.*

In countries like China, though, less than 6 percent of women are daily smokers compared to 56 percent of men (Table 4) these differences reflect different stages of the smoking epidemic in each country. Prevalence rates of smoking vary considerably across developed and developing countries from as much as 58 percent in Nepal to just half of this in UK (Table 5).

*Table 5: Prevalence of cigarette smoking among women in selected conuntries*

| *Region/Country* | *Prevalence (%)* | *Year of Survey* |
|---|---|---|
| **AMERICAS** | | |
| Bolivia | 38 | 1986 |
| Brazil | 33 | 1990 |
| Guyana | 4 | - |
| Honduras | 11 | 1988 |
| Jamaica | 27 | 1988 |
| Trinidad | 5 | 1986–89 |
| United States | 26 | 1990 |
| **EUROPE** | | |
| Denmark | 45 | 1988 |
| France | 30 | 1991 |
| Germany | 27 | 1988 |
| Poland | 35 | 1989 |
| Portugal | 12 | 1988 |
| Spain | 28 | 1988 |
| United Kingdom | 28 | 1992 |
| **AFRICA** | | |
| Ivory Coast | 1 | 1981 |
| Guinea | 1 | 1981 |
| Nigeria | 10 | 1990 |
| Swaziland | 7 | 1989 |
| South Africa | 17 | 1995 |
| Zambia | 4–7 | 1984 |
| **EASTERN MEDITERRANEAN** | | |
| Bahrain | 20 | 20 |
| Egypt | 2 | 2 |
| Sudan | 19 | 19 |
| Tunisia | 6 | 6 |
| **SOUTH-EAST ASIA** | | |
| India | 0–67* | – |
| Indonesia | 10 | 1990 |
| Nepal | 58 | 1991 |
| Thailand | 4 | 1988 |
| **WESTERN PACIFIC** | | |
| Australia | 27 | 1986–1989 |
| China | 5 | 1991 |
| Japan | 14 | 1990 |
| Malaysia | 5 | 1990 |
| New Zealand | 24 | 1986–1989 |
| Singapore | 2 | 1988 |

***Source:*** *Amos A: Women and Smoking, British Medical Bulletin. 52 (1): 74–89, 1996.*

Table 6 shows the number of cigarettes smoked per day for men and women aged 15 and above in selected countries. It can be seen that in several countries the smoking rates are identical for men and women, notably Hong Kong, Ireland, Italy, Singapore, South Korea and Spain.

***Table 6: Number of cigarettes smoked per smoker per day by gender***

| *Country* | *Men* | *Women* |
|---|---|---|
| Australia | 21.3 | 19.7 |
| Austria | 19.2 | 15.7 |
| Bahamas | 14.0 | 12.0 |
| Belgium | 17.6 | 15.1 |
| Canada | 24.6 | 21.6 |
| Denmark | 12.8 | 11.3 |
| Finland | 15.4 | 12.9 |
| France | 14.2 | 11.2 |
| Germany | 19.5 | 17.8 |
| Hong Kong | 14.1 | 14.1 |
| Ireland | 20.9 | 20.9 |
| Italy | 15.1 | 15.1 |
| Israel | 21.0 | 15.0 |
| Japan | 24.9 | 21.6 |
| Netherlands | 15.7 | 13.7 |
| New Zealand | 17.4 | 16.0 |
| Norway | 11.7 | 10.3 |
| Portugal | 20.8 | 17.8 |
| Singapore | 18.7 | 18.7 |
| South Korea | 24.8 | 24.8 |
| Spain | 12.5 | 12.5 |
| Sweden | 15.3 | 14.3 |
| Switzerland | 22.1 | 19.6 |
| United Kingdom | 18.4 | 16.9 |
| United States of America | 24.3 | 22.5 |

***Source:** Ranson K; Jha P; Chaloupka F., and Yurekli A.: Effectiveness and cost effectiveness of price increases and other tobacco control policy interventions. In: Jha P and Chaloupka F (eds) Tobacco Control Policies in Developing Countries. Oxford University Press, New York, 2000.*

A recent national survey in Singapore has shown that since the start of the National Smoking Control Programme in 1986, there has been an overall decrease in smoking prevalence from 20 % (37% males and 3% females) in 1984 to 15% (26.9% males and 3.1% females) in 1998. Of concern is the increase in the smoking among young women aged 18–24 years. The smoking prevalence among women in this age group has increased from 0.8% in 1984 to 2.8% in 1992 and 5.9% in 1998 as depicted in table 7 (Aghi *et al.,* 1999).

**Table 7: Prevalence of daily smoking among age groups in Singapore by gender, 1998.**

| | Male (%) | | Female (%) | | Total (%) | |
|---|---|---|---|---|---|---|
| AGE (Years) | 1992 | 1998 | 1992 | 1998 | 1992 | 1998 |
| 18–24 | 29.0 | 25.5 | 2.8 | 5.9 | 16.1 | 15.8 |
| 25–44 | 35.2 | 27.2 | 2.4 | 2.6 | 19.0 | 15.0 |
| 45–64 | 31.5 | 27.0 | 4.7 | 2.5 | 18.1 | 14.8 |
| 18–64 | 33.2 | 26.9 | 3.0 | 3.1 | 18.3 | 15.0 |

***Source:*** *Aghi M; Asma S; Vaithinathan R and Chng CY (1999) Initiation and Maintenance of Tobacco Use. Presented at Kobe International Conference on Women and Tobacco. Kobe, Japan.*

Cigarette smoking in women is not widely accepted in Indian society. Prevalence of smoking habit or chewing habit differs in various parts of the country. Types of smoking habits, such as *beedi, chutta, chillum, hookah,* and chewing habits such as *khaini, mawa,* betel quid, *Zarda, paan masala,* differ in various parts of the country. In general., men smoke as well as chew tobacco. In the coastal areas of Andhra Pradesh and Orissa, women smoke *cheroot* or *chuttas* in a reverse manner (i.e. with the burning end inside the mouth), and in some northern parts of India, women often smoke *hookah* (described in details later).

There is a varied profile of rural women in India using tobacco; they are generally housewives or farm-labourers with low literacy rate. The main reason of initiation of tobacco use was found to be accepted norms, beliefs and use as medicinal aid (to cure toothache, during labour, etc). In Kerala (a southern state in India), where literacy rate is highest and women are by and large financially independent, chewing tobacco with betel leaf and areca nut is quite common. Several population-based studies from different parts of the country during late 1970s reveal the consumption rates ranging from 33–80 percent among men and 15–67 percent among women.

Trade liberalization has contributed significantly to rise in women cigarette consumption, particularly in the low and middle-income countries of which India is no exception. The entry of a multi-national tobacco company into these markets accompanied by aggressive advertising and promotional activities targeting the women as potential customers has eroded the age-old stigma associated with women tobacco smoking in traditional societies. In India where women cigarette smoking was frowned upon earlier, it is not an uncommon phenomenon according to a study conducted in the urban population of India in 1998, which has found 2–5 percent women smoking cigarettes (Kalia, 1998). Studies suggest that cigarette smoking in women will lead to increased burden of disease over the next few years (GYTS, 2003).

Other Asian countries show similar trends. Recent increases in female smoking prevalence have been reported from Cambodia, Malaysia and Bangladesh[13]. Figures for 1998 reveal that 4% of the Chinese women smoked as compared to 3% in 1991[14]; this figure has risen to 6% in 2000.

## Global Tobacco Consumption and Age

Most affected age group is between 30 to 39 years (Table 8). Individuals who avoid smoking in adolescence or young adulthood are unlikely to ever become smokers. Majority of smokers start before 25 years of age, often in childhood or people under the age of 18 began smoking daily. Nearly 10 percent of these begin smoking even before 13 years and more than one third of high school students report almost daily smoking.

During adolescence, in the high-income countries, eight out of ten begin to smoke in their teens. In the United States, 90% of adult smokers begin smoking by 18 years of age (Pierce *et al.*, 1991).

***Table 8: Global prevalence of smoking and number of smokers, by age and gender, 1995.***

| | *Males* | | *Females* | | *Total* | | |
|---|---|---|---|---|---|---|---|
| *Age in years* | *Prevalence %age* | *Number of smokers (millions)* | *Prevalence %* | *Number of smokers (millions)* | *Prevalence %* | *Number of smokers (millions)* | *Total smokers %age* |
| 15–19 | 33 | 86 | 5 | 13 | 19 | 98 | 8 |
| 20–29 | 42 | 212 | 12 | 58 | 27 | 271 | 23 |
| 30–39 | 57 | 234 | 15 | 61 | 36 | 295 | 26 |
| 4049 | 58 | 181 | 15 | 46 | 37 | 227 | 20 |
| 50–59 | 51 | 107 | 12 | 25 | 31 | 132 | 11 |
| 60+ | 40 | 101 | 11 | 34 | 25 | 134 | 12 |
| Total | 47 | 921 | 12 | 236 | 30 | 1157 | 100 |
| % of total | | 80 | | 20 | | 100 | |

***Source:*** *Ranson K; Jha P; Chaloupka F and Yurekli A (2000) Effectiveness and cost-effectiveness of price increases and other tobacco control policy interventions. In: Jha P and Chaloupka F (eds) Tobacco Control Policy in Developing countries; Oxford University Press, New York.*

A decline in the starting age of smoking has been observed in the high-income countries. In one of the surveys[15] it was noted that in 1998, each day in the US more than 2000

[13] U S Federal Trade Commission (FTC) Cigarette Report for 2002; http://www.ftc.gov/reports/cigarette/041022cigar etterpt.pdf

[14] The Tobacco epidemic: A Global Public Health Emergency. WHO, 2003. WHO urges countries to prevent a tobacco epidemic among women and girls: Press release, WHO/27, May, 2001.

adolescents began to smoke. The US is currently witnessing a new harmful trend amongst teenagers in the form of *beedi* smoking. Small filter-less, flavoured tobacco sticks, imported primarily from India have become quite popular among American adolescents[16]. Several studies[17] conducted in school population in the age range of 7 to 14 years reveal the prevalence of *beedi* smoking among the US students to be alarmingly high. Investigators have found that 3.8 to 31% school students smoke *beedis.* Starting to smoke at younger ages increases the risk of death from a smoking related cause and those who continue to smoke throughout their lives, about half can expect to die from a smoking-related cause, with half of those deaths occurring in the middle age. In France and Spain where more than 40% of young people aged 18–24 smoke, a very heavy future death toll from tobacco use can be expected[18].

**Table 9: Tobacco-use among children aged 13–15 years (%)**

| *Country/State* | *Cigarette* | *Other Tobacco Product* | *Any Tobacco Product* |
|---|---|---|---|
| **India** | | | |
| Bihar | 7.2 | 51.8 | 58.9 |
| Assam | 7.7 | 28.6 | 36.1 |
| Meghalaya | 7.0 | 37.3 | 43.9 |
| Goa | 0.4 | 4.1 | 4.5 |
| Tamil Nadu | 20.4 | 4.1 | 4.5 |
| Maharashtra | 0.5 | 12.4 | 12.9 |
| West Bengal | 3.5 | 10.8 | 14.3 |
| **Sri Lanka** | 4.0 | 7.2 | 9.9 |
| **Indonesia** | 20.4 | 2.5 | 20.8 |

***Source:*** *Prevalence of Tobacco use in school-going children aged 13 to 15 years in the selected countries of South East Asia Region, 1999–2001. WHO/SEARO, Malaria Unit 2002. http://www.whosea.org/eip/TAB69.htm*

In middle income and low income countries, most smokers start by early twenties, but the trend is toward younger ages. In China, between 1984 and 1996, there was a significant increase in the number of young men, aged between 15 and 19 years, who took to smoking. Tobacco consumption among 13–15 year old students is studied worldwide through the

15 National Household Survey on Drug-abuse (1999) USA.

16 Cancer Cause, Control and Prevention (2000) Kluwer Academic Publication, printed in the Netherlands; 11:577-578.

17 Centre for Disease Control and Prevention (2000), Tobacco Use among Middle and High school students in the USA, Morbidity, Mortality Weekly Reporter, 49:49-53.

18 The Tobacco Epidemic: A Global Public Health Emergency WHO, 1999.

Global Youth Tobacco Survey (GYTS, 2003) incorporating Global School Personnel Survey (GSPS). Prevalence of tobacco use among school-going children aged 13–15 years in the selected countries of the South East Asian Region between 1999–2001 is shown in Table 6. Prevalence of smoking and use of other forms of tobacco is highest in India's Eastern states of Bihar, Assam, and Meghalaya; however, smoking alone is higher in the State of Tamil Nadu. Smoking prevalence in Indonesian children is quite high even in the age group of 13–15 years (Table 9).

In India, every year, about 55,000 children take up the smoking habit. Those who start smoking at an early age generally hail from lower socio-economic strata, have poor social support, are illiterate, and victims of broken homes, and deprivations and discriminations. Use of intoxicants including tobacco smoking in erstwhile lower castes of Hindu social hierarchy of Indian society is most prevalent (Briggs, 1920). Two-third of the country's smokers begin at an early age. By the time they realize the risk they become addicted to it[19].

Evidence is quite clear that in most countries, the median age of smoking initiation is under 15 years. It is also observed that the individuals who start to smoke at a young age are likely to become heavy smokers, and are also at increased risk of dying from smoking-related diseases in later life such as cancer, pulmonary or cardiac diseases.

## Socio-economic Status and Global Smoking Pattern

Historically, as incomes have risen within populations, the number of smokers has risen too. In the earlier decades of tobacco epidemic, in high-income countries, smokers were more likely to be affluent than poor. But in the last three or four decades this pattern seems to have reversed, at least among men. Affluent men in the high-income countries have increasingly abandoned tobacco, whereas poorer men have not done so. For example, in Norway, the percentage of men with high income who smoked fell from 75% in 1955 to 28% in 1990. Over the same period, the population of men with low income who smoked declined much less steeply from 60% in 1955 to 40% in 1990. Today, in most high-income countries, there are significant differences in the prevalence of smoking between different socio-economic groups. In UK, for instance, only 10% women and 12% men in the highest socio-economic group are smokers; in the lowest socio-economic groups the corresponding figures are three folds greater, i.e., 35% and 40%. More than 55 percent of men in the United States smoked at the peak of consumption

[19] Legislation goes up in smoke, The Times of India, 16th May, 2005.

in the mid-twentieth century, but the proportion has fallen to 28 percent by the mid 1990s. Per capita consumption in high-income countries as a whole has decreased, however, among women and adolescents in these countries, smoking has grown in 1990s. Overall then, the smoking epidemic is spreading from its original focus among men in high-income countries, to men in low-income countries and women in both high- and low-income countries.

***Table 10: Smoking prevalence by socio-economic status, gender & number of smokers 15 years & above***

| *Geographical location* | *Male %* | *Female %* | *Overall* | *Millions* | *% Smokers* |
|---|---|---|---|---|---|
| Low/Middle Income Countries | 49 | 10 | 30 | 948 | 82 |
| High Income Countries | 39 | 22 | 30 | 209 | 18 |
| Total world | 47 | 12 | 30 | 1157 | 100 |

***Source:*** *World Bank (1999) Development in Practice-curbing the Epidemic – Governments and Economics of Tobacco Control: Washington DC.*

Table 10 depicts socio-economic aspects of tobacco use. 82 percent (948 million) smokers hail from middle and low-income countries. 49 percent males from these countries are smokers as compared to 39 percent males smoking from higher income countries. The situation is reversed among women; 10 percent of women from low-income countries and 22 percent from high-income countries smoke tobacco. These data may, of course, reflect some under-reporting of smoking among women particularly from countries where it is socially and culturally unacceptable for women to smoke.

An inverse relationship is found between education levels (a marker for socio-economic status) and smoking. In general, individuals who have received little or no education are more likely to smoke than those who are more educated. In China, individuals with no schooling were 6.9 times more likely to smoke than individuals with a college degree while uneducated adults in Brazil were 5 times more likely to smoke than adults who had received at least a second grade education.

The most recent research concludes that lower and middle-income men of developing countries are more likely to smoke than those of high socio-economic status. Educational status is a clear determinant of smoking in Chennai (India) (Figure 1). Studies in Brazil, China, South Africa, Vietnam and several Central American nations confirm this pattern.

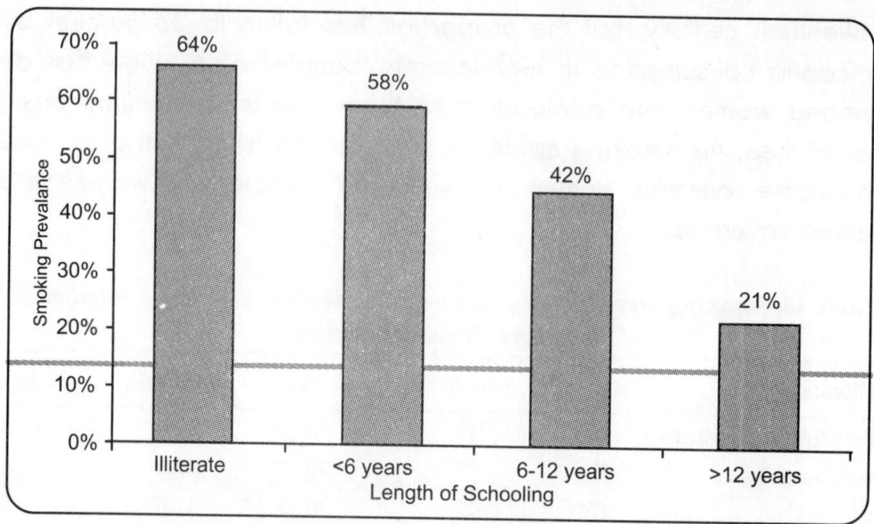


***Figure 1: Smoking and educational level in Men in Chennai (India)***

***Source:*** *Gajalakshmi, Jha, Nguyan and Yusekli (2000) Patterns of Tobacco Use and Health Consequences. In: Jha P; Chaloupka F (Eds) Tobacco Control Policies in Developing Countries. Oxford University Press.*

In India where not surprisingly, smokers with college level education tend to consume more cigarettes, which are relatively more expensive, while smokers with low levels of education consume larger number of the inexpensive *beedis.*

It is clear that the prevalence of smoking is higher among the poor and less educated worldwide. There has been a clear association between tobacco intake and poverty. The contribution of tobacco to death and disease is well documented. However, tobacco consumption itself leads to poverty. Not much attention is given to the ways in which tobacco increases poverty. Damage is done to the financial status of the family when scarce family resources are spent on tobacco products instead of food and other essential needs such as schooling and nutrition. The money that poor households spend on tobacco products (between 4 to 5% of all their disposable income) has very high opportunity costs, diverting scarce resources from food and other basic needs. In developing countries, the proportions of household expenditures used to purchase tobacco products are often very high. For example, if two-third of the money spent on cigarettes in Bangladesh were spent on food instead, it could save more than 10 million people from malnutrition.[20] In India, tobacco use is linked with the worst nutrition and child health outcomes. In Bulgaria, low-income households with at least one smoker spend 10.4% of their total income on tobacco products. In China, smokers surveyed in the Minhang district reported spending 17% of their household income

20 file://C:/WINDOWS/desktop/The Tobacco Epidemic A Global Public Health Emergency.htm

on cigarettes[21]. WHO's "No Tobacco Day" theme for the year 2004 is Tobacco Control and Poverty. The theme is very relevant to the association between tobacco use and poverty with its determinants such as illiteracy, malnutrition, poor housing, overcrowding and disease.

## Per Capita Cigarette Consumption

In high-income countries, with some exceptions, poor and less educated men smoke more cigarettes per day than the richer, more educated men. Per capita consumption of cigarettes is more in people from developed countries as compared to those of the developing world (Figure 2). In general, smokers with low levels of education consume equal or slightly larger number of cigarettes than those with higher levels of education.

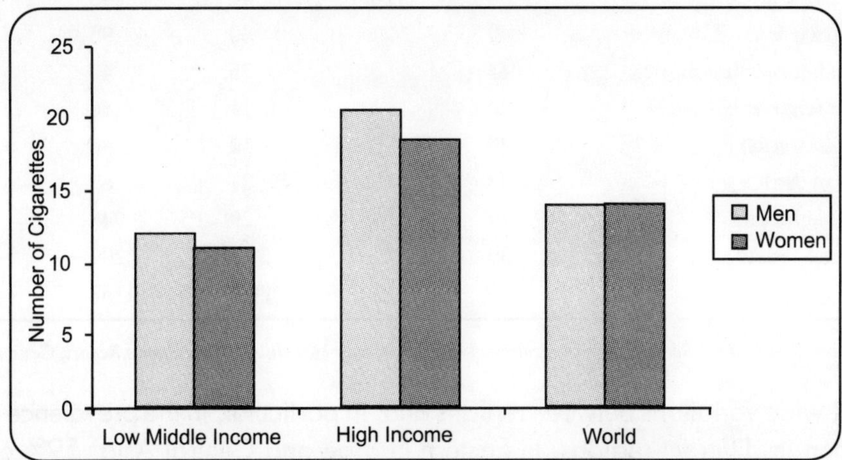


***Figure 2: Number of cigarettes smoked per capita***

***Source:*** *World Health Organization (1997) Tobacco or Health: A Global Status Report, Geneva, Switzerland.*

There are specific characteristics of the spending pattern of Indian consumers influencing the structure of domestic market that reflects the differences existing between the socio-economic groups in the country, with the upper and middle class segments preferring filtered cigarettes, while the lower socio-economic groups are the consumers of the other types of tobacco products. Almost 182 million Indians smoke – representing 17% of all consumers world-wide (Shimkhada and Peabody, 2003).

## Regional Patterns

As per the 1995 data, of the 1.157 billion people above 15 years of age using tobacco all over the globe, 47% are males and 12% females constituting 29–30% of the world's population are scattered differently in different regions of the globe. The populations of the low and middle-income countries have been increasing their cigarette consumption

[21] Curbing the Epidemic, Governments and the Economics of Tobacco Control: The World Bank Report, 1999.

since about 1970. The per capita consumption in these countries climbed steadily between 1970 and 1990, although the upward trend may have slowed a little since the early 1990s.

*Table 11: Regional Patterns of Smoking: Estimated smoking prevalence by gender and number of smokers in population aged 15 or more, by World Bank Region, 1995*

| World Bank Region | Smoking Prevalence (%) | | Total (%) | Smokers Millions | % |
|---|---|---|---|---|---|
| | M | F | Total | | |
| East Asia and Pacific | 59 | 4 | 32 | 401 | 35 |
| Eastern Europe & Central Asia | 59 | 26 | 41 | 148 | 13 |
| Latin America & Caribbean | 40 | 21 | 30 | 95 | 8 |
| Middle East & North America | 44 | 5 | 25 | 40 | 3 |
| South Asia (cigarettes) | 20 | 1 | 11 | 86 | 8 |
| South Asia (Beedis) | 20 | 3 | 12 | 96 | 8 |
| Sub-Saharan Africa | 33 | 10 | 21 | 67 | 6 |
| Low/Middle Income | 49 | 9 | 29 | 948 | 82 |
| High Income World | 39 | 22 | 30.5 | 209 | 18 |
| | 47 | 12 | 29.5 | 1157 | 100 |

***Source:*** *Calculations based on World Health Organization, 1997. Tobacco or Health: A Global Status Report, Geneva, Switzerland.*

There are wide variations between regions and, in particular, in the prevalence of smoking among women in different regions. In Eastern Europe and Central Asia, 59% of men and 26% of women smoked in 1995, which was more than any other region. In East Asia and the Pacific, where the prevalence of male smokers is equally high, at 59%, just 4% of the women were smokers (Table 11). This gap between men and women smokers is an opportunity, but one that must be grabbed quickly to prevent the epidemic of tobacco deaths among women as being seen among men today[22]. Tobacco related diseases are on rise among women, particularly young women. It is not only because more and more women are starting to use tobacco products but also due to the fact that millions are exposed to second hand smoking on daily basis. Women are exposed to second hand smoking particularly in the Asian region where significant number of men smokes. Millions of women and children are exposed to second hand smoking.

---

22 WHO Press Release No. 27, 30th March, 2001.

## Cigarette Consumption in South-east Asian Countries

In 1999, South Asia region accounted for 3.4% of world's total cigarette consumption, of which 54% is consumed in India alone (Figure 6). In fact, in India, use of other tobacco products is much higher than cigarette smoking alone. In India, cigarettes account only for 14% of tobacco consumption and the rest of the tobacco consumption is either in the form of *Beedi, hookah, chillum* and various forms of smokeless tobacco, which account for the largest forms of tobacco consumption. In other South Asian (SA) countries too, use of smokeless tobacco products is quite common. Therefore, it is not surprising that all SA countries show very low cigarette consumption per person 15 years and older. In 1999, Pakistan had the highest per capita consumption of 30 packs of cigarettes amongst SA countries. On an average, per capita consumption was 10 packs in all SA countries. In South Asia (SA) region 25% of adult population smoke cigarettes (including *beedis*) which is lower than the global prevalence (30%) because of use of other forms of tobacco products. Of all SA countries, prevalence of smoking is highest in India at 26% (Figure 4). Total number of cigarettes smoked was highest in India in 1999. 54% of the total cigarettes smoked in SA region during that year were consumed in India alone (Figure 3).

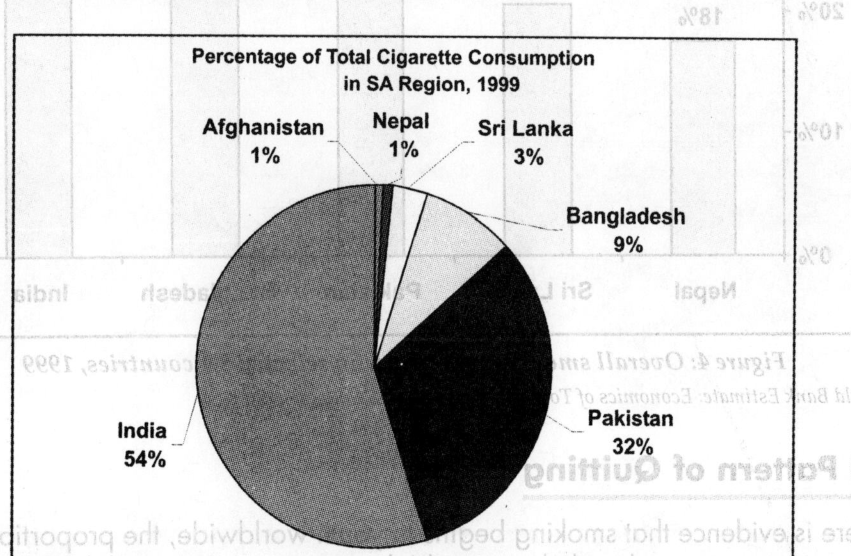


***Figure 3: Percentage shares of SA cigarette consumption, SA, 1999***

***Sources:** USDA and ILO. Note: Bhutan and Maldives are not included in the MNA total consumption due to lack of information. Regional report South Asia: Economics of Tobacco for the South Asia (SA) Region, 2001.*

## Tobacco Use and Health Professionals

Role of health professionals is significant as far as tobacco use in community is concerned. They are the role models for people in community. As the dangers of smoking become better known to health care professionals, a decrease in the prevalence of smoking will occur earlier in the medical community than in the general population, indicating that health professionals have a major role in influencing smoking (Pierce 1989, Dekker et al 1993). Smoking prevalence among Greek physicians was about 39%, which is comparable to that of the general population (Sotiropoulos 2007). In India, the prevalence of tobacco use in medical students, medical professionals and community health specialists is lower than general population but still a major concerned if this problem needs to be eradicated (Kishore 1994, Tessier et al 1992).

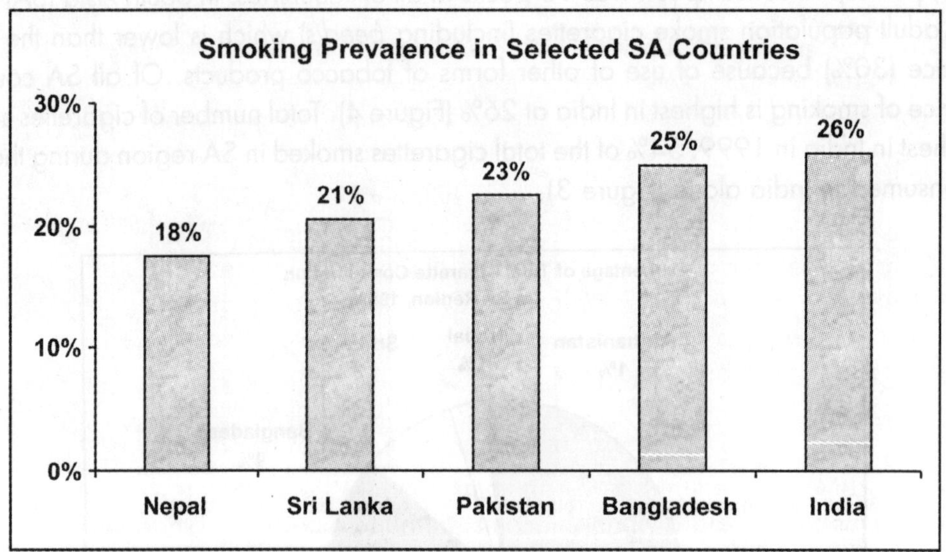


*Figure 4: Overall smoking prevalence in selected SA countries, 1999*

***Source:*** *World Bank Estimate: Economics of Tobacco, South Asia (SA) Region, 2001.*

## Global Pattern of Quitting

While there is evidence that smoking begins in youth worldwide, the proportion of smokers who quit appears to vary sharply between high-income countries and the rest of the world. The prevalence of smoking has gradually fallen and a significant number of former smokers have accumulated over the decades. In most high income countries, about 30% of male populations are former smokers. In contrast, only 2% of Chinese males had quit in 1993, only 5% of Indian males at around the same period, and only 10% of the Vietnamese males had quit in 1997. Since 1970, population of cigarette smokers in low and middle income countries is increasing[23].

The per capita consumption of cigarettes increased between 1970 and 1990 and then declined. Smoking is more in males in low and middle-income countries; however, there is overall decline in the males of high-income countries during the same period. In USA, more than 55% males smoked in the mid-fifties and the proportion has fallen to 28% in the mid-nineties. Per capita consumption has also fallen in higher income countries.

## Tobacco-related Global Mortality

Currently, about 5 million deaths occur every year due to tobacco-related diseases of which about 1 million deaths occur in China alone. Worldwide, the only two major causes of death whose effects are now increasing rapidly are HIV and tobacco and if tobacco prevalence continues to increase with the same pace there will be about one billion deaths during the 21st century compared with 100 million during the 20th century.

Most of the tobacco attributed deaths worldwide in 1990s have occurred in developed countries to the tune of 2 million annually and around 1 million per year in the developing countries (3 million tobacco related deaths globally). However, the situation is changing rapidly now. With the current rate of tobacco consumption, it is expected that 650 million people alive today will eventually be killed by tobacco related diseases (WHO, 2003) half of them in productive middle age, each losing 20 to 25 years of life.

Among persons of both genders, the proportion of all deaths attributed to smoking increased overtime. However, the increase was relatively greater in women, resulting in narrowing of gender gap. In the age group 35–69 years, the proportion of all deaths due to smoking among women increased from 2% in 1955 to 13% in 1995, while among men it increased from 20% to 36%. One in eight female deaths (13%) between the ages of 35 and 69 in developed countries in 1995 was due to smoking, and for men and women combined, each smoker who died in this age group lost significant numbers of life expectancy due to smoking (WHO, 1996).

## Smoking Devices, Smokeless Products and Tobacco Quality

A smoker takes into his mouth and the lungs the quantities of smoke through a smoking device specifically designed for the purpose. There are several devices available that are in use either universally or specifically in a particular culture. Of these, cigarette is the most

23 World Health Organization, Global Status Report, Geneva, 1997.

prevalent form of tobacco smoking used almost all over the world. Manufactured cigarettes and hand rolled cigarettes such as *Kreteks* (clove flavoured cigarettes, particularly popular in Indonesia) and *beedis* — common in South East Asia and India —account for up to 65 to 85% of all tobacco consumption worldwide while 15–35% of tobacco is consumed in the form of all other tobacco products particularly popular in the Indian sub-continent. Apart from cigarette and *beedis*, cigar, *hookah, chillum, cheroot* etc. are common devices used in smoking practices.

After cigarette had appeared in mass-manufactured form, its availability became easier, cheaper and common which helped in rapid spread of its use across cultures. Mechanical production of cigarette provided an ample scope to manipulate the device in accordance with the smokers' needs. Cigarette acquired different characteristics not only as with or without filter, variations in tobacco contents, shape of cigarette, quality of tobacco and paper used and content of smoke have also occurred from time to time. In 1923, *du Maurier* – Britain's first filter cigarette in response to the rising importance of female smokers who disliked conventional soggy cigarette ends, economized on the expansively taxed tobacco leaves by preserving the cigarette length while avoiding wastage of tobacco in the un-smoked cigarette butt (Corina, 1975). Many early filter brands, in fact, yielded more nicotine and tar in their smoke than some non-filter brands and there was suspicion that the manufacturers were taking the opportunity presented by use of filter to use high-yielding but poorer quality grades of tobacco. In most countries where tobacco blends with air cured (burley) tobacco are used, the nitrate content of the cigarette tobacco is higher. In the United States, nitrate content in the cigarette tobacco rose from 0.3–0.5% to 0.6–1.35%, thereby enhancing the combustion of tobacco. More complete combustion decreases the carcinogenic polycyclic aromatic hydrocarbons (PAH), yet the increased generation of nitrogen oxide enhances the formation of carcinogenic N-nitrosamines, especially the tobacco-specific nitrosamines (TSNA) in the smoke[24].

Since 1950, the make up of cigarettes and composition of cigarette smoke have gradually changed. In the United States, the sale-weighted average "tar" and nicotine yields have declined from a high of 38 mg "tar" and 2.7 mg nicotine in 1954 to 12 mg and 0.95 mg in 1992, respectively. A significantly lower frequency of precancerous histological abnormalities were observed in smokers who used cigarettes with low-tar as compared to the smokers of 1950s when the tar content of cigarettes was higher (Auerbach, Hammond and Garfinker 1979). In the United Kingdom, the same figures declined from about 32 and 2.2 to less than 12 and 1.0 respectively per cigarette. During the same time, the other smoke constituents changed correspondingly. These reductions of smoke yields were primarily achieved by the introduction of filter tips, with or without perforation, selection of tobacco

24 Frequently asked questions: tobacco control in 21st century, University of Sydney, 2001.

types, and varieties, utilization of high porous cigarette paper, incorporation of reconstructed tobacco into the tobacco blend, opened and cut ribs, and "expanded tobacco". Use of low nicotine cigarette has also led to change in the pattern of smoking. Recent smoking assays have demonstrated that most smokers of cigarettes with low nicotine yield take between 2 and 4 puffs per minute with volume up to 55 ml to satisfy their needs for nicotine (Hoffmann and Hoffmann, 1997).

When the scientific inquiry began associating cigarette smoking with lung cancer in the early 1950s, most US smokers were smoking unfiltered cigarettes. With the growing awareness of the health-risks of cigarette smoking, filter cigarettes became more popular, as they were designed to reduce the tar inhaled in the smoke. Later, low-tar cigarettes were marketed; however, many smokers compensated by smoking more intensely and by blocking the filter's ventilation holes. Cigarette smoking posed much greater danger to health than earlier forms of tobacco use.

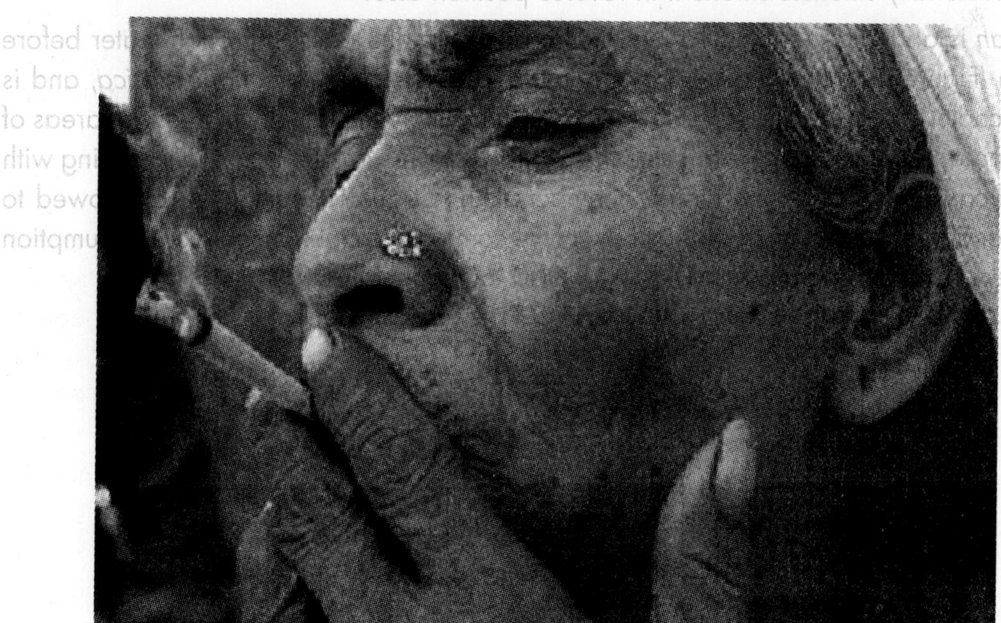

*Figure 5: An Indian woman smoking beedi*

In India, *cigarette* smoking is the second most popular form of tobacco smoking after *beedis.* Cigarette use seems to be confined to manufactured cigarettes; there are no reports on the use of roll-your-own cigarettes. The prevalence varies greatly among different geographic areas and subgroups such as rural-urban. Only 14% of the total domestic tobacco consumption is in the form of cigarettes while the rest is consumed in the form of other smoke and smokeless tobacco products.

Non-cigarette forms of tobacco products are largely produced in the unorganized sector which offers lower rates of tax and ineffective enforcement. Consequently, the tax base of tobacco sector is rapidly shrinking. *Beedi* smoking constitutes 40% of total tobacco consumption in India and it is more popular in the lower socio-economic strata of the society. Since *beedi* manufacturing falls under the domain of the unorganized sector, unlike cigarettes beedis are lowly taxed and are within the purchasing power of the poor people (Figure 5).

*Chutta* smoking is wide spread in the coastal areas of Andhra Pradesh, Tamil Nadu and Orissa. Reverse *chutta* smoking is practiced extensively by the women in the rural areas of Visakhapatnam and Srikakulam districts of Andhra Pradesh. *Chutta* is a coarsely prepared *cheroot.* It is usually manufactured by the cottage and small scale industry, or made at home. Nearly 9% of the tobacco produced in India is used for making *chuttas*. It is estimated that nearly 3000 million pieces of *chutta* are made annually in India.

*Dhumti* is prepared by the smokers themselves. It is a kind of conical cigar made by rolling tobacco leaves in the leaf of another plant. *Dhumti* is smoked in the rural areas of Goa. Occasionally smokers smoke it in reverse position also.

*Hookah* is an Indian water-pipe in which tobacco smoke passes through water before inhalation (Figure 6). *Hookah* tobacco is derived from the plant *Nicotiana rustica,* and is grown in cooler climates. *Hookah* smoking in Indian society (especially in the rural areas of northern India) is a community affair and the one who shares common *hookah* smoking with others indicates his equality with other members. An ostracized person is not allowed to share water and *hookah* with other members of the community. *Hookah* tobacco consumption is estimated to be between 17, 000 and 18,000 tons annually.

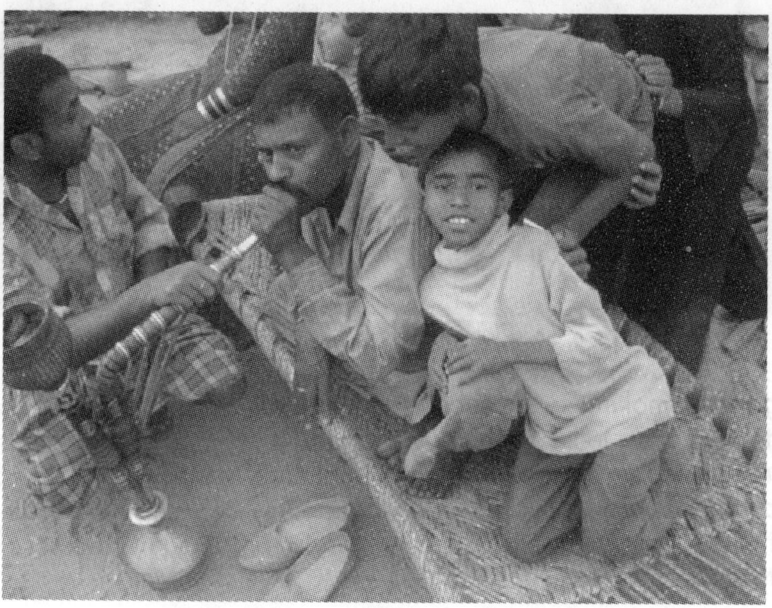

*Figure 6: Hookah smoking in an Indian family*

*Chillum* smoking is exclusively a male practice; like *hookah* smoking it is limited to the northern states of India, predominantly in the rural areas. *Chillum* is a straight, conical pipe made of clay; 10–14 centimeters long, held vertically, *Chillum* smoking requires a deep pulmonary effect. Often one chillum is shared by a group. *Chillums* are made locally, are inexpensive and easily available in the villages. *Chillum* probably predates the introduction of tobacco to India and was used for smoking opium and other narcotics (Wahi, 1968). Even today, cannabis is commonly smoked by *sadhus* and those who have renounced the world filled in *chillum* and often mixed with tobacco. To inhale smoke with a chillum, the smoker uses a piece of cloth through which smoke is filtered into the mouth and the lungs.

*Smokeless tobacco:* The term 'smokeless tobacco' is used to describe tobacco that is consumed without heating or burning at the time of consumption. Smokeless tobacco can be used orally or nasally. Smokeless tobacco products are often made at home but are also manufactured. Recently, varieties of smokeless tobacco products have been produced industrially on a large scale, commercially marketed and are available in small plastic or aluminum foil packets (Figure 7).

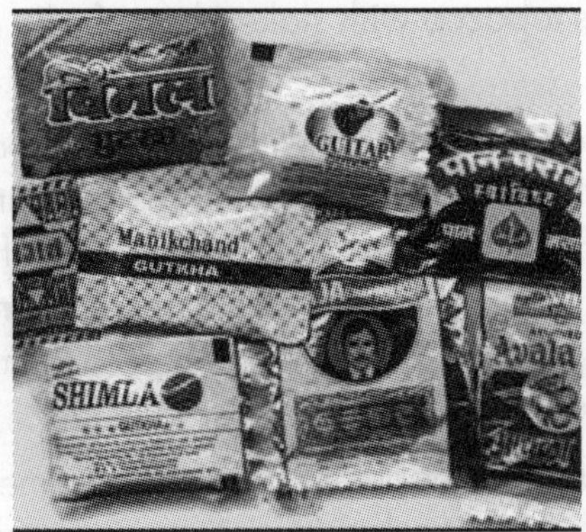


*Figure 7: Smokeless tobacco products consumed in India*

Chewable tobacco leaves are generally rich in flavour, tough, gummy and have qualities to absorb flavouring materials that are added during their processing. Their usage is widespread in India, and is classified into *Zarda*, or flake type and *dana,* or minced type. The third type in the form of pasties called *kimam*. It is mostly consumed by the rural and the economically backward classes of Indian society. The annual production of chewable tobacco ranges from 65,000 to 75,000 tons.

*Paan* chewing or betel quid chewing is often erroneously referred to as 'betel nut chewing'. *Paan* consists of four main ingredients – betel leaf (*piper betle*), areca nut (areca catechu), slaked lime $[Ca(OH_2)]$ and catechu (acacia catechu). Betel leaves contain volatile oils such as eugenol and terpenes, nitrates and small quantities of sugar, starch, tannin and several other substances (Gowda, 1951). Condiments and sweetening agents may be added as per regional practices and individual preferences. Sometimes after its introduction, tobacco has become an important ingredient of *paan*, and currently most habitual *paan* chewers include tobacco. *Chewing tobacco* consists of small pieces of raw or commercially available finely cut tobacco.

Tobacco is the most important ingredient of *paan* for regular users. It is used in the raw state (as in Kerala) as well as after processing. Depending upon the processing and additives used, tobacco is variously referred to as *kaddipudi* and *hogesoppu* in Karnataka, *kadapaan* in Orissa and West Bengal, and *pattiwala* in Uttar Pradesh. *Zarda* and *kiwam* are commercially manufactured varieties often used as ingredients of *paan*.

*Paan masala* is a commercial product containing areca nut, slaked lime, *catechu* and condiments, with or without powdered tobacco. *Paan masala* contains almost all the ingredients that go into the making of a *paan*, but are dehydrated so that the final product is not perishable. *Paan masala* is very popular in urban areas and is fast becoming popular in rural areas too. Its popularity can be gauged by the production figures: according to commercial estimates, the Indian market for *paan masala* is now worth several hundred million US dollars.

*Mainpuri* tobacco contains tobacco with slaked lime, finely cut areca nut, camphor and cloves.

*Mawa* contains thin shavings of areca nut with the addition of some tobacco and slaked lime. Its use is becoming popular in Gujarat, especially among the youth. *Mawa* use is also prevalent in other regions of the country. The prevalence of *mawa* use has increased significantly in the recent years. Its magnitude can be assessed from the fact that the Bhavnagar (Gujarat) city administration appealed to the people not to litter the streets with cellophane wrappers of *mawa*, as they clogged the city drains.

*Khaini* is the mixture of sun-dried tobacco and slaked lime used in Maharashtra and several states of Northern India. A regular *khaini* user may carry a double-ended metal container, one side of which is filled with tobacco and other with slightly moistened slaked lime. A small quantity of tobacco is taken in the palm and a little slake lime is added. The ingredients are then mixed vigorously with the thumb and placed in the mouth. In Maharashtra and Gujarat, *khaini* is placed in the premolar region of the mandibular groove, whereas in Bihar and Uttar Pradesh, it is generally held in lower labial groove.

Swedish snuff called *snus* is available in teabag like pouches. The pouch can be kept in buccal or labial groove and sucked. It is marketed in India by the Swedish Match Company under the name of *Click*.

*Tobacco products for application:* Several smokeless tobacco preparations are intended primarily to clean the teeth. Such use, however, soon becomes an addiction. Some people, in Indian society carry a misconception that tobacco is good for teeth. Many companies take advantage of this misconception by packaging and positioning their products as dental care products without explicitly stating so (by law, oral care products cannot contain tobacco). Following tobacco products are used for application:

*Mishri,* a roasted, powdered preparation made by baking tobacco on a hot metal plate until it is uniformly black, is used to clean the teeth. Women, who use it to clean their teeth initially, soon apply *mishri* several times a day. This practice is common in Maharashtra. It is also reportedly used in Goa. *Gul* is a pyrolysed tobacco product. It is marketed under different brand names in small tin cans and used as a dentifrice in the eastern parts of India. In the Global Youth Tobacco Survey (GYTS) *gul* use was reported to be 6% in Bihar, 3% each in Arunachal Pradesh and Nagaland and 2% each in Assam, Uttar Pradesh and Uttaranchal. *Bajjar* is dry snuff applied commonly by women in Gujarat on the teeth and gums. *Lal Dantmanjan* is a dentifrice; a red-coloured tooth powder. Traditionally it contained tobacco but tobacco having been legally banned in oral care products, the listing of tobacco as an ingredient is stopped by the manufacturers. *Gudhaku* is a paste made of tobacco and molasses. It is available commercially and is carried in a metal container but can be made by the user himself. It is commonly used in Bihar, Orissa, Uttar Pradesh and Uttaranchal. It is applied to the teeth and gums mainly by women. Creamy snuff, tobacco water etc. are the other tobacco products available for use.

The National Sample Survey (NSS) reveals that use of tobacco and its various products appears to have declined in India over the period from 1987–1988 to 1999–2000. According to the National Sample Survey (NSS) data, consumption of tobacco in all recorded forms has reduced (NSS, 2001). This declining trend is faster among the urban population. Since *Gutka* is a recent introduction, the trend of oral tobacco consumption in Indian population is not clearly documented.

## REFERENCES

Aghi M., Asma S., Vaithinathan R. and Chng C.V.: *Initiation and Maintenance of Tobacco Use*, presented at Kobe *International Conference on Women and Tobacco*, Kobe, Japan, 1999.

Amos A: Women and Smoking. *British Medical Bulletin*, 52(1): 74-89, 1996.

Auerbach O, Hammond E.C. and Garfinkel L.: Changes in Bronchial Epithelium in Relation to Cigarette Smoking, 1955–56 vs 1970–77. *New England Journal of Medicine*, 300(8):381–386, 1979

Briggs GW: *The Chamars: Religious Life of India Series*, Association Press, Calcutta, 1920.

Chandler W: *Banishing Tobacco*, World-watch Institute, Washington. D.C., 1986.

Corina M: *Trust in Tobacco: The Anglo-American Struggle for Power*, Michael Joseph, London, 1975.

Gajalakshmi C.K., Jha P., Nguyen S. and Yurekli A.: *Patterns of Tobacco Use and Health Consequences.* In: Jha P and Chaloupka F (Eds.) Tobacco Control Policies in Developing Countries. Oxford University Press, New York, 2000.

Global Youth Tobacco Survey (GYTS) Collaborating Group: Differences in Worldwide Tobacco use by Gender: Findings from Global Youth Tobacco Survey. *Journal of School Health*; 73 (6): 2007–215, 2003.

Gottsegen J.J.: *Tobacco: A Study of Its Consumption in the United States*, Pitman Publishing Corporation, Chicago. 8–10, 28,87,147, 153, 155, New York, 1940.

Gowda M: *The Story of Paan Chewing in India, Botanical Museum Leaflets*;14: 181–214, 1951.

Hoffmann D. and Hoffmann I.: *The Changing Cigarette:1950–1995*, Journal of Toxicology and Environmental Health; 50:307–364, 1997.

Juliet L. and Hatcher, M. P. H.: Encourage Teens to Adopt Safe, Healthy Life-style: A Foundation for Improving Future Adult Behaviour. Children Trends: Washington D.C., 2001.

Kalia H. L.: Research on Smoking among Women. In: Smoking Among Women, New Delhi, India, 1998.

Luthra U; Sreenivas V; Menon G; Prabhakar AK and Chaudhry K (1992) Tobacco Control in India: Problems and Solutions. In: Gupta PC; Hamner JE; and Murti PR (Eds) Cotrol of Tobacco Related Cancers and Other Diseases, International Symposium 1990. Oxford University Press: Bombay.

National Sample Survey (NSS).: *Consumption of Some Important Commodities in India: 1999–2000, 55th Round. Department of Statistics and* Programme Implementation, Government of India, 2001.

Mackay J. and Eriksen J. The Tobacco Atlas, World Health Organization, Geneva, Switzerland.

Pierce J. P., Naquin M., Gulpin E.: *et al Smoking Inhalation in United States A Role for Worksite and College Smoking Bans*, Journal of National Cancer Institute 83:1009–1013, 1991.

Ranson K., Jha P., Chaloupka F. and Urekli A.: Effectiveness and Cost-effectiveness of Price Increases and Other Tobacco Control Policy Interventions. In: Jha P and Chaloupka F (Eds.) *Tobacco Control Policies in Developing Countries*. Oxford University Press: New York, 2000.

Simkhada R. and Peabody J.W.: *Tobacco Control in India*, Bulletin of the World Health Organization; 81: 48 52. Available from URL: http://wwwscielops.org

Townsend J. L., Roderick P. and Cooper J.: Cigarette Smoking by Socio-economic Group, Sex and Age: Effects of Price, Income, and Health Publicity. *British Medical Journal*. 309 (6959): 923–926, 1994.

Tunistra T.: Editorial, Tobacco Reporter, *Summer*, 1998.

Wahi P.N.: The Epidemiology of Oral and Oropharyngeal Cancer. A Report of Study in Mainpuri district, Uttar Pradesh, India. *Bulletin of World health Organization*; 38: 495–521, 1968.

The World Bank: *Curbing the Epidemic: Governments and Economics of Tobacco Control*, Washington D.C. 1999.

World Health Organization: *The Tobacco Epidemic: A Global Public Health Emergency*, Geneva WHO, 1996.

World Health Organization: *Global Status Report on Tobacco*, Geneva, Switzerland, 1997.

World Health Organization: *Tobacco and Heath in Developing World*, Background Paper for the High Level Round Table on Tobacco Control and Development Policy, Brussels.

Wickstrom B: *Cigarette Marketing in the Third World*, In: L M Ram Stroom (Eds.) The Smoking Epidemic: The Proceedings of the 4th World Conference on Smoking and Health. Almqvist and Wicksell International: Stockholm, 1980.

CHAPTER 3

# Tobacco: Cultivation, Curing and Commerce

*The tobacco plant is the most loved and hated member of plant kingdom.*

— Ashton Heather and Stepney Rob, 1982.

The plant from which tobacco is obtained belongs to *Solanaceae* family of the plant kingdom. Unlike other members of this family, such as tomato and potato, which have an uncontroversial nutritional role, or winter cherry and petunia, which have undoubted decorative value, tobacco plant carries in its leaves quantities of an alkaloid, nicotine, which gives it instead, power over man's mind (Ashton and Stepney, 1982). Cultivation of tobacco plant forms an important commercial crop all over the world due to its use in one form or another by the consuming populations (Chojar, 2002). It is a hardy, tall, tender and shrubby flowering plant which may be annual or perennial and is a native of the Americas; some varieties are found on the islands of the Pacific Ocean.

## Tobacco Cultivation

There are many types of tobacco plant, but all are grown similarly. Tobacco seeds are very minute and 10,000 seeds typically weigh just one gram. To grow tobacco plants, the tiny seeds are spread across sterilized seedbeds in light soil and they need light to sprout. The tiny tobacco seeds germinate just about anywhere and quickly grow into very tall and robust plants. In the regions where the growing season is fairly long, they may be sown directly outside in early spring. When they are large enough to be handled, they should be transplanted into the flats, where they should be spaced 2-inches apart and should be filled with sandy fertile soil. They are generally transplanted when they are a few inches high (Figure 1).

Successful tobacco growing depends on a good support of well developed, healthy seedlings transplanted at the right time. For seedlings to grow well, they need to be free from weeds, disease and insects. Seedbeds need to be shielded from the wind and should have an ample supply of water.

Tobacco plant has a well developed fibrous root-system which is required to supply the great leaf area with water and nutrients. The leaves are large and pubescent (hairy) and are carefully tended while growing the plant in the field. The plants can grow to around ten feet high, are "topped" i.e. the flowers are cut off, to encourage the leaves to grow further down the stem. This is done for commercial purposes so that large leaves on the main axis are produced. The number of the leaves left on the plant after "topping" depends upon the type of tobacco grown, soil fertility, soil moisture, weather and the strength of the plant.

The leaf weight of the tobacco plant increases from the bottom upwards hence plants are reaped from the bottom to top.

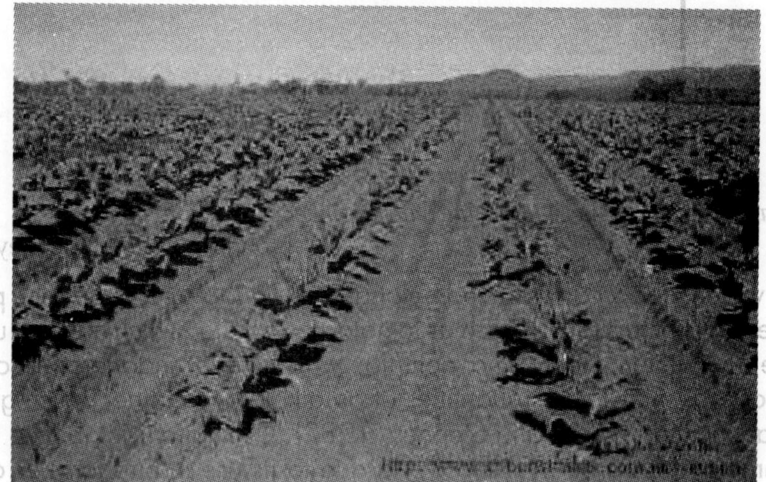

*Figure 1: Tobacco plantation*

## Types of Tobacco Plant

There are 65 known species of the tobacco plant of which the one that is grown commercially and widely as a source of tobacco is *Nicotiana tobaccum* (Figure 2) having at least 100 horticultural varieties. However, much of the tobacco from Northern India and Afghanistan comes from the species *Nicotiana rustica* (Figures 3 and 4).

To begin with, *Nicotiana tobaccum* was a tropical species. It has, over a period of time, become adapted to sub-tropical and temperate regions. It is an annual variety of tobacco, un-branched, and generally 3–6 feet tall. Its leaves are large, attractive, alternate, numerous, somewhat decurrent, ovate, lanceolate, viscid, pubescent, pale-green, brittle, narcotic in odour and bitter acrid in taste. It has rose pink flowers, which have swollen corolla tubes. The whole plant is fuzzy and somewhat clammy when handled. On the other hand, *Nicotiana rustica* is a smaller and hardier plant with its origin believed to be in Mexico, and still grown in wild, in parts of North America. *Nicotiana sylvestris* (Figure 5) and *Nicotiana alata*

(Figure 6) are taller and 3–5 feet high. Their leaves are oval, heart-shaped or elliptical; more towards the base and 5–12 inches long. *Nicotiana acuminata* (Figure 7) is an annual plant that bears white flowers. *Nicotiana tobaccum* and *Nicotiana rustica* are the two main varieties used for preparation of tobacco products.

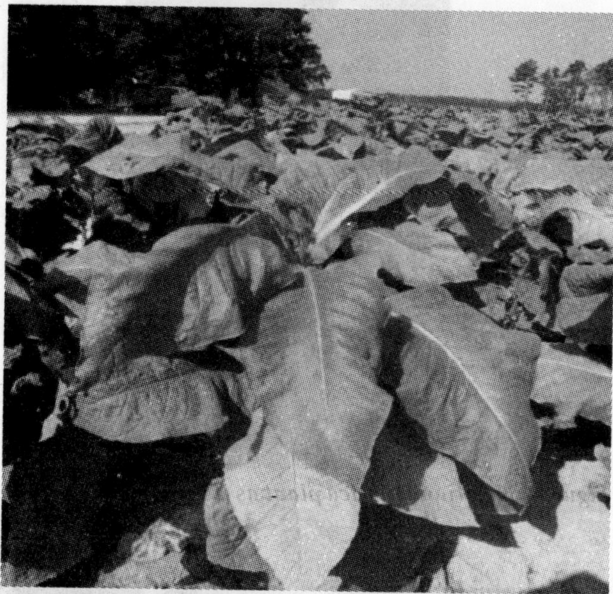

*Figure 2: Nicotiana tobaccum*

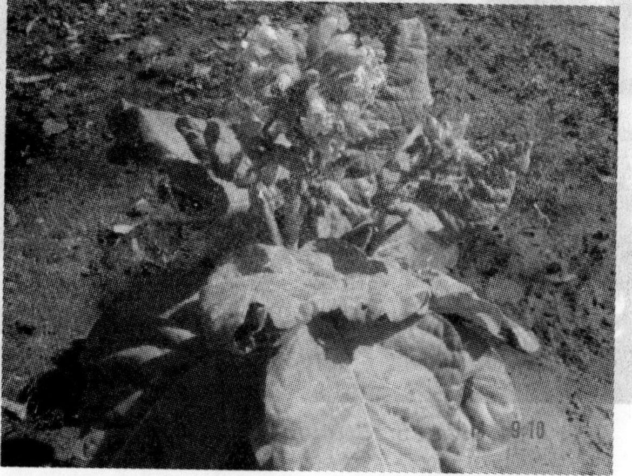

*Figure 3: Nicotiana rustica (from north India)*

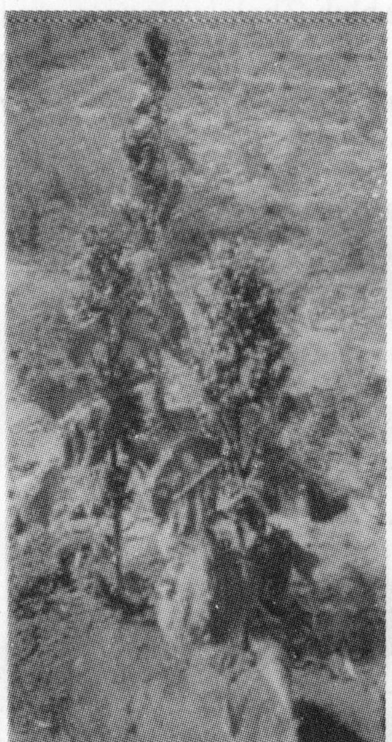

*Figure 4: Nicotiana rustica plant as it is grown in north India*

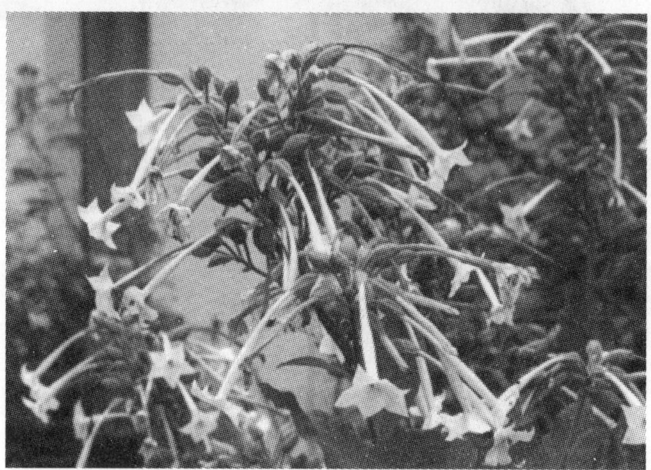

*Figure 5: Nicotiana sylvestris*

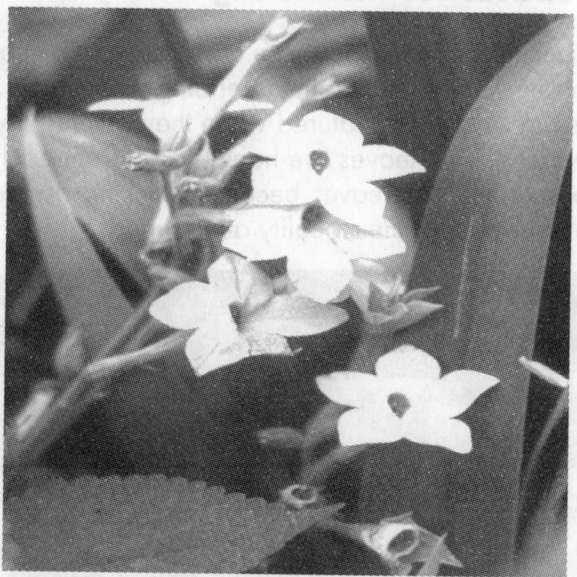

*Figure 6: Nicotiana alata*

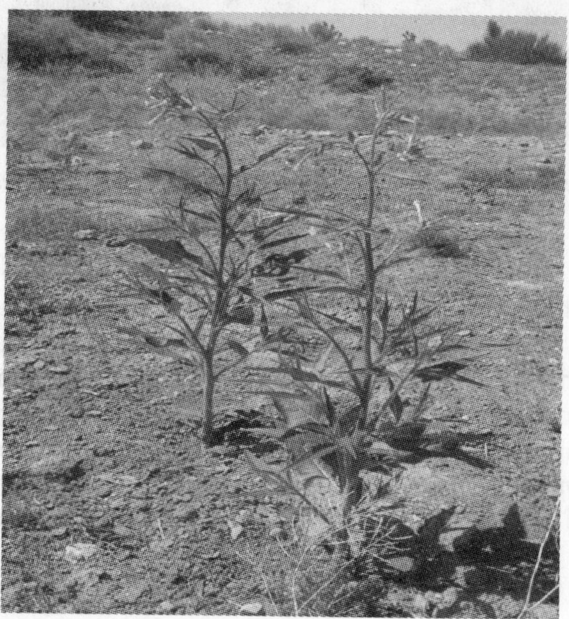

*Figure 7: Nicotiana acuminata*

## Preparation of Tobacco for Marketing

Unlike many other agricultural products, tobacco crop needs to be carefully handled during harvesting. Maturity of the leaves occurs in ascending order, and the lowermost leaves mature first. The leaves are said to be matured when they assume a yellowish green colour (Figure 8). During harvesting, 3–4 leaves are hand-picked from each plant. Care needs to be exercised during plucking of the leaves because plucking of over-mature or immature leaves can result in deterioration of their quality after curing.

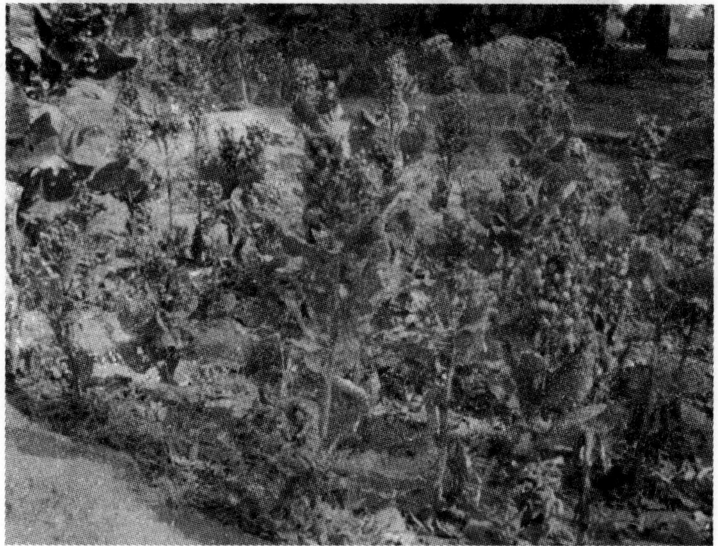

*Figure 8: A field with matured tobacco plants (from north India)*

## Harvesting

Tobacco crop is often topped and de-suckered to remove flowers in order to concentrate growth in leaves, which are the main inputs used in tobacco industry. Upon maturity, tobacco plants are harvested either by priming leaves from the stalk or cutting the tobacco crop stalks. Priming is in fact leaf to leaf harvesting of the mature leaves starting from lower leaves in ascending order. Virginia tobacco crop is harvested by the priming method. In the stalk-cut method, when maximum number of leaves mature, tobacco plants are cut from their stalks close to the ground and are generally left in the fields for leaves to wilt.

## Curing

After harvesting, the next step is curing. After being picked, tobacco leaves which contain 80–85% water need to be dried out to make them usable for manufacturing tobacco products. This process is called curing. Curing brings about rapid destruction of chlorophyll,[1] giving

[1] Chlorophyll is a green pigment present in leaves.

leaves their yellow appearance, converting starch into sugar and removing moisture. Curing brings out the aroma and flavour in all varieties of tobacco. After the curing cycle is completed, there is essentially no water left in the leaves. There are many factors which influence curing schedule including soil, position of the leaves on the stalk and weather.

***Stages of curing:*** Curing involves three essential steps:

(a) Yellowing
(b) Leaf drying
(c) Stem drying

(a) *Yellowing*: is a continuation of the ripening process and is thought to be the most important part of the curing process. The leaf is still alive during the yellowing phase, which allows it to carry on certain biological processes needed to convert starch into sugar and breakdown chlorophyll. When tobacco leaves are harvested, they are high in starch and low in sugar. As starch decreases through the process of hydrolysis and respiration, the amount of sugar increases.

(b) *Leaf drying:* occurs when the leaf tissue is dried to a particular moisture level.

(c) *Stem drying:* is referred to as the "killing out stage" because all moisture is removed from the stem and leaf and it is ready for further processing.

The curing environment can be manipulated by controlling heat, humidity and air movement. There are four common methods of curing (Table 1) and the method used depends upon the type of tobacco and its intended use. These are:

1. Air curing
2. Sun curing
3. Fire curing
4. Flue curing

### *1. Air Curing*

Air-curing is a relatively slow process and generally takes 4–8 weeks. Tobacco leaves are sheltered from wind and sun in a well ventilated barn where they air-dry for four to eight weeks. Air-cured tobacco is low in sugar and high in nicotine content. Cigar and Burley tobacco are air-cured. In India, the cigar tobacco grown in West Bengal and the burley tobacco cultivated in Andhra Pradesh, are air-cured.

### *2. Sun Curing*

Here, the tobacco is dried uncovered in the sun for 2–3 weeks. This method is used in Turkey, Greece, and other Mediterranean countries to produce oriental tobacco. Sun-cured tobacco is low in sugar and is used in cigarettes. In India, tobacco used in *beedi, natu,* chewing, cigar, snuff and *hookah,* is sun- cured.

### 3. Fire Curing

Fire curing is done with smoke from low burning fire on the barn floor which permeates the leaves. This gives the leaves a distinct smoky aroma and flavour. Methods vary considerably; however, all fire-cured tobaccos are subjected to wood smoke to dry the leaves. It is the type of wood which is used to smoke the tobacco leaves and it is the amount of smoke exposure that lends fire-cured tobacco leaves their distinct flavour. As heat is generally not introduced into the curing process fire-curing takes longer than flue-curing – typically a few weeks.

At the end of the process, air is released into the barn to allow some moisture to be reintroduced into the leaves; a dark colour is acquired by the leaves. Fire-curing takes three to ten weeks and produces tobacco low in sugar and high in nicotine content. Pipe tobacco, chewing tobacco and snuff are fire- cured. This method is practiced for curing few varieties of chewing tobacco in Tamil Nadu state of India.

*Table 1: Methods of tobacco curing*

| *Curing type* | *Method* | *Contents* | *Tobacco type* |
|---|---|---|---|
| Air Curing | Slow process, takes 4-8 weeks, leaves dried in well ventilated barns avoiding wind and sun | Low in sugar and high in nicotine content | Cigar and Burley tobacco are air cured |
| Sun Curing | Dried uncovered in the sun for 2-3 weeks | Low in sugar | Used in cigarette, in India it is used in *beedi*, *natu*, *hookah*, chewing, cigar and snuff. |
| Fire Curing | Curing is done with wood smoke from low burning fire on the barn floor, heat from the barn floor. The process takes three to ten weeks. | Low in sugar and high in nicotine content | Pipe tobacco, chewing tobacco and snuff are fire-cured. |
| Flue Curing | Artificial heat is applied by using flue-pipes under controlled conditions of humidity and temperature without the use of fumes or smoke coming in direct contact of tobacco leaves. It is the shortest process of curing tobacco leaves taking three to seven days. | Has highest level of dextrose (sugar) thus giving a sweet flavour. | Pipe tobacco |

### 4. Flue Curing

Application of artificial heat by using flue-pipes to convey heat in an air-tight barn is called flue-curing. This technology was developed in 1860s and unlike many other agricultural commodities, farmers have to take great care in harvesting and picking flue-cured tobacco. In the flue-curing process, tobacco leaves are dried under controlled conditions of humidity and temperature without the use of smoke and fumes coming in direct contact with the tobacco leaves. During flue-curing, the colour of the harvested leaves changes to bright yellow. While doing so the leaves must retain commercial qualities with respect to the body, texture, aroma, and elasticity/plasticity. It not only involves the drying of the leaves but also involves physical and chemical changes which are essential for manufacturing process. Flue-curing is carried out in "barns" made of bricks with roofing material consisting of corrugated iron sheets. Barn size varies from area to area and depends upon when they were constructed. Buildings used for flue-curing generally have a larger height in comparison with the floor space, hence acting as a sort of chimney. Humidity within the building is regulated carefully to allow the leaves to dry out over the required time period. Inside the barn are the layers of tiers or sticks which run horizontally in a desired direction (Figure 9).

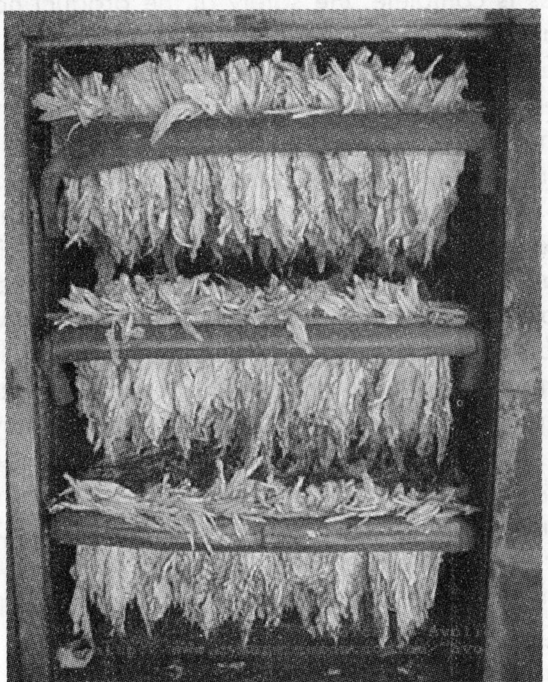

*Figure 9: Flue curing of tobacco leaves*

Sticks are used for tying the leaves which are arranged in these air tight barns with controlled sources of heat and ventilation. For heating, wood-based or coal-based furnace is used, which is connected to the flue-pipe system from the bottom of the barn. At higher temperature inside the barn, the water holding capacity of air goes up, and consequently the capacity of air to remove moisture from the leaves also increases. The heating system should be capable of operating between 90° F and 160° F. During the curing process, the role of air-temperature, humidity and air movement is very important. The flue-curing process is carried out in three stages. In the *first stage*, leaves are wilted upside down in "hogsheads" tied to the sticks in the drying barn to *reduce the water content* from 80–85% to 20%. In this process, the colour of the leaf changes from green to yellow, a breakdown of proteins into amino-acids takes place and starch is converted into sugar. Yellowing of the leaves occurs because of the breakdown of the green pigment, chlorophyll. The *second* stage is the *colour fixation* stage, which takes place after the yellowing has occurred. In the *third* stage, *drying of the leaves* and stems is accomplished by increasing the temperature and ventilation of the barn. After flue-curing, ventilation and doors are opened as barn is allowed to cool down. During the process, the leaves absorb moisture from the atmosphere and become soft. Flue-curing is the shortest process to cure the leaves for marketing, taking only 4–7 days.

## Bulking, Grading and Packing

After the curing process is complete, the safety of the product has to be ensured while unloading tobacco leaves from the sticks with which they were tied during the curing process. The leaves are then folded, bundled and kept in piles or small heaps on the floor for 2–3 days, and covered to avoid moisture losses. The bulk is turned over regularly once or twice a day or remade so that leaves remain in good physical condition and there is uniformity in leaf colour. Afterwards, there is more aging, blending and addition of other flavours, i.e. sugar or sorbitol and moisturizers in the development of the final aroma. After bulking, leaves are graded. Grading specification of black soil raised tobacco differs from flue-cured Virginia tobacco (FCV) raised in light soil. After the grading of tobacco is completed, the leaves of the same grade are packed into bundles which are called *bales*. The compactness of a *bale* is achieved by exerting the body-weight on the plank kept on the heap of leaves; some farmers even process the mechanical screw technique for that purpose. Tobacco is a hygroscopic commodity because of its ability to absorb moisture, it is therefore essential to maintain uniform moisture level. Before re-drying, moisture levels range between 15–18%. In many threshing and re-drying plants, leaf-stems are first separated from the lamina, moisture levels are then raised to 20–22%; the lamina portion is then threshed and cut into small pieces. The re-drying operation usually brings down the moisture level in un-manufactured tobacco leaf to 11–12%, before packing it for export or domestic manufacturing.

## Types of Tobacco

As it has already been discussed earlier, the tobacco plant is a native of tropical America and its cultivation spread to North America before the arrival of Europeans to claim this part of the world. Spanish settlers took up cultivation of tobacco on a commercial basis by 1531 and by the middle 16th century, it was introduced in Europe. By 1605, it reached the Far East countries of China and Japan, other Asian countries, Africa and even to Australia. Today, tobacco is the most widely grown non-food crop. It grows in every inhabited continent of the world, in almost 100 countries. There are several forms of tobacco grown world-wide, of which important ones are:

### 1. *Virginia Tobacco*

When the English settlers of the North America arrived at Virginia coast, they found that the natives grew a smaller and hardier plant of tobacco which was later identified as *Nicotiana rustica*. Neither the settlers nor the people in Europe could develop a taste for this variety of tobacco when they tried it for smoking purposes. The English preferred *Nicotiana tobaccum* for which had they already developed a liking even before the Virginia colony came up. As a result of this, the English settlers of Virginia acquired the seeds of the desired variety from West Indies and began its cultivation in Virginia. Its production increased rapidly and so did the demand for consumption. This came to be known as Virginia tobacco.

Very soon it became the most important item the settlers of Virginia colony could produce in exchange for the required manufactured goods from Europe. Today, this is the most common variety of tobacco used world over. Virginia tobacco is by far the most popular tobacco type in pipe tobacco. It is the mildest of all blended tobaccos and has the highest level of dextrose (sugar), which basically gives it a light sweet taste. Virginia tobacco is virtually used in all blends, it is a good burner and aids in lighting. Virginia tobacco is "flue-cured" and is golden in colour. It is believed that China is the largest producer of Virginia tobacco, followed by United States of America. Other prominent producers of Virginia tobacco are: Brazil, Japan, Korea, India, Zimbabwe, Philippines, Thailand, Taiwan, Pakistan, Tanzania, Malawi, Zambia, South Africa, Argentina, Indonesia, Italy and Australia.

### 2. *Burley Tobacco*

The world's second most popular tobacco is Burley tobacco or white Burley tobacco. The Burley leaf is very light and fluffy and lends itself to the production of favoured, blended cigarettes commonly referred to as "Americans."

It contains almost no sugar which gives it a much dryer and full aroma than Virginia tobacco. Burley tobacco is used in many aromatic blends because it absorbs the flavourings. Burley tobacco burns slowly and gives a cool smoke, which makes it a nice addition to the stronger blends that tend to burn faster. This tobacco is air-cured and the curing is done in large open barns by the natural air flow, for one or two months. The colour ranges from light brown to mahogany. The United States of America is the world's largest producer of Burley tobacco. Other large producers include: Korea, Mexico, Greece, Brazil, Japan, Spain, and some Southern European countries.

### 3. *Oriental Tobacco*

It is the sole constituent of Turkish cigarettes. A highly labour-intensive product to harvest, Oriental tobacco is characterized by high aroma from small leaves which are mostly "sun-cured". Usually, the larger the leaf, the milder the aroma, and hence Oriental tobacco is regarded expensive to harvest by many tobacco manufacturers. It is a variety of tobacco that is grown in Turkey, the Balkans and Russia. The best known types are Izmir, Samsun, Yedidje, Cavella, and Bursa. A common characteristic is a dusty dry and somewhat slightly sourish aroma. Some of them are also used in "exotic" cigarettes from Egypt and other Arabian countries.

### 4. *Spice Tobacco*

Spice tobacco is actually not one type of tobacco, but rather a broad variety of more special types, used in small amounts to create an interesting blend. These would include: Oriental, Latakia, Perique, and Kentucky among others. Most of them are frequently used in English blends.

*(i) Latakia*

Latakia is the result of a curing process involving fire-curing the leaves over controlled fires of aromatic woods and fragrant herbs. It is probably the most well known spice tobacco and is mainly grown in Cyprus and Northern Syria. After the leaves are harvested and dried, they are hung in tightly closed barns and smoke-cured. Small, smouldering fires of oak and pine fill the barn with smoke, and cover the leaves with smoke particles.

Latakia produces a very rich, heavy taste, with an aroma that has a "smoky" characteristic. Latakia is an indispensable ingredient of traditional English mixtures. The content can vary from a small percentage to about 40–50%, or even more.

*(ii) Perique*

It is a red burley type of tobacco, grown and processed in St. James, Louisiana near New Orleans. Perique is a rare, slow burning, strong-tasting tobacco. The production is small, so its value is quite high. Perique is cured like Burley, but for a short time. Thereafter, leaves are put in large oak barrels or cypress logs under heavy pressure, which squeezes out some juice fermenting the entire lot. Once in a while the leaves are taken out for a short period and then repacked and re-fermented. This process takes one full year, sometimes even longer. The aroma of tobacco treated by this method is full-bodied. The nicotine content is overwhelming, thus perique can be smoked by itself. Due to its full-bodied nature, perique is used on a limited basis in blends. It is usually blended with Virginias to give it more body.

*(iii) Kentucky*

This is actually a specially treated Burley tobacco, produced in Kentucky. Unlike Burley, it is fire cured. Its aroma is not as heavy as Latakia, but very unique. The nicotine content tends to be rather high, and therefore is used in limited amounts.

*(iv) Havana*

Cuban and other cigar tobaccos are used in a limited range in Virginia blends and mixtures.

*(v) Cavendish*

It is more a method to treat tobacco than a type. English Cavendish uses a dark flue or fire-cured Virginia steamed and then stored under pressure to permit it to cure and ferment for several days to several weeks. When done well, this tobacco is really a fine stuff. Cavendish can be produced from any tobacco type.

## World Tobacco Scenario

More than 100 countries grow tobacco, of which about 80 are from the developing world. Two-third of world's tobacco is produced by just four countries. In 2003–2004, China was responsible for the production of 39.2% of all tobacco grown world-wide, with India, Brazil and the United States, producing about 25% among them. More than 75% of the total tobacco is produced by the top 10 countries (Table 4). In 2002–2003, the world production of un-manufactured tobacco was 6,024,689 tons (as against 8,048000 tons in 1997) of which 2,365,988 tons (39.3% of the world tobacco) was produced by China and 592,000 tons were produced by India, constituting 9.8% of the world tobacco (Tables 2 and 4). For the year 2003–2004, China's estimated contribution to the world market is the maximum, to the tune of 2,224,481 tons (39.2%) while that of India is 595,000 tons (10.5%). For the last few years India's contribution of raw tobacco to the world market has been consistently increasing. Thus, India has become the world's second largest producer of tobacco after China, leaving USA and Brazil behind (Tables 2, 3, and 4). Though, India's enhanced tobacco production in the recent years has brought it to the second position[2] yet India's share in the international trade continues to be less than 1%.[3]

Table 2 depicts the tobacco position of 30 countries in its various aspects during the year 1997. 42.12% of total world tobacco was produced by China alone using maximum geographical area for its cultivation. However, tobacco export from China has been much less (2.9%) meaning thereby that the domestic tobacco consumption is very high. Hence China stands first in tobacco consumption as well. Table 3 depicts the position of the top six tobacco growing countries during 13 years between 1984 and 1997, the total production and their share in the international market. Table 4 depicts the position of raw tobacco production by 11 prominent tobacco producing countries and their share in the world market in the years 1998–1999, 2002–2003 and 2003–2004.

Whereas China uses most of its tobacco crop for its domestic market (Table 5), other major producers export a large proportion of their tobacco. Brazil, Turkey, Zimbabwe,

---

2 Medium-term Export Strategy 2002-2007 for tobacco and tobacco products. Tobacco Board: Ministry of Commerce, Government of India. http://www.indiantobaccc.com

3 Countdown to Budget 2003-04, http://www.capitalmarket.com

Malawi, Greece and Italy all export more than seven-tenth of their crop. Growing tobacco itself has become a major part of the economy of many countries such as Malawi and India. Two countries are largely dependent on raw tobacco for their export earnings — Zimbabwe (23%) and Malawi (61%). A few other countries — Bulgaria, Moldova, the Dominican Republic, Macedonia, Kyrgyzstan, and Tanzania — rely heavily on the tobacco-growing market as a source of foreign exchange, although their share of the global tobacco-growing market is small. Tobacco is a major earner for a few countries with heavily agrarian economies, including Malawi, Zimbabwe, India and Turkey.

The total geographical area used for tobacco growing world-wide during 1995 was 4.32 million hectares which increased to 4.89 million hectares (Table 2) in 1997 at the cost of many food crops. The total global tobacco production during 1995 was 6.45 million metric tons which increased to 8 million metric tons during 1997. Of the total world area, amongst all types of tobacco in 1995, flue-cured Virginia (FCV) tobacco accounted for 2.39 million hectares, with a harvest of 4.036 million tons. Thus Virginia tobacco was the most important type of tobacco grown, accounting for 62% of the total tobacco production, harvested from 55% of the total tobacco plantation area. China, USA, Brazil, Zimbabwe, India, Canada, Afghanistan, Japan and South Korea are the main producers of FCV tobacco in the world. In 1995, India's share of FCV tobacco in the total world area and production was around 5% and 3% respectively.

*Table 2: The top 30 raw-tobacco-producing countries in 1997*

| *Country* | *Production 1,000 Metric Tons.* | *Production Change Over 1994–1997* | *World Shar≥ % (Tobacco)* | *Area 1000 Hectares* | *World Share (Area)* | *Export Ratio%* | *Import Ratio%* |
|---|---|---|---|---|---|---|---|
| China | 3,390.0 | 54.5 | 42.12 | 1880.0 | 38.4 | 2.9 | 4.7 |
| U.S.A. | 746.4 | 4.0 | 9.27 | 328.4 | 6.7 | 38.5 | 7.4 |
| India | 623.7 | 18.1 | 7.75 | 420.2 | 8.6 | 23.2 | |
| Brazil | 576.6 | 30.5 | 7.16 | 329.5 | 6.7 | 77.0 | 0.2 |
| Turkey | 296.0 | 57.7 | 3.68 | 323.0 | 6.6 | 89.3 | 0.5 |
| Zimbabwe | 192.1 | 8.0 | 2.39 | 99.7 | 2.0 | 109.7 | |
| Indonesia | 184.3 | 15.2 | 2.29 | 217.5 | 4.4 | 10.2 | 27.6 |
| Malawi | 158.6 | 61.7 | 1.97 | 122.3 | 2.5 | 74.2 | |
| Greece | 132.5 | –2.2 | 1.65 | 67.3 | 1.4 | 74.5 | 12.8 |
| Italy | 131.4 | 0.3 | 1.63 | 47.5 | 1.0 | 78.7 | 18.3 |
| Argentina | 123.2 | 50.3 | 1.53 | 71.0 | 1.5 | 60.6 | 5.1 |
| Pakistan | V86.3 | –14.0 | 1.07 | 45.9 | 0.9 | 1.6 | |
| Bulgaria | 78.2 | 124.3 | 0.97 | 48.5 | 1.0 | 532.5 | 58.3 |
| Canada | 71.1 | | 0.88 | 28.5 | 0.6 | 24.0 | 12.6 |

*Contd...*

| Country | Production 1,000 Metric Tons | Production Change Over 1994–1997 | World Share % (Tobacco) | Area 1000 Hectares | World Share (Area) | Export Ratio% | Import Ratio% |
|---|---|---|---|---|---|---|---|
| Thailand | 69.3 | 17.4 | 0.86 | 47.0 | 1.0 | 48.5 | 15.3 |
| Japan | 68.5 | –13.8 | 0.85 | 25.6 | 0.5 | 0.5 | 145.4 |
| Philippines | 60.9 | 8.7 | 0.76 | 29.4 | 0.6 | 17.2 | 18.3 |
| South Korea | 54.4 | –44.8 | 0. 68 | 27.2 | 0.6 | 8.4 | 26.2 |
| Mexico | 44.3 | –35.1 | 0.55 | 25.4 | 0.5 | 31.8 | 8.3 |
| Bangladesh | 44.0 | –26.7 | 0.55 | 50.3 | 1.0 | | 16.1 |
| Poland | 41.7 | –3.3 | 0.52 | 19.0 | 0.4 | 6.9 | 66.4 |
| Spain | 42.3 | 0.1 | 0.53 | 13.3 | 0.3 | 53.9 | 126.7 |
| Cuba | 37.0 | 117.6 | 0.46 | 59.0 | 1.2 | 13.5 | 0.8 |
| Moldova | 35.8 | –15.8 | 0.45 | 17.2 | 0.4 | 61.4 | 6.7 |
| Vietnam | 32.0 | n.a. | 0.40 | 36.0 | 0.7 | N.a. | n.a. |
| Dominican Rep | 30.3 | 41.7 | 0.38 | 21.2 | 0.4 | 58.1 | 2.2 |
| Macedonia | 30.0 | n.a. | 0.37 | 22.0 | 0.4 | N.a. | n.a. |
| Kyrgyzstan | 30.0 | –33.3 | 0.37 | 12.0 | 0.2 | 76.7 | 3.3 |
| South Africa | 29.0 | –1.4 | 0.34 | 14.9 | 0.3 | 41.5 | 55.5 |
| Tanzania | 25.1 | 15.1 | 0.31 | n.a. | n.a. | 55.8 | |
| World Total | 8,048.8 | | 100.0 | 4893 | 100 | | |

***Source:*** *van der Merwe, Rowena and others. The supply-side effects of Tobacco Control Policies. Background paper having data, are compiled from US Department of Agriculture, Food and Agriculture Organization, and other sources.*

**Table 3: Total unmanufactured tobacco – major producers in the world: 1984 – 1997**

| Country | 1984 | 1985 | 1986 | 1987 | 1988 | 1989 | 1990 | 1991 | 1992 | 1993 | 1994 | 1995 | 1997 |
|---|---|---|---|---|---|---|---|---|---|---|---|---|---|
| China | 1789.0 | 685.6 | 1707.1 | 1943.0 | 2734.0 | 2830.4 | 2627.1 | 3031.0 | 3498.6 | 3468.0 | 2257.0 | 23330.0 | 3390.0 |
| | (27.4) | (9.7) | (28.4) | 31.5) | (39.9) | (40.1) | (37.2) | (40.6) | (43.5) | (41.5) | (34.4) | (36.2) | (42.1) |
| USA | 784.0 | 485.9 | 528.0 | 539.3 | 621.2 | 621.2 | 620.2 | 737.7 | 757.2 | 780.9 | 731.8 | 718.0 | 603.0 |
| | (12.0) | (6.9) | (8.8) | (8.7) | (9.1) | (8.8) | (10.5) | (10.1) | (9.7) | (8.8) | (10.9) | (9.4) | (9.2) |
| India | 493.0 | 410.5 | 441.2 | 441.2 | 367.4 | 491.4 | 551.6 | 555.9 | 584.4 | 596.5 | 562.9 | 587.1 | 623.7 |
| | (7.6) | (5.8) | (7.3) | 7.3) | (5.4) | (7.0) | (7.8) | (7.4) | (7.3) | (7.1) | (8.6) | (9.1) | (7.8) |
| Brazil | 414.0 | 170.5 | 386.8 | 386.8 | 431.0 | 446.0 | 445.5 | 413.8 | 575.7 | 655.0 | 519.0 | 453.0 | 576.6 |
| | (6.4) | (2.4) | (6.4) | (6.4) | (6.3) | (6.3) | (6.3) | (5.5) | (7.2) | (7.8) | (7.9) | (7.0) | (7.1) |

*Contd...*

| | | | | | | | | | | | | | |
|---|---|---|---|---|---|---|---|---|---|---|---|---|---|
| Turkey | 178.0 | 107.9 | 158.5 | 158.5 | 219.1 | 269.9 | 296.0 | 240.9 | 334.3 | 338.8 | 187.0 | 210.0 | 296.0 |
| | (2.7) | (1.5) | (2.6) | (2.6) | (3.2) | (3.8) | (4.2) | (3.2) | (4.2) | (4.1) | (2.8) | (3.3) | (3.7) |
| Zimbabwe | 125.0 | 107.9 | 116.5 | 116.5 | 114.7 | 130.4 | 130.4 | 178.6 | 130.4 | 205.0 | 182.0 | 198.0 | 192.1 |
| | (1.9) | (1.5) | (1.9) | (1.9) | (1.7) | (1.8) | (1.8) | (2.4) | (1.8) | (2.5) | (2.8) | (3.1) | (2.4) |

***Source:*** 1. *United Nations Conference on Trade and Development (UNCTAD) Commodity Year Books, 1990 and 1994 editions, Geneva.*

2. *Food and Agriculture (FAO) production yearbook, 1995, Rome.*

3. *FAO Agro stat Database, December, 1995, Rome.*

***Notes:*** 1. *Unmanufacuterd tobacco production data is on farms sales weight basis.*

2. *Bracketed figures depict percentage.*

Many countries are net importers of tobacco leaf and tobacco products, and lose millions of dollars each year in foreign exchange as a result. In 2002, two-third of the 161 countries surveyed imported more tobacco leaf and tobacco products than they exported. Nineteen countries had a negative balance of trade in tobacco products of over $100 million or more, including Cambodia, Malaysia, Nigeria, Romania, the Russian Federation, South Korea and Vietnam[4].

Globally, in the international market, tobacco prices remain relatively stable and tobacco, a highly attractive crop for farmers, provides a higher net income yield per unit of land than most cash crops and substantially more than the food crops. In the best tobacco-growing areas of Zimbabwe, tobacco is approximately 6.5 times more profitable than the next best alternative crop.

***Table 4: World unmanufactured tobacco consumption (in tons)***

| | *Production in tons* | | | *Share in world production* | | |
|---|---|---|---|---|---|---|
| | *1998–1999* | *2002–2003* | *2003–2004* | *1998–1999* | *2002–2003* | *2003–2004* |
| China | 2,010,250 | 2,365,988 | 2,224,481 | 32.2 | 39.3 | 39.2 |
| USA | 604,131 | 358,363 | 339,241 | 9.7 | 5.9 | 5.9 |
| India | 572,200 | 592,000 | 595,000 | 9.2 | 9.8 | 10.5 |
| Brazil | 373,150 | 551,250 | 515,720 | 5.9 | 9.2 | 9.1 |
| Turkey | 217,570 | 133,812 | 142,190 | 3.5 | 2.2 | 2.5 |
| Indonesia | 123,653 | 144,700 | 135,000 | 1.9 | 2.4 | 2.4 |

*Contd...*

[4] Figures calculated from FAO database.<http://apps.fao.org>

| | | | | | | |
|---|---|---|---|---|---|---|
| Malawi | 95,996 | 124,301 | 122,580 | 1.5 | 2.1 | 2.2 |
| Greece | 127,000 | 120,000 | 121,000 | 2.0 | 1.9 | 2.1 |
| Italy | 112,225 | 108,460 | 106,250 | 1.8 | 1.8 | 1.9 |
| Argentina | 98,100 | 106,000 | 97,700 | 1.6 | 1.8 | 1.7 |
| Pakistan | 84,636 | 84,721 | 86,389 | 1.4 | 1.4 | 1.5 |
| Others | 1,815,686 | 1,335,000 | 1,187,016 | 29.1 | 22.2 | 20.9 |
| World Total | 6,234,577 | 6,024,689 | 5,672,567 | 100 | 100 | 100 |

***Source:*** *United States Department of Agriculture (USDA) estimates for February, 2004.*

***Table 5: World un-manufactured tobacco consumption (in tons)***

| | *Production in tons* | | | *Share in world production* | | |
|---|---|---|---|---|---|---|
| | *1998–1999* | *2002–2003* | *2003–2004* | *1998–1999* | *2002–2003* | *2003–2004* |
| China | 2,341,761 | 2,772,904 | 2,897,554 | 33.4 | 42.0 | 44.3 |
| India | 483,360 | 481,130 | 488,130 | 6.9 | 7.2 | 7.5 |
| Russia | 180,460 | 309,300 | 293,100 | 2.6 | 4.7 | 4.5 |
| Germany | 142,651 | 180,000 | 162,000 | 2.0 | 2.7 | 2.5 |
| Japan | 172,700 | 149,000 | 149,000 | 2.5 | 2.3 | 2.3 |
| Indonesia | 133,300 | 155,400 | 142,491 | 1.9 | 2.4 | 2.2 |
| Turkey | 108,850 | 120,10 | 123,000 | 1.6 | 1.8 | 1.9 |
| Brazil | 155,925 | 112,525 | 107,700 | 2.2 | 1.7 | 1.7 |
| UK | 136,750 | 100,750 | 100,750 | 1.9 | 1.5 | 1.5 |
| USA | 616,835 | 463,190 | 444,190 | 8.8 | 7.0 | 6.8 |
| Philippines | 74,690 | 94,120 | 96,320 | 1.1 | 1.4 | 1.5 |
| Others | 2,472,732 | 1,663,606 | 1,536,574 | 35.2 | 25.2 | 23.2 |
| World Total | 7,020,012 | 6,601,765 | 6,540,809 | 100.0 | 100.0 | 100.0 |

***Source:*** *United States Department of Agriculture (USDA) estimates for February, 2004.*

Farmers also find tobacco to be an attractive crop for more practical reasons: (i) the global price of tobacco is relatively stable compared with other crops. The stability allows farmers to plan ahead and obtain credit for other enterprises as well as tobacco farming. (ii) In addition to the cash revenue, strong support in kind is also provided by the tobacco industry in the form of material and advice. (iii) the industry often gives farmers loan. (iv) other crops may cause farmers problems with storage, collection and delivery. Tobacco is less perishable than many crops, and the industry may assist with its delivery or collection; by contrast, late collection, late payment, and price fluctuations may blight other crops.

Currently, the situation in the global tobacco market is transforming into a favourable market environment for tobacco exports due to several reasons. Brazilian export prices have almost leveled the most expensive American tobacco prices. Zimbabwean farm prices have also been higher than Brazilian prices. Because of increased cost of production and imposition of significant amount of export cesses on tobacco exports by the Government of Zimbabwe and Malawi recently their tobacco became further expensive. However, because of consistent decline in tobacco consumption in the developed world, the tobacco demand in these countries is decreasing.

## Tobacco in India

Arrival of the Portuguese in India in the sixteenth century brought many European usages in this subcontinent. They introduced from the New World the cultivation of potato, maize and tobacco into India (Burke and Quraishi, 1999). Within a few years of its introduction, tobacco cultivation began in many parts of the country though not yet for commercial purposes. It was with the establishment of British colonial rule, however, that the commercial dimension of India's tobacco production and consumption grew to be greatly magnified. Initially the British traders imported American tobacco into India to finance the purchase of the Indian commodities. When the American colonies declared independence in 1776 and here in India, the East India Company settled comfortably to exercise its political powers after the Battle of Plassey to exploit the rich resources of this country, the English found it to be in their benefit to use India's fertile agricultural land for the cultivation of their own crops. Tobacco plant was then a recent introduction to the European soil from the Americas and the increasing tobacco demand the world over motivated the English to experiment its growing in the Indian soil at the cost of local food-crops. The East India Company and its successor, the British *Raj,* used tobacco as an important cash crop, both for domestic consumption and foreign trade. In 1787, the British tried to produce quality tobacco in the botanical gardens of Sibpur, Calcutta. In 1829, Maryland and Virginia tobacco imported from the United States of America was introduced in the provinces of Bombay, Madras and Bengal. Samples of tobacco produced from these provinces were sent to England for evaluation which failed to gain acceptance because of shortcomings in curing, handling and packing. In 1875, trials were repeated in United Province (Uttar Pradesh), and Pusa farms in Bihar. Seeds and curers were brought from the United States. Still the produce failed to gain acceptance. In 1901, the British and American Tobacco Company expanded their trade into India and set up three companies, which later together became the Imperial Tobacco Company, India (which is currently known as Indian Tobacco Company (ITC) Limited). In 1903, the Imperial Agricultural Research Institute and College at the Pusa farms were established and the cultivation of new varieties of tobacco was initiated. The Indian Leaf Tobacco Development (ILTD) division of Imperial Tobacco Company conducted trials of cultivating Virginia tobacco in 1920s in Guntur area of South India. The trials were completed in 1929 and the results were desirable. Thus, the cultivation of Virginia tobacco got established in the black soil of

South India unlike other countries where it was cultivated under light soil areas. As a result, Virginia tobacco produced in black soils was characteristically different from other tobaccos.

After a series of successful trials, the Indian Leaf Tobacco Development (ILTD) division of the Imperial Tobacco Company (ITC) decided to introduce large scale production of Virginia tobacco in Andhra Pradesh (a state in South India). Four leaf curing barns were established in Guntur, Nambur, Parchoor, and Chilakalupewriket for demonstration purposes. These barns were managed by the Imperial Tobacco Company and provided training to the farmers. The Company also provided financial help to the farmers who wished to establish their own barns and needed other inputs such as fertilizers, seeds, fuels etc; with these promotional activities, cultivation of tobacco spread to the coastal districts of Andhra Pradesh as well. Mysore Tobacco Company was formed in 1937 and with its efforts Virginia tobacco cultivation was introduced in the light soil of Karnataka state of South India in 1937.

Gradually, cultivation of tobacco became an integral part of India's agricultural activities and currently, a wide variety of tobaccos are grown in 16 different States of India under diverse agro-climatic conditions. However, most of the varieties grown (other than Virginia, Burley and Oriental) are of the non-cigarette type.

India's agriculture sector encompasses a wide spectrum of agricultural practices, ranging from traditional village farming approaches to the farms on which modern agricultural equipment are utilized and techniques applied. An indication of the continuing importance of agriculture to Indian economy is that around two third of India's labour force is employed in the agriculture sector.

The importance of tobacco industry within the agricultural sector is small reflecting the large size of the Indian economy. At the same time, it is important to note that tobacco industry in India is integral to the economies of a number of Indian states and regions. To this extent, the industry, and particularly the growing and curing of tobacco make an important contribution to employment prospects and incomes of many thousands of employees and their dependents throughout these regions. A combination of strong prices of tobacco, good export demand, and low prices of other crops results in increased tobacco plantation every year. In 2001, India's share was 5.6% of world's tobacco export occupying world's 5th position after Brazil (17%), USA (10%), Zimbabwe (9%), and China (6%).

## Tobacco Status in India Since Independence

India is a major player in the international tobacco market. It is the second largest tobacco producer in the world, next only to China. In 1997, India cultivated over 420,200 hectares of tobacco, producing 604,500 metric tons, a 2% increase over 1995 (Christopher Bickers, 1997). Around 70% of this was used in the production of b*eedis* and other non-cigarette tobacco products. It was further increased in 1998 and India became second only to China in terms of the area of land, on which tobacco was grown, with more than 432,000 hectares of land used for tobacco plantation. Around 633,000 FSW tons[5] of tobacco was produced during 1998. The total value of tobacco leaves produced in India in 1998 was of the order of $US 635 millions.

*Table 6: Tobacco economy in the post-independence India*

| Year | Area (1000 Hectare) | Production (Million Kg) | Excise Revenue (Rs. in Million) | Export Revenue (Rs. in Million) | Consumption (Million Kg) |
|---|---|---|---|---|---|
| 1950–51 | 360 | 260 | 258 | 150 | 245 |
| 1960–61 | 400 | 310 | 540 | 160 | 328 |
| 1970–71 | 450 | 360 | 2284 | 320 | 367 |
| 1980–81 | 450 | 480 | 7553 | 1400 | 360 |
| 1990–91 | 410 | 560 | 2,5957 | 2630 | 474 |
| 2000–01 | 290 | 490 | 8,1824 | 9034 | 470 |
| 2001–02 | – | 601 | – | 8885 | – |

***Source:*** *Tobacco Board 2002; Directorate of Tobacco Development, 1997.*

From 1951 to 2001, there has been an increase in tobacco production by 130%, in excise revenue by 31614%, in export revenue by 5823% and in consumption 92% (Table 6). The area under tobacco cultivation increased within the first 20 years of independence. Although there was a steep reduction in the area of cultivation in 1975–1976, it increased by 20% in 1980–1981. However, there was a drastic reduction in the tobacco cultivation area in 2000–2001 because of various reasons. These fluctuations apart, overall, the area under tobacco cultivation has been limited to 4 lakh hectares, because of non-suitability of the soil for tobacco cultivation in other parts of India. With the increase in tobacco production, there has been corresponding increase in revenue generated from its domestic sale as well as export to other countries.

Excise revenue has increased from 258 million rupees in 1950–1951 to 81824 million rupees in 2000–2001. Similarly, with the increased tobacco export, there has been a many fold increase in the revenue generated from tobacco export touching 8885 million rupees in 2001–2002 from a small amount of 150 million rupees in 1950–1951. Consumption has almost doubled during this period.

## Types of Tobacco Cultivation in India

India produces a wide range and variety of tobacco in different agro-climatic zones. As a result, the plant characteristics of different types of tobacco, their cultivation

5 It is important to be aware that two different units of weight can be used for tobacco: Farm Sales Weight (FSW) and Dry Weight. In the majority of instances, farms sales weight is used. The weight being used in particular situation needs to be indicated. For conversion purposes, dry weight equals farms sales weight multiplied by 0.842.

practices, harvesting and curing techniques and leaf chemistry are different. A special feature of domestic tobacco production scene in India is the varietal composition of the produce. India is the only country where the bulk of production consists of numerous non-smoking types of tobacco. Usually, there are seven broad types of un-manufactured tobacco, based on the end-use and curing methods. These are: (i) FCV, (ii) Burley, (iii) Oriental, (iv) Dark air/Sun-cured, (v) Light air-cured, (vi) Dark air-cured and (vii) Dark fire-cured. Between 1980–1981 and 1995–1996, Flue-cured Virginia (FCV) tobacco generally accounted for 20–25% of total un-manufactured tobacco production, and one-fourth to one-third of the total area planted under all types of tobacco. The main non-flue-cured or non-FCV types of tobacco grown in India include *beedi, natu*, cigar, *cheroot*, chewable variety and snuff and *hookah* tobacco besides Burley tobacco varieties. FCV tobacco leaves are usually bright, and have orange or lemon yellow colour, and a fruity smell with sugar-nicotine ratio of around 10. Non-FCV tobaccos are usually dark brown, copper brown, dark green and have sugar-nicotine ratio of about 1. FCV tobacco is the chief cigarette tobacco grown in India followed by some quantities of non-FCV types of cigarette tobacco such as *Natu* (sun-cured country tobacco), air-cured Burley and HDBRG (Harvel de Baexo Rio Grandie) variety which is similar to Burley. On an average, *beedi t*obacco accounts for the highest production among different types of tobacco cultivated in India (Table 7 and 8). Its annual production ranges from 170,000 to over 200,000 tons, followed by flue-cured Virginia tobacco (FCV), whose average production ranges from 100,000 to 150,000 tons on annual basis. Products such as *beedi,* chewing tobacco, *hookah* tobacco, snuff etc. are mostly cottage industry based, and cater to different segments of the Indian society which are either rural or economically backward.

In mid-nineties India was ranked 5$^{th}$ among the top FCV tobacco exporting countries in the world. India accounted for 4.2% share of the world's total un-manufactured tobacco export during 1995.

Currently, India produces 600 million kilograms (dry weight) of tobacco on average. Of this FCV tobacco accounts for 185 million kilograms (31%) as against 175 million kilograms in 2002 (Table 8).

*Table 7: Area and production of unmanufactured tobacco in India*

| *TYPE* | *1990–1991* | | *1991–1992* | | *1992–1993* | | *1993–1994* | | *1994–1995* | | *1995 1996* | |
|---|---|---|---|---|---|---|---|---|---|---|---|---|
| | *Area* | *Prod* | *Area* | *Prod* | *Area* | *Prod* | *Area* | *Prod* | *Area* | *Prod* | *Area* | *Prod* |
| FCV | 118.9 | 112.9 | 156.6 | 164.7 | 155.2 | 165.5 | 133.2 | 123.8 | 125.9 | 122.6 | 127.6 | 127.8 |
| natu | 50.0 | 55.2 | 50.0 | 72.8 | 38.1 | 62.2 | 38.2 | 60.1 | 36.2 | 57.7 | 54.1 | 72.0 |
| bidi | 128.3 | 197.1 | 113.3 | 167.1 | 123.8 | 188.3 | 118.6 | 188.2 | 130.8 | 218.5 | 125.5 | 185.7 |
| cigar | 13.7 | 14.4 | 13.0 | 14.1 | 11.7 | 16.8 | 11.9 | 16.0 | 14.5 | 16.8 | 10.7 | 16.8 |

| TYPE | 1990–1991 | | 1991–1992 | | 1992–1993 | | 1993–1994 | | 1994–1995 | | 1995 1996 | |
|---|---|---|---|---|---|---|---|---|---|---|---|---|
| | Area | Prod | Area | Prod | Area | Prod | Area | Prod | Area | Prod | Area | Prod |
| Hookah | 32.9 | 82.7 | 29.3 | 72.3 | 31.8 | 78.9 | 29.3 | 97.3 | 24.6 | 89.7 | 25.4 | 82.7 |
| Chewing | 58.7 | 87.8 | 54.7 | 79.0 | 52.2 | 71.2 | 48.5 | 65.7 | 50.2 | 68.8 | 57.6 | 76.8 |
| Snuff | 8.5 | 11.8 | 8.1 | 14.4 | 6.0 | 13.3 | 5.1 | 11.8 | 8.0 | 127.7 | 5.4 | 14.4 |
| Total | 410.8 | 555.9 | 427.0 | 554.4 | 418.5 | 596.5 | 384.8 | 562.9 | 391.1 | 587.1 | 406.3 | 576.2 |

**Source:** *Directorate of Tobacco Development, Government of India, Chennai.*
**Note:** *Area in thousand hectares and production in thousand tons.*

FCV, Burley and *Natu* tobacco are the three main varieties of cigarette tobacco. FCV tobacco is the primary ingredient in the manufacture of cigarettes. It is mainly cultivated in Andhra Pradesh and Karnataka, whereas *beedi* tobacco is grown in Gujarat. Tobacco in India is grown mainly in Andhra Pradesh, Karnataka, Gujarat and Uttar Pradesh. Regional resource endowments tend to determine the type of the leaf that is produced. Growers in Andhra Pradesh and Karnataka have traditionally produced flue cured Virginia tobacco (FCV).

India is not only the second largest tobacco producer, it is also the second largest country in consumption of un-manufactured tobacco. It is also a major exporter of un-manufactured tobacco. About 40–50% of flue-cured Virginia tobacco (FCV) production in India is normally consumed by the domestic industry, and the remaining quantity is exported. It is cultivated mostly in the southern states of the country like Andhra Pradesh and Karnataka. A small area in Maharashtra bordering Andhra Pradesh also cultivates to FCV tobacco.

The two major leaf types are dark air and sun cured, which are widely used in tobacco products other than cigarettes, and flue cured which is required for making cigarettes. The preference for air and sun cured leaf demonstrates the desire for strong flavour in tobacco products. An advantage with air and sun curing for Indian farmers, however, is the lower level of investment required to produce these leaf types (Table 10 and 11).

*Table 8: Types of tobacco produced in India in 2002*

| Type of tobacco | Quantity (million kilograms) |
|---|---|
| Cigarette tobacco: | |
| FCV | 175 |
| Dark air/sun-cured | 40 |
| Burley | 8 |
| HDBRG | 20 |
| DWFC | 0.1 |
| Sub-total | 244.1 |

| | |
|---|---|
| *Non-cigarette tobacco* | |
| *Beedi* | 200 |
| Chewing | 65 |
| Cigar | 22 |
| *Hookah* | 60 |
| Snuff | 10 |
| Sub-total | 357 |
| TOTAL | 601.1 |

**Source:** *www.Indiantobacco.com*

It is evident from Tables 10 and 11 that during 1998, India's use of major leaf type (dark air and sun cured leaf) exceeded production by about 26,000 tons. On the other hand, the production of each of the other 3 main leaf types exceeded the volume used in domestic production.

***Table 9: Area, production and yield of total un-manufactured and flue-cured virginia (FCV) tobacco in India between 1980–81 and 1995–99***

| *Year* | *Area (Hectares)* | | | *Production (Metric Tons)* | | | *Yield (Kg/Hec)* | |
|---|---|---|---|---|---|---|---|---|
| | *Total un-manufac-tured tobacco* | *FCV Tobacco* | *(% of the total)* | *Total un-manufac-tured tobacco* | *FCV tobacco* | *(% of the total* | *Total tobacco* | *FCV* |
| 1980–81 | 451500 | 142400 | (31,54) | 480800 | 11700 | (24.33) | 1065 | 822 |
| 1981–82 | 443800 | 150900 | (34.00) | 520100 | 125500 | (26.05) | 1172 | 898 |
| 1982–83 | 502700 | 202600 | (40.30) | 581600 | 188700 | (32.44) | 1157 | 937 |
| 1983–84 | 439700 | 152300 | (34.64) | 492500 | 130000 | (26.40) | 1120 | 854 |
| 1984–85 | 436600 | 133100 | (30.49) | 485900 | 110000 | (22.64) | 1113 | 826 |
| 1985–86 | 397000 | 116205 | (29.27) | 441200 | 98085 | (22.23) | 1111 | 844 |
| 1986–87 | 369200 | 106037 | (28.72) | 461800 | 113730 | (24.64) | 1251 | 1073 |
| 1987–88 | 318000 | 68375 | (21.50) | 367400 | 59353 | (16.16) | 1155 | 868 |
| 1988–89 | 375300 | 105219 | (28.04) | 491400 | 116210 | (23.65) | 1309 | 1104 |
| 1989–90 | 413100 | 109900 | (26.60) | 551600 | 109400 | (19.83) | 1335 | 995 |
| 1990–91 | 410800 | 118900 | (2894) | 555900 | 112900 | (20.32) | 1353 | 950 |
| 1991–92 | 427000 | 158600 | (37.14) | 584400 | 164700 | (28.18) | 1369 | 1038 |
| 1992–93 | 418500 | 155200 | (37.08) | 596500 | 165800 | (27.80) | 1425 | 1068 |
| 1993–94 | 384800 | 133200 | (34.62) | 562900 | 123800 | (21.99) | 1464 | 929 |
| 1994–95 | 391100 | 125900 | (32.19) | 587100 | 122600 | (2088) | 1501 | 974 |
| 1995–96 | 406300 | 127600 | (31.41) | 576200 | 127800 | (22.18) | 1418 | 1002 |

**Source:** 1. *Tobacco Board, Government of India, Guntur.*
2. *Directorate of Tobacco Development, Chennai.*

**Note:** *From 1985–1986 to 1988–1989, Tobacco Board Data for FCV tobacco area & production have been used due to inconsistencies in Directorate of Tobacco Development Data.*

*Table 10: Tobacco production – 1998*

| *Leaf type* | *Volume (in tons)* | *Producer price — $US/Kg* | *Value of crop — $US'(000)* |
|---|---|---|---|
| Dry air and sun cured | 434,000 | 0.95 | 412,300 |
| Flue cured | 162,000 | 1.23 | 199,260 |
| Light air cured | 27,400 | 0.61 | 16,714 |
| Burley | 9,800 | 0.69 | 6,762 |
| TOTAL | 633,200 | | 635,036 |

*Table 11: Tobacco consumption – 1998*

| *Leaf type* | *Volume (tons FSW)* |
|---|---|
| Dark air and sun cured | 459,400 |
| Flue cured | 95,070 |
| Light air cured | 13,060 |
| Burley | 6,530 |
| TOTAL | 1,589,900 |

*Source: FAOSTAT, FAO 1998.*

As already stated, India has recorded a strong growth in tobacco leaf production in recent years. This trend appears to be partially in response to the growing demand in export market for flue cured leaf. Indian tobacco is exported to more than 80 countries. Of the total export, 80% of the tobacco is un-manufactured, while 20% of the manufactured tobacco is exported. India exports a reasonable volume of tobacco each year especially flue cured Virginia (FCV) tobacco. Of the un-manufactured tobacco exports, Flue-cured Virginia (FCV) tobacco is the single largest item accounting for 75–80% of the total exports. During 1998, more than 71,000 tons of FCV was exported, along with smaller amounts of other types. The other varieties exported are Burley, HDBRG (Harvel de Baexo Rio Grandie), *Natu*, DWFC, Top Leaf and Jutty – all of which are cigarette tobaccos. Non-cigarette tobaccos exported are *Lal chopadia, Judi, Rustica* for chewing purposes and *beedi* tobacco in small quantities. 8–10% of the total export constitutes non-cigarette tobacco. Contrary to the international trend, India's tobacco production is dominated by non-cigarette tobaccos.

In spite of India being an important producer and exporter of FCV tobacco in the international market, Indian FCV tobacco continues to face competition from other countries. It is on account of increased production and export of flavourful and semi-flavourful tobaccos from countries like Brazil, Argentina, Zimbabwe and Malawi. Tobacco industry sources opine that larger supplies and various styles/grades of FCV tobacco are available for exports from these countries at average prices. Indian FCV tobacco is generally neutral filler type tobacco which is used mainly for blending purposes. In addition to the quality parameters,

FCV tobacco production in these countries ranges from 2000 to 2500 kilograms/hectare, which is 2–3 times higher than Indian FCV tobacco cultivated in different soil types.

The newly opened East European and CIS markets are not in a position either to absorb high cost tobacco or cigarettes made with high conversion cost. Phasing out of the farm subsidies by the European Union will further enhance price competitiveness of Indian tobacco. Under these circumstances, India can play an important role in the global tobacco market if it can harness the emerging opportunities and enhances its exports to the major import markets.

The advantages for Indian tobacco are: a low unit production cost; average export price of Indian FCV tobacco is more competitive than that of Brazil, United States of America, Zimbabwe; low conversion cost of tobacco into cigarettes of 0.80 US $/10000 pieces in 1999 in India compared to 3.50 in UK and 4.0 in USA; low to medium nicotine to suit the current requirement of world market; anticipated decline in production in China, USA, Zimbabwe, EU in the next five years due to declining consumption in USA and Europe, government controls to restrict production in China, phasing out of Agri subsidies by EU and land invasions and land acquisition in Zimbabwe i.e. change of tobacco farms from White farmers to Native farmers; and phasing out of agricultural subsidies in European Union and Argentina, etc.

## Cigarette Industry in India

Cigarette is the most preferred form of tobacco consumption all over the world except India where *beedi* smoking is more common. Cigarette smoking in India is limited to educated, urban and relatively affluent people of the society. The first cigarette factory was established in 1906 at Monghyr in Bihar by the Indian Tobacco Company of what is now known as ITC (formerly Imperial Tobacco Company). In 1912, the first brand '*scissors*' was launched. Indian Leaf Tobacco Development Division (ILTD) (ITC's research subsidiary) had increased the area under the cultivation of Virginia Tobacco by 1928[6].

In 1950–1951, India was producing just 20.7 billion sticks of cigarettes which reached a peak of 96.1 billion pieces in 1984–85 and then declined. It recovered again in 1990. In 1994–1995, sale of cigarettes in India amounted to 84 billion sticks, which represented 1.6% of the world cigarette output level of 5.44 trillion sticks in 1994. Cigarette sale, however, rebounded to 95.6 billion sticks in 1995–1996, 13.85 higher than 1994–1995. In 1998–99 production increased to 101 billion sticks of which 2543 million sticks were exported. 35 million cigarettes were imported that year (Table 12).

At present, many national and multinational companies together manufacture 100 cigarettes brands (Bhosle *et al.,* 1990).

6 Technology Information, Forecasting and Assessment Council. Nicotine and its derivatives from tobacco waste. Available from URL: http://www.tifac.org.in/offer/tlbo/rep/TMS158.htm (8th August 2004).

About 17 factories are operated by 11 cigarette companies in India. The manufacturing industry is capital intensive, which provides employment to those working in manufacturing units besides indirect employment to many more who are employed in distribution network, advertising etc. Currently there are four major cigarette manufacturers in India – ITC Limited (formerly, Imperial Tobacco Company); VST Industries Limited (formerly, Vazir Sultan Tobacco Company); Godfrey Philips India Limited and GTC Industries Limited (formerly, Golden Tobacco Company). There are a couple of small sized cigarette companies with manufacturing facility. ITC is the dominant cigarette manufacturer with its market share being 66%, followed by Godfrey Phillips, GTC and VST (Table 13).

Cigarette industry generally uses light coloured tobacco leaf, which is obtained either from flue-cured Virginia (FCV) tobacco, or a combination of light air-cured tobacco types such as Burley and Harvel de Baexo Rio Grandie (HDBRG) tobacco. Additionally sun-cured country tobacco, *natu* is also used in cigarette manufacturing, particularly for marketing cheaper brands. In India, FCV type tobacco is the chief tobacco type used in cigarette manufacturing, as Burley and HDBRG tobaccos are generally exported because their use in the American type blended cigarettes.

***Table 12: Production, export and import of cigarettes in India***

| *Year* | *Production** | *Import** | *Export** |
|---|---|---|---|
| 1950–51 | 20,700 | | |
| 1960–61 | 35,000 | | |
| 1970–71 | 63,100 | | |
| 1980–81 | 78,600 | | |
| 1981–82 | 90,600 | | |
| 1982–83 | 89,100 | | |
| 1983–84 | 87,300 | | |
| 1984–85 | 96,100 | | |
| 1985–86 | 82,400 | | |
| 1986–87 | 81,100 | | |
| 1987–88 | 77,800 | | |
| 1988–89 | 80,300 | | |
| 1989–90 | 83,500 | | |
| 1990–91 | 86,100 | | 800 |
| 1991–92 | 85,700 | | 6428 |
| 1992–93 | 80,800 | 51 | 2410 |
| 1993–94 | 78,800 | 25 | 3456 |
| 1994–95 | 84,000 | 86 | 3463 |
| 1995–96 | 95,600 | 134 | 1461 |
| 1996–97 | 102,300 | 157 | 1206 |
| 1997–98 | 104,600 | 252 | 1446 |
| 1998–99 | 101,000 | 35 | 2543 |

**Source:** *Union Budget and Foreign Trade Data from Directorate General of Commercial Intelligence.*
** Figures are in million pieces.*

*Table 13: Leading cigarette brands available in India**

| *Type* | *ITC* | *VST* | *GPI* | *GTC* |
|---|---|---|---|---|
| **Major Filter brands** Premium | India King, Classic State Expess, 555 Benson & Hedges | Kingston Legend Buton | Rothmans, Jaisalmer, Chestenfield, Marlboro | Chancellor, Harvard, Craven, Dunhill, Cartier |
| Medium | Wills, Navy Cut | Charms mini King, Gold Premium, Charms Viginia filter | Four Square Red & White | Panama Filter, King Baton |
| Popular | Gold Flake Bristol Capstan | Charminar Gold filter | Red & White filter, Commando, Originals | Panama Filter |
| **Major non-filter brands** | | | | |
| Upper | Scissors | Charminar Gold | Red & White | Flair, Style |
| Lower | Hero | Charminar, Charms Standard | Cavenders | Panama |

***Source:** *Measures to Reduce the Supply of Tobacco. Economics of Tobacco Control, World Bank Groups, 2003.*

The tobacco industry in India is subject to a range of taxes imposed by the Central and State Governments. The Union Government raises revenue from the sales of all types of tobacco products predominantly through the imposition of excise duty calculated on an ex-factory basis. During 1998–1999, a sum of Rs. 532,460 million was collected by the Indian Government from excise taxes. The total excise duty generated by tobacco products was Rs. 57,680 million which is 10.8% of the total excise revenue collected. In 2000–2001, the contribution of tobacco to Indian economy was to the extent of Rs 81,820 million, which accounted for about 12% of the total excise collections. Foreign exchange earned during this period was Rs 9030 million accounting for 4% of India's total agricultural exports. Tobacco excise has become a particularly important source of revenue for the national budget.

However, the contribution of tobacco to the excise revenue has reduced from 14% in 1960–1961 to 12% in 2000–2001. The slowdown in the share of excise revenue is partly due to the excise rates over time. The bulk of tobacco consumption in India is in traditional forms such as *beedi* and chewing and other nonsmoking products, whereas the excise revenue from tobacco is largely dependent on cigarettes, which account for less than one-fifth of tobacco consumption but contribute nearly four-fifth of the excise revenue. Irrespective of the large contribution of cigarette industry to excise revenue, it has shown an increasing trend of profit. The profit of cigarettes and cigarette products industries reached 78.2% of the total profit of all tobacco industries in 1997–1998 from 61.2% in 1979–1980[7]. Similarly, the profit share of *paan masala* and *catechu* industry has also increased substantially over the years. However, the profit margin of the *beedi* industry has been declining over the years.

It is estimated that the total tobacco market in India is in the order of $US 6.2 billion a year[8]. With cigarette consumption of around 100 billion sticks a year, the value of this segment of tobacco market is around $US 2.4 billion. The magnitude of non-cigarette form of tobacco products in India is in the order of $US 3.8 billion. The overall market for tobacco products in India is increasing over the last 15 years; growing at 3% or more each year since 1988.

The growth in the domestic market reflects overall population growth, increased consumption and increased financial well-being of the people in India. Per capita tobacco consumption in India is 0.9 kg compared to the world average of 1.8 kg. Per capita consumption of tobacco in Indians is among the lowest in the world[9].

Domestic un-manufactured tobacco consumption has increased from 483,360 tons in 1998–1999 to 488,130 tons in 2003–2004 (Table 11). Tobacco usage in India is contrary to world trend since chewing tobacco and *beedi* are the dominant forms of tobacco consumption, whereas internationally, cigarette is the dominant form of tobacco use. The notable feature of consumer market for tobacco products in India, however, is a very high consumption of tobacco in forms other than manufactured cigarettes.

## Beedi Industry in India

*Beedi* is unprocessed tobacco wrapped in a *tendu* leaf and tied with a string. *Tendu* leaf accounts for 74% by weight of *beedi*. *Beedi* tobacco is the major sun-cured tobacco grown in non-Virginia tobacco category in India. 30–35% of the total area used for tobacco cultivation is used for production of *beedi* tobacco and accounts for 34–40% (34% at present) of the total tobacco produced in the country. Gujarat is the main *beedi*-tobacco producer followed by Karnataka and Maharashtra. In India, *beedi* is the major competitor of the cigarette industry with its annual outturn being 6–8 times more than that of the cigarettes.

*Beedis* are made by rolling a dried rectangular piece of *tendu* leaf with 0.15–0.25 gram of sun-cured, dried flake tobacco (Bhosle, Murti and Gupta, 1992). The collection of *tendu* leaf that is used to wrap *beedis* forms an important link for the *beedi* industry. *Tendu* leaf is almost wholly grown on government owned forest land, with around 62% of *tendu* leaf being grown in Madhya Pradesh alone. There are about 290,000 growers of *beedi* tobacco in India.

---

7 Price Waterhouse Coopers, Economic Studies and Strategies Unit, Canberra, Australia, August, 2000.

8 Indian Institute of Foreign Trade (IIFT), (2002) Medium term plan for tobacco exports from India and strategies for the next five years, New Delhi.

9 United States Department of Agriculture (USDA) estimates for February, 2004.

*Beedis* are the most popular form of smoking tobacco in India. *Beedis* are puffed more frequently than cigarettes to prevent them from going out. *Beedis* are also consumed in other Asian countries such as Bangladesh, Pakistan, Sri Lanka, Nepal, Singapore and Malaysia. India accounts for 85% of world *beedi* production. Recently, *beedis* have gained popularity among youth in United State of America, exported from India.

Toxicological findings indicate that mainstream smoke from *beedi* (and other forms of tobacco such as "chutta") is higher in nicotine than smoke from US and Indian made cigarettes. (Pakhale and Maru, 1998). The health risk from *beedis* as from other tobacco products, is substantial (Gupta, Murti and Bhonsle, 1996).

*Cigars are* made of air-cured, fermented tobacco, usually in factories, and are generally expensive. Cigar smoking is predominantly an urban practice. This tobacco product is on the decline due to popularity of cigarettes and *beedis* in India. *Cheroot* is a roll made from tobacco leaves.

## REFERENCES


Ashton H. and Stepney R.: *Smoking: Psychology and Pharmacology,* Travistock Publications, London, 1982.

Bhosle R.B., Murti P.R. and Gupta P.C.: Tobacco Habits in India. In: Gupta PC, Hamner J III, Murti P (Eds). *Control of Tobacco-related Cancers and Other Diseases.* Proceedings of An International Symposium, 15–19 January 1990; Mumbai:TIFR, Oxford University Press;1992:25–46, 1992.

Burke S.M. and Quraishi S.A.D.: *The British Raj in India: An Historical Review.* Oxford University Press, Delhi, 1999.

Chojar A.K.: *Tobacco Cultivation and Marketing,* Deep and Deep Publications Private Limited, New Delhi, 2002.

Christopher Bickers: Exporting Growth, *Tobacco International,* 1997.

Gupta P.C., Murti P.R. and Bhosle R.B. Epidemiology of Cancer by Tobacco Products and the Significance of TSNA. *Critical Review in Toxicology;* 26:183–198, 1996.

Gowda M.: *The Story of Paan Chewing in India, Botanical Museum Leaflets;*14:181–214, 1951.

National Sample Survey (NSS). (2001) *Consumption of Some Important* Commodities in India: 1999–2000, 55th Round. Department of Statistics and *Programme Implementation,* Government of India.

Pakhale S.S. and Maru G.B.: Distribution of Major and Minor Alkaloids in Tobacco Mainstream and Side-stream of Popular Indian Smoking Products. *Food and Chemical Toxicology;* 36:1131–1138, 1998.

CHAPTER

# 4 Nicotine: Pharmacokinetics, Metabolism and Pharmacodynamics

*Nicotine, a major pharmacological constituent of tobacco is a powerfully toxic and highly addictive substance and just one drop of free nicotine placed on the tongue or the skin is sufficient to kill a dog (or a man) within minutes.*

— Larson *et al.*, 1961

Tobacco smoke and smokeless tobacco both contain a large number of chemicals which have their impact on the body in various ways. Nearly 3000 chemicals have been identified in smokeless tobacco, while close to 4000 are present in tobacco smoke. Tobacco plant, in its leaves, carries several alkaloids of which nicotine is the most prominent and other prominent ones are nornicotine, cotinine, anatabin, anabasin etc. Aliphatic hydrocarbons present in the waxy leaf-coating and hundreds of isoprenoids that give the aroma to tobacco constitute important ingredients of tobacco chemistry. Phytosterols such as cholesterol, campesterol, etc. and alcohol, phenolic compounds, chlorogemic acid, rutin, carboxylic acid and several free amino acids are found in tobacco. In addition, a wide range of toxic metals including mercury, lead, cadmium, chromium and other trace elements have been detected in Indian tobacco (Mishra and Shaikh, 1983).

Dependence on tobacco is related to the pharmacological effects of nicotine present both in tobacco leaves and tobacco smoke. Nicotine contains Carbon, Hydrogen and Nitrogen, in the proportion $C_{10}H_{14}N_2$, combined together to form a double ring-like structure (Figure 1).

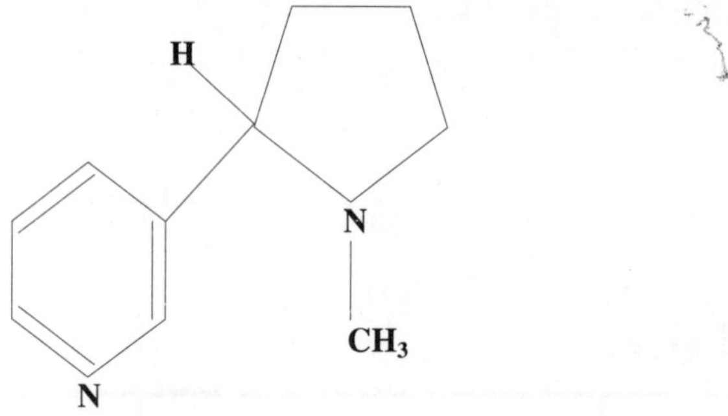


*Figure 1: Chemical structure of nicotine*

Nicotine is a tertiary amine composed of a pyridine and a pyrrolidine ring (Figure 2). Nicotine may exist in two different three-dimensionally structured shapes called stereoisomers. Since tobacco is a plant product, there are differences in the amount of nicotine among and within different types and strains of tobacco plant, including variations in different parts of the plant as well as differences due to the growing conditions (Table 1). Within a tobacco plant, leaves harvested from higher stalk positions have higher concentrations of nicotine as compared to leaves from lower stalk positions; ribs and stems of the leaves have the least nicotine concentrations (Rathkamp *et al.*, 1973).

Biologically, production of nicotine requires nicotinic acid (niacin) and an N-methyl-pyrrolinium cation, which is diverted from ornithine (a non-protein amino acid derivative from Kreb cycle intermediates) (Figure 2). Nicotine production is induced by Jasmonic acid signals in response to leaf damage (Baldwin and Schmelz, 1996; Baldwin and Schmelz, 1994). Synthesis occurs in the roots of the plant followed by transport via the xylem to the leaves and throughout the plant. By using Jasmonic acid as a chemical signal, the defense becomes inducible. Induced plants have about 6% of the total nitrogen content locked and the synthesis diverts fixed carbon out of the TCA (a- ketoglutarate is an ornithine precursor).

In its pure state, nicotine is a dense, oily, colourless, volatile and strongly alkaline liquid, which turns pale yellow to dark brown on exposure to air and gives off a characteristic tobacco smell. Nicotine is isolated from tobacco by a variety of methods like supercritical $CO_2$ extraction in which $CO_2$ is compressed to a supercritical state (between a liquid and a gas) under high pressure and thus making a non-polar solvent. When extraction is done, the $CO_2$ evaporates, leaving behind nicotine.

Nicotine is a powerfully toxic and highly addictive substance and just one drop of free nicotine placed on the tongue or the skin is sufficient to kill a dog (or a man) within minutes (Larson *et al.*, 1961). As little as 4 mg can produce symptoms of toxicity in a subject whose body is not used to the drug and 60 mg proves to be an absolutely lethal dose. Food and Drug Administration (FDA) of the United States has approved it as an insecticide and its effectiveness is similar to that of an organophosphorus compound and it is one of the few poisons for which bugs have not evolved resistance to (Geiger, 1993).

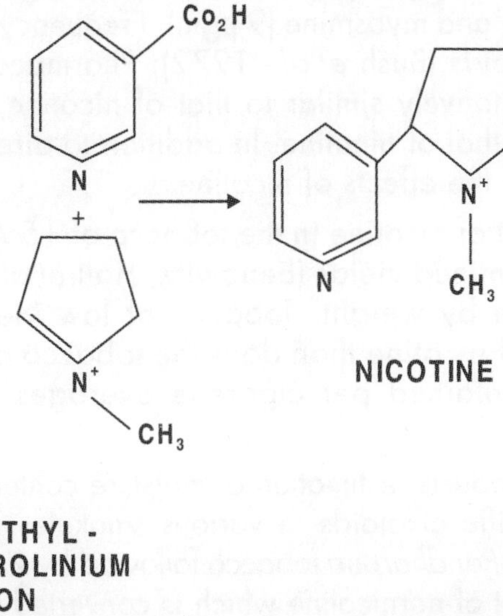

$CO_2H$

N
+

$N^+$

$CH_3$

N-METHYL - PYRROLINIUM CATION

$N^+$

N

$CH_3$

NICOTINE

*Figure 2: Synthesis of nicotine from nicotinic acid and ornithine precursors*

Use of nicotine in human beings is usually from cigarette smoking and use of other tobacco products. In the cigarette smoke, free nicotine is suspended on minute droplets of tar. These droplets are so small (less than one thousandth of a millimeter) that, if inhaled, they can reach the smallest passages and alveoli in the interior of the lungs. In an unlit cigarette, nicotine is dissolved in the moisture of tobacco leaf as a water-soluble salt. Those who inhale smoke of the cigarette are likely to absorb more nicotine than those who do not inhale smoke (Armitage *et al.*, 1975). Pictec and Crepienx first synthesized pure nicotine in 1893; however, the first laboratory synthesis was reported in 1904.

Nicotine is the major cause of the predominant behavioural effects of tobacco and some of its physiological consequences. Development of tolerance to its own actions is similar to that produced by other addictive drugs. Although, nicotine has long been considered as a primary pharmacological reason and a source of a number of physiological effects for tobacco use, the effects of nearly four thousand chemical constituents detected in tobacco smoke cannot be underestimated since many of these have significant pharmacological activity and trigger profound and damaging changes in the body.

As already mentioned, other than nicotine, a number of pharmacologically active alkaloids have been isolated from tobacco smoke namely nornicotine, anabasine, myosmine, nicotyrine, anatabine, N-methylanabasine, N′-methylanatabine, 2-3-Dipyridyl, N′-nitrosonornicotine, metanicotine, nicotine-N-oxide, cotinine, 6-oxoanabasine, pseudo-oxynicotine, nornicotyrine etc. (Figure 3). These substances make up 8 to 12 percent of total alkaloid content of tobacco products (Piade and Hoffmann, 1980) (Tables 1 and 2). In some varieties of tobacco, nornicotine concentrations exceed those of nicotine (Schmeltz and Hoffman, 1977). In the smoke of a cigarette, quantities of minor alkaloids are: nornicotine (27 to 88 μgms.), cotinine (9 to 50 μgm), anabasine (3 to 12 μgm), anatabine (4 to 14 ugm) and myosmine (9 μgm). Frequency of puff influences the delivery of the component alkaloids (Bush *et al.,* 1972). Pharmacological action of nornicotine and anabasine is qualitatively similar to that of nicotine, with potencies of 20 to 75 percent compared with that of nicotine. In addition to direct activity, some of the minor alkaloids may influence the effects of nicotine.

In a study of amount of nicotine in the tobacco of 15 American cigarette brands of different machine-determined yields (Benowitz, Hall *et al.,* 1983), tobacco contained average 1.5% nicotine by weight. Tobacco of low yield cigarettes tends to have higher concentration of nicotine than does the tobacco of high-yield cigarettes. Total amount of nicotine contained per cigarette averages 8.4 mg similar in different brands (Table 2).

In Indian tobacco products, estimation of moisture content, pH, nitrite, nitrate, nicotine and other tobacco-specific alkaloids in various smokeless tobacco products, maximum concentration is found in *Pandharpuri* tobacco followed by *Zarda* (Table 3). These two types also show a high content of nornicotine which is converted to N-nitrosonornicotine during curing process which is a carcinogenic compound. Alkaloid levels are also two-fold higher in *beedi* tobacco filter than cigarettes tobacco filter. Nitrate content is two times higher in cigarette tobacco.

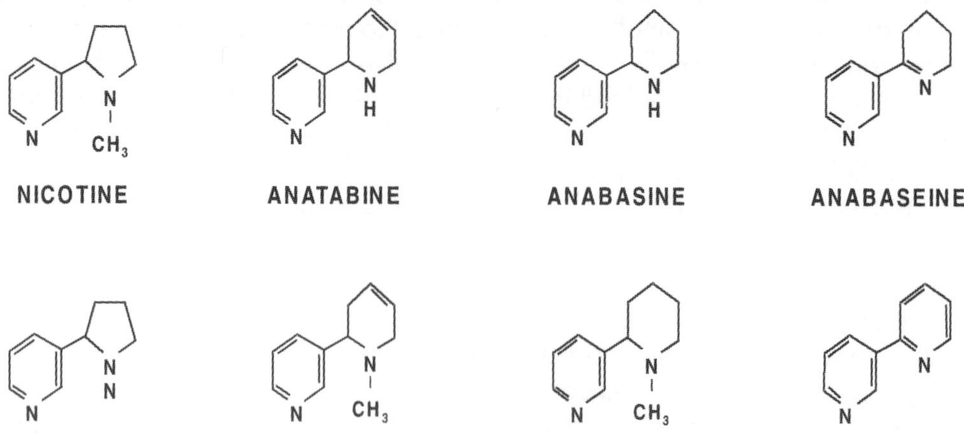

N-NITROSONORNICOTINE NICOTYRINE NORNICOTYRINE METANICOTINE

NICOTINE N-OXIDE (OXYNICOTINE) COTININE 6'-OXOANABASINE PSEUDOOXYNICOTINE

*Figure 3: Structure of nicotine and other alkaloids*

*Table 1: Alkaloid contents of various tobaccos (mg/kg, dry basis)*

| *Alkaloids* | *Dark Commercial Tobacco* | | *Burley* | *Bright* |
|---|---|---|---|---|
| | *A* | *B* | | |
| Nicotine | 11,500 | 10,000 | 15,400 | 12,900 |
| Nornicotine | 550 | 200 | 630 | 210 |
| Anatabine | 360 | 380 | 570 | 600 |
| Cotinine | 140 | 150 | 90 | 150 |
| Myosmine | 195 | 140 | 90 | 40 |
| 2,3′- Dipridyl | 100 | 110 | 30 | 10 |
| N′-Formyl-nornicotine | 175 | 210 | 140 | 40 |

**Source:** *Piade and Hoffman (1980)*

*Table 2: Nicotine content of various tobacco products*

| *Product* | *No. of brands tested* | *Concentation of nicotine (mg/gm tobacco)* | *Typical single dose* (gm Tobacco)* | *Nicotine in a single dose* (mgs)* | *Nicotine in dose typically consumed in a day* |
|---|---|---|---|---|---|
| Cigarette | 15 | 15.7 (13.3–26.9) | 0.54 | 8.4 | 168 mg/20 cigarettes |
| Moist snuff | 8 | 10.5 (6.1–16.6) | 1.4 | 14.5 | 157 mg/15 gms |
| Chewing tobacco | 2 | 16.8 (9.1–24.5) | 7.9 | 133 | 1176 mg/70 gm |

**Single dose refer to a cigarette or an amount of smokeless tobacco placed in the mouth.* ***Source:*** *Benowitz, Hall, et al., (1983).*

## Pharmacokinetics and Metabolism of Nicotine

The scientific study of drugs and chemicals in the body - their absorption, distribution in the body and their elimination from the body is called Pharmacokinetics. In the following pages pharmacokinetics of nicotine is discussed.

### Absorption

From the incandescent tip of the lighted cigarette, burning at a temperature of 800 °C, the smoker with each puff draws along the tobacco rod and into his mouth a hot potpourri of gases and many-sized particles. Nicotine is distilled from burning tobacco and is carried proximally on tar droplets (mass median diameter 0.3 to 0.5 μm) and also probably in vapor phase (Eudy *et al.,* 1985), which are inhaled. Nicotine from cigarette smoke is absorbed rapidly through the lungs similar to that after intravenous administration (Tutka *et al.,* 2005).

*Table 3: Moisture, pH and alkaloid content of chewing tobacco products*

| Tobacco Product | Moisture (%) | pH | Nitrate (mg/g) | Nitrite (ug/g) | Nicotine (mg/g) | Nornicotine (mg/g) | Anabasin (mg/g) | Anatabin (mg/g) | Cotinine (mg/g) |
|---|---|---|---|---|---|---|---|---|---|
| Pandharpuri | 3.99 | 5.15 | 4.66 | 23.05 | 55.25 | 17.11 | 0.31 | 0.63 | 0.37 |
| Zarda | 11.58 | 5.02 | 5.00 | 30.80 | 25.79 | 10.23 | 0.09 | 0.92 | 0.15 |
| Masheri Br 1 | 7.69 | 6.33 | 6.49 | 11.07 | 5.52 | 0.46 | 0.05 | 0.04 | 0.10 |
| Masheri Br 2 | 5.80 | 7.12 | 2.26 | 9.25 | 18.90 | 3.66 | 0.07 | 0.38 | 0.43 |
| Rawa tobacco | 9.52 | 5.18 | 8.56 | 9.01 | 14.35 | 4.23 | 0.72 | 0.91 | 0.09 |
| Rawa Masheri | 4.29 | 5.89 | 4.49 | 16.40 | 5.60 | 0.34 | 0.74 | 0.09 | 0.11 |

*Source: Pakhale et al., 1997.*

Absorption of nicotine across membranes depends upon pH (London 1999). Nicotine is a weak base with a pKa (index of ionic dissociation) of 8.0 (aqueous solution, 25 °C). This means that, at pH 8.0, 50 percent of nicotine is ionized and the rest 50 percent is nonionized. In its ionized state, such as in acidic environment, nicotine does not rapidly cross membranes. At an acidic pH of smoke from cigarette (pH 5.5) nicotine is mostly ionized and does not readily permeate the cell membrane (Zevin *et al.,* 1998). Absorption of nicotine from different sites of the body is determined by the pH of cigarette smoke. The pH of individual puffs of the cigarette made of flue-cured tobacco is acidic and decreases with sequential puffs from pH 6.0 to pH 5.5 (Brunnemann and Hoffmann, 1974). At these pHs', the nicotine is almost completely ionized and thus there is little buccal absorption from cigarette smoke, even when it is held in mouth (Gori *et al.,* 1986). This is partly because most cigarette smoke is acid and for physicochemical reasons, dissolved nicotine is not well absorbed in acid conditions. Moreover, the surface area available in mouth and nose for absorption is limited. In the lungs nicotine is buffered to a physiological pH and rapidly crosses membranes. Nicotine from smokeless tobacco is absorbed through the oral mucosa. An alkaline pH of smoke from tobacco in pipes, nicotine is mostly non-ionized and well absorbed from the mouth. Air cured tobacco smoke is alkaline with progressive puffs increasing its pH from 6.5 to

7.00 or higher (Brunneman and Hoffmann, 1974). At alkaline pH, nicotine is largely nonionized and readily crosses the membranes. Nicotine from products, which deliver smoke of alkaline pH, is well absorbed through the mouth (Armitage *et al.*, 1978; Russel, Raw and Jarvis, 1980).

There is a vast surface area in the lungs for absorption in the regions where thousands of small blood vessels course under the linings of the air sacs into which the smoke is drawn. The surface fluid into which nicotine is dissolved is slightly alkaline and, therefore, absorption of nicotine is efficient and rapid when cigarette smoke is inhaled. Rapid absorption occurs because of the huge surface area of the alveoli, small airways and also due to dissolution of nicotine at physiological pH (approximately 7.4) that facilitates transfer across cell membranes.

When a cigarette is smoked and smoke inhaled, blood nicotine levels rise very rapidly and the peak level is achieved by the time the entire cigarette is smoked. It is believed that 90% of nicotine present in the inhaled smoke is absorbed (Creeighton, 1973). The levels of nicotine in plasma rise over 30 minutes and slowly decline over the next hours. The increase in plasma nicotine concentration following repeated puffs from a cigarette closely parallels with that found with bolus intravenous injection of similar dose (Russell and Feyerabend, 1980). If cigarettes are smoked at frequent and regular intervals (e.g. one cigarette every hour), the effect is cumulative so that even in 'trough' periods, nicotine levels are higher than the baseline. Each inhalation of smoke produces a peak of its own and repeated inhalation has a cumulative effect. On the contrary, non-inhaled cigarette smoke has very little effect on blood nicotine levels (Haines *et al.*, 1974; Armitage *et al.*, 1975). In a study, little absorption of nicotine in non-inhaling cigar smokers was observed (Turner *et al.*, 1977) and similar absence of nicotine absorption was seen in non-inhaling pipe smokers (Turner *et al.*, 1975). However, the intermediate alkaline effect of smoke held in the mouth persists (Armitage *et al.*, 1978), which is similar to the one found in chewing of the nicotine gum (Russell, Feyerabend and Cole, 1976) *'pan-masala' 'gutka'* etc. Nicotine absorbed in this manner is sufficient to attain the blood level observed in an average cigarette smoker. The regular use of smokeless tobacco results in the plasma concentration of nicotine comparable to those seen in cigarette smokers (Benowitz *et al.*, 1988). Blood-levels of nicotine with fine ground nasal snuff rises almost as fast as those observed after cigarette smoking (Russell *et. al.*, 1981). At an alkaline pH of smoke from tobacco in pipes, nicotine is mostly nonionized and well absorbed from the mouth (Westman, 1995).

Chewing tobacco is absorbed more gradually and poorly in the stomach due to acidity of gastric fluid (Travell, 1960). Chewing tobacco, snuff etc. are of alkaline pH as a result of tobacco selection. The alkaline pH facilitates absorption of nicotine through mucous membranes. The rate of absorption from smokeless tobacco depends upon the product and the route of administration. Nicotine gum and nicotine trans-dermal patch used in smoking-cessation treatment as a substitution therapy, deliver nicotine more slowly than smoking. Absorption of nicotine from the gum is gradual and the total amount of absorbed nicotine is significantly lower compared to the amount of nicotine contained in the gum. Plasma levels after chewing the gum are lower than the levels after cigarette smoking. Frequent dosing is necessary to achieve adequate nicotine absorption from the oral mucosa. However it is well absorbed in the small intestine (Jenner, Gorrod and Beckett, 1973), which has more alkaline pH and large surface area. Bioavailability of nicotine from the gastro-intestinal tract is incomplete because of pre-systemic metabolism, whereby, after absorption into the portal venous circulation, the liver metabolizes nicotine before it reaches the systemic venous circulation. Nicotine from the trans-dermal patch is slowly absorbed; its plasma concentration rises gradually over 6 to 8 hours and declines slowly over the final 6 hours.

With the nicotine nasal spray, nicotine is absorbed through the nasal mucosa. The absorption is very rapid and the peak arterial plasma levels are reached in about 5 minutes after administration (Zevin *et al.*, 1998).

Nicotine base can also be absorbed through the skin and there have been case reports of poisoning after skin contact with pesticides containing nicotine (Faulkner, 1933; Benowitz, Lake *et al.*, 1987). There is evidence of cutaneous absorption of and toxicity from nicotine in tobacco field-workers (Gehlbach *et al.*, 1975). Dose of nicotine taken is determined by measuring the nicotine blood levels and the rate of its elimination from the body.

## Distribution

After entering the blood stream (which is at pH 7.4) through the lungs, some of the absorbed nicotine immediately enters the lung tissue and the rest, through the blood stream, reaches the left side of the heart from where it is pumped rapidly to the all parts of the body. After the first puff of cigarette smoke, nicotine reaches the brain in about seven seconds and the big toe within 15–20 seconds. About 31 percent of the nicotine flowing in the blood stream exists in a free form (non-ionized) and the rest 69 percent of nicotine exists as dissociated salts (ions). Binding to plasma proteins is less than 5 percent (Benowitz, Jacob *et al.*, 1982). Nicotine in its free form is exceedingly lipophillic and since the membranes surrounding the cells of the body are largely composed of lipids, it can easily penetrate through these membranes into tissue cells. That is how the major part of nicotine can easily reach the vital cellular structure of most organs - including those of the fetus, in a pregnant smoker. On the account of its fat dissolving property, nicotine can pass through dermal tissue and blood-brainbarrier. Penetration of nicotine across the blood-brain barrier occurs by both passive diffusion and active transport by the choroids plexus (Spector and Goldberg, 1982).

Nicotine is unequally and extensively distributed to body tissues, with a steady state volume of distribution averaging 180 litres (2.6 times the body weight) (Figure 4). This means that when nicotine concentrations have fully equilibrated, the amount of nicotine in the body tissue is 2.6 times the amount predicted by the product of blood concentration and body weight and over time, there is a variation in nicotine concentration in different body tissues. In experimental animals, nicotine is taken up with great rapidity by the brain and other nervous tissues (Larson and Silvette, 1975; Maziere *et al.*, 1976). After rapid intravenous injection, concentration of nicotine declines rapidly because of tissue uptake of the drug. Shortly after intravenous injection, concentration in arterial blood, lungs and brain are high while concentration in tissues such as muscle and adipose are low. The consequence of this distribution pattern is that uptake into the brain is rapid, occurring within 1 or 2 minutes and blood level falls because of the peripheral tissue uptake after 20 or 30 minutes of administration. Rapid nicotine uptake into tissues and its intensive metabolism lead to quick disappearance from the plasma.

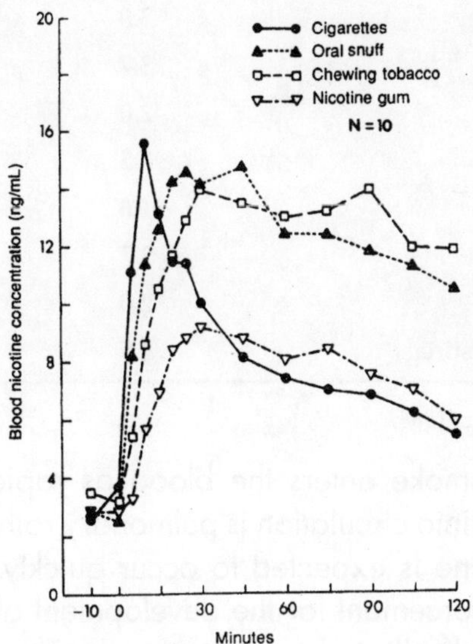


*Figure 4: Blood nicotine concentrations during and after smoking cigarettes (11/3 cigarettes), using oral snuff (2.5 gm), using chewing tobacco (avg. 7.9 gm), and chewing nicotine gum (two 2 mg pieces)*

In a mouse, maximum brain concentration of nicotine is reached within one minute of injection or direct application of nicotine to the respiratory tract and at this time, the concentration of nicotine in the brain is more than five times greater than that in the blood. This avid sequestration of nicotine by the brain is in no doubt important in determining its swift psychological effects. Other parts of the nervous system, which quickly take up nicotine from the blood, are the medulla of the adrenal glands and the sympathetic ganglion cells - both parts of the autonomic nervous system concerned, among other things, with the control of circulation. The early entry of nicotine in these structures, as well as into the brain and the cells of the heart itself, account for the rapid onset of circulatory changes associated with smoking of cigarette.

*Table 4: Human pharmacokinetics of nicotine and cotinine*

| | *Nicotine* | *Cotinine* |
|---|---|---|
| Half-life | 120 min. | 18 hrs |
| Volume of distribution | 180 L | 88 L |
| Total clearance | 130mL/min | 72 mL/min |
| Renal clearance | 200 mL/min | 12 mL/min |
| Non-renal clearance | 1,100 mL/min | 60 mL/min |

***Source:** Average value based on data from Benowitz, Jacob et al., (1982) and Benowitz, Kuyt et al., (1983).*

*Table 5: Steady state distribution of nicotine*

| Tissue | Tissue to blood ratio |
|---|---|
| Blood | 1.0 |
| Brain | 3.0 |
| Heart | 3.7 |
| Muscle | 2.0 |
| Adipose | 0.5 |
| Kidney | 21.6 |
| Liver | 3.7 |
| Lung | 2.0 |
| Gastrointestinal | 3.5 |

*Source: Benowitz (1986)*

Nicotine inhaled in tobacco smoke enters the blood as rapidly as after intravenous injection except that the entry point into circulation is pulmonary rather than systemic venous. After smoking, the action of nicotine is expected to occur quickly. Rapid onset of effects, after a puff, provides optimal reinforcement for the development of drug dependence. The effect of nicotine declines as it is distributed to other tissues. The distribution half-life that describes the movement of nicotine from the blood and other rapidly perfused tissues, such as brain, to other body tissues is about 9 minutes (Feyerabend *et al.*, 1985). Distribution kinetics rather than elimination kinetics determine the time course of actions in the central nervous system after smoking a single cigarette.

Nicotine is secreted into saliva (Russell and Feyerabend, 1978). Passage of saliva containing nicotine into the stomach, combined with trapping of nicotine in the acidic gastric fluid and re-absorption from small bowel, provides a potential route for enteric nicotine re-circulation. This re-circulation may account for some of the oscillations in the terminal decline phase of nicotine blood levels after intravenous nicotine infusion or cessation of smoking (Russell, 1976).

As nicotine freely crosses the placenta, it is found in amniotic fluid and umbilical cord blood of the neonates (Hibberd, O'Connor and Gorrod, 1978· Luck *et al.*, 1982). Nicotine is found in breast milk and the breast fluid of non-lactating women (Petrakis *et al.*, 1978) and cervical mucous secretion (Sasson *et al.*, 1985). Nicotine is also found in freshly shampooed hair of smokers and nonsmokers who are environmentally exposed to tobacco smoke (Haley and Hoffmann, 1985).

Intake of nicotine by nervous system depends upon various factors - like high lipid concentration, abundance of blood flow and the ability to take up certain substances from the blood stream, even against a concentration gradient, by enzymatic process. Those areas of the body, which are less richly supplied with these attributes, take up correspondingly less nicotine. High lipid solubility of nicotine permits it to diffuse out from the cells as readily as it can enter them. The stream of blood, which brings nicotine to the brain cells, is equally capable of carrying it away. The speed of exit of nicotine is equally dramatic as the speed of its entry into the brain cells. In an experimental mouse, an injection of nicotine causes its peak concentration in the brain within a minute and within five minutes, level falls down to 50% of the maximum and only 1% is left after 60 minutes.

Distribution of nicotine in different regions of the brain also varies over time. Experiments show that ten minutes after nicotine injection, its concentration in hippocampus – an area concerned with emotions, learning and memory may be 30% higher than the rest of the brain. It seems that nicotine first goes to the gray matter and then to the white matter in the brain before finally getting eliminated.

Studies related to the nicotine's passage in and out of the brain have been largely carried out in small mammals in which circulation time is undoubtedly shorter than that in human beings. However, the same general pattern is applicable to the human beings as well - the nicotine entering the lungs, concentrates in the brain within a matter of minutes, and soon thereafter, starts getting eliminated.

Smoking of nicotine does not deliver nicotine in a steady stream to the smoker; rather, he receives a series of intermittent 'shots' or 'slugs' of nicotine coinciding with each inhaled puff (Russell, 1978). However, this discrete configuration does not last for long as these intermittent 'shots' become mixed by churning of the heart and travel in and out of organs along tortuous vascular channels. The intermittent nature of nicotine presentation by smoking, along with almost instantaneous uptake of nearly all the nicotine presented ensure that, in the first passage of nicotine round the body after each puff, tissues are briefly exposed to a high concentration — much higher than if the same amount of nicotine were evenly mixed with the whole blood volume. The body tissues, which receive quickest and most direct blood supply (e.g. Brain cells), get the highest concentration of nicotine.

Action of nicotine depends upon its intermittent high concentration in the tissue. In the experimental animals, to get the equivalent effect of inhaled puffs of nicotine by intravenous injection of nicotine, it is necessary to give multiple small, separate and quickly injected shots, rather than giving the same dose smoothly (Armitage, Hall and Sellers, 1969).

## Metabolism

Nicotine metabolism has been extensively studied both *in vivo* and *in vitro*. Various models used *in vitro* include intact cell, hepatocytes and perfused isolated organ systems. Of these models, hepatic microsomal enzymatic system is a popular and valuable mode. Hepatic microsomes are incubated with nicotine and its principle metabolite, cotinine under physiological conditions. Formation of nicotine or cotinine metabolites is assayed in the samples after incubation by gas chromatography/mass spectrometry which leads to identification and quantitation of nicotine metabolites as well as characterization of new pathways of nicotine biotransformation. By using microsomes, it is possible to examine the role of each factor influencing nicotine metabolism independently, and to determine dose-response relationships.

*In vivo,* studies are performed on animals and have many limitations. It is questionable whether the studies conducted on animals can be extrapolated on human beings. Moreover, nicotine metabolism may differ among species (Jenner *et al.,* 1988). In contrast to rats, rabbits seem to be a good model for studying human nicotine metabolism.

As nicotine is a highly lipid soluble alkaloid, it rapidly and extensively metabolizes in the body (Turner *et al.*, 1975). Enzymes responsible for breakdown of nicotine into many pharmacologically inactive substances are contained in several body organs *(Figure 5).* The main metabolites are cotinine and nicotine–N–oxide. Nicotine is mainly metabolized in the liver. The studies have shown conversion of nicotine to the nicotine-iminium ion catalysed by cytochromes P-450, and numerous studies have indicated that CYP2A6 enzyme is responsible for this reaction (Messina *et al.,* 1997). Nicotine is converted into cotinine in a two-step process. The first step involves oxidation of position 5 of the pyrrolidine ring in a cytochrome P-450 mediated process to Nicotine D1 (5) iminium ion (Peterson, Trevor and Castagnoli, 1987). In the second step the iminium ion is metabolized by a cytoplasmic aldehyde oxidase to cotinine (Hibberd and Gorrod, 1983). Though the second step, the metabolism of the iminium ion to cotinine, is mediated by cytosolic aldehyde oxidase, a microsomal enzyme may also be involved. CYP2B6 may also inactivate nicotine to cotinine but it has lower affinity and variable expression in human liver (Yamazaki *et al.,* 1999). Cotinine, itself, is also extensively metabolized with only about 17 percent excreted unchanged in the urine (Benowitz, Kuyt *et al.*, 1983). Several metabolites of cotinine have been reported, including trans-3′-hydroxycotinine, 5′-hydroxycotinine, cotinine-N-oxide, and cotinine methonium ion, however, little is known about the quantitative importance of these metabolites. Nicotine-1′ N-oxide is quantitatively a minor metabolite of nicotine. Oxidation of nitrogen atom of the pyrrolidine ring depends on a microsomal flavoprotein system and produces a mixture of the two diasterisomers. After intravenous injection, 100 percent of nicotine-N-oxide is excreted unchanged in the urine indicating no further metabolism. However, after oral administration, only 30 percent is recovered in the urine; remainder is recovered as nicotine and its metabolites.

Recent studies have discovered several nicotine metabolites and pathways of its biotransformation such as N-oxidation, N-demethylation and glucronidation (Kyerematen and Vesell, 1991). N-oxidation is an important route of nicotine biotransformation. Approximately 4% of nicotine is metabolized to nicotine-1′-N-oxide, a main product of N-oxidation. The nicotine-1′-N-oxide formation occurs through a reaction catalyzed by flavin-containing monooxygenase. It has been suggested that nicotine-1′-N-oxide administered intra-peritoneally in rabbit could be reduced back to nicotine and could represent a reservoir for sustained generation of nicotine (Duan *et al.*, 1993). Similarly, nicotine-1′-N-oxide can influence pharmacokinetics of nicotine in humans. Although nicotine-1′-N-oxide is generally regarded as non-toxic, it has been proposed that it may be converted to the tobacco-specific nitrosamines (TSNA).

The main product of N-demethylation of nicotine is nornicotine (Kyerematen and Vesell, 1991). The majority of nornicotine excreted by cigarette smokers is derived from nicotine metabolism even though 40% of nornicotine may come from tobacco *per se*. Small amounts of nornicotine is also found in human urine. Nornicotine exerts some pharmacological and toxic activity contributing to the neuropharmacological effect of nicotine.

Another pathway of nicotine biotransformation is N-glucronidation which accounts for 4% of total nicotine metabolism in humans (Benowitz *et al.*, 1994). The involvement of UDP-glucronosyltransferase1A1 and 1A9 as well as 1A4 isoforms in nicotine glucronidation has been suggested, although the contribution of each isoforms have not been determined conclusively (Kuehl and Murphy, 2003). To a smaller extent nicotine is also metabolized in the lungs and the kidneys.

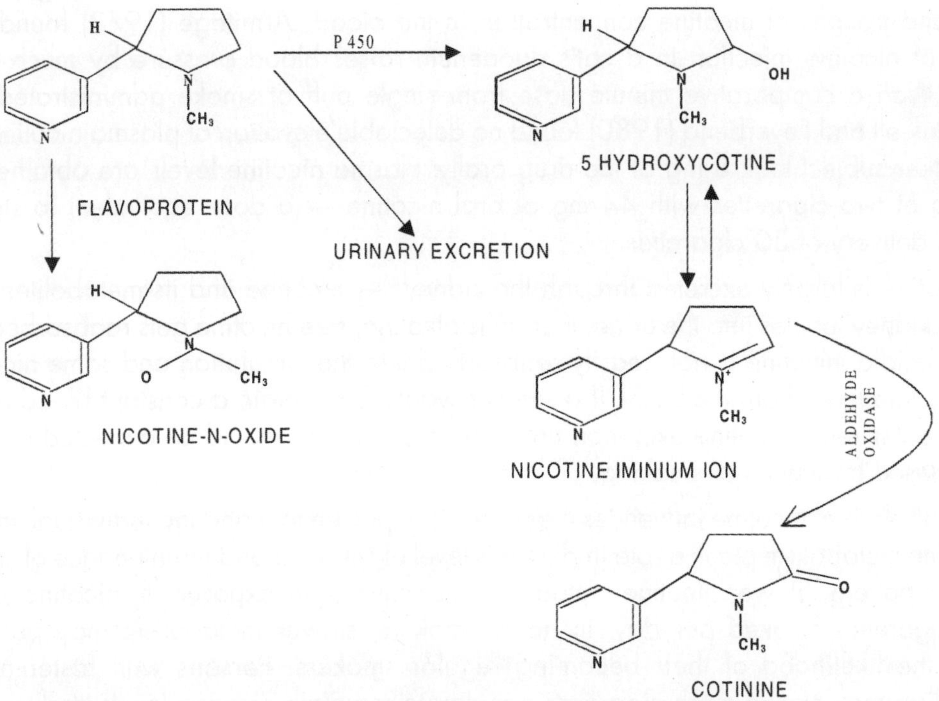


*Figure 5: Major pathways of nicotine metabolism*

Some metabolism occurs in other organs, like lungs and kidneys, but not in the brain. Formation of different metabolites depends upon the individual and his/her sex (Beckett, Gorrod and Jenner, 1971). Metabolism in habitual smokers is more efficient than in casual smokers and cotinine may begin to appear in the blood within minutes of the start of smoking.

Renal excretion of unchanged nicotine depends on urinary pH and urine flow and may range from 2 to 35 percent and it typically accounts for 5 to 10 percent of total elimination (Benowitz, Kuyt *et al.*, 1983). Nicotine is eliminated primarily by hepatic metabolism by way of C-oxidation to cotinine. Nicotine has shorter half-life of 2 hours while cotinine has half-life of about 20 hours. Therefore, cotinine provides a more stable marker of exposure in the person since there is less variability in cotinine throughout the day than that observed for nicotine. Nicotine taken orally in a tablet form might provide levels of the drug adequate to replace smoking (Jarvik, Glick and Nakamura, 1970), though it reaches the general circulation of the blood after getting absorbed through the gastro-intestinal tract into the blood vessels via the liver. It is because of this reason that most of the ingested nicotine gets inactivated by hepatic metabolism before it gets distributed around the body and any nicotine emerging from the liver is already mixed and diluted in a considerable pool of blood. It may be because of this reason that the swallowing of a potentially lethal dose of nicotine is without serious ill effects, for example, small children who have eaten cigarettes containing several milligrams of nicotine have survived unharmed. Swallowed tobacco does not give rise to peaks and troughs of nicotine concentration in the blood. Armitage (1973) found that 1 mg/kg of nicotine injection in a cat's duodenum raises blood pressure by much smaller amount than a comparative minute dose from single puff of smoke administrated to the lungs. Russell and Feyerbend (1980) found no detectable elevation of plasma nicotine when a volunteer subject took 8 mg of the drug orally. Plasma nicotine levels are obtained after smoking of two cigarettes with 44 mg of oral nicotine — a dose equivalent to standard nicotine delivery of 30 cigarettes.

Nicotine is largely excreted through the kidneys — nicotine and its metabolites diffuse through kidney tubules into the urine. If urine is alkaline, free nicotine gets reabsorbed. If the urine is acidic, nicotine is not easily reabsorbed into the circulation and some nicotine is removed unaltered from the body. If a smoker wants to maintain a constant blood nicotine level, greater renal nicotine excretion under acid conditions would be expected to lead to an increased frequency of smoking.

Metabolism of nicotine influences the person's exposure to it and the individual variation in nicotine metabolism plays a role in person's level of smoking and maintenance of smoking behavior pattern. Slower nicotine metabolism permits longer exposure to nicotine yielding fewer cigarettes smoked per day. In naïve smokers, slower metabolism may potentially reduce the likelihood of their becoming regular smokers. Persons with faster nicotine metabolism may smoke more cigarettes per day to maintain nicotine levels and would be more likely to develop and maintain a smoking pattern.

The rate of nicotine metabolism can be determined by measuring blood levels after administration of a known nicotine dose. In one study, cigarette smokers were given intravenous infusion of nicotine for 30 to 60 minutes and their total and renal clearance were computed (Benowitz, Jacob *et al.*, 1982). Total clearance was found to be 1,300 mL/minute on an average and non-renal clearance was 1,100 ml/minute which represented 70% of the liver blood flow. On an average, 85 or 90 percent of nicotine is metabolized by the liver and due to this reason, about 70 percent of the drug is extracted from the blood in each pass through the liver.

## Factors Influencing Nicotine Metabolism

Nicotine metabolism leads to formation of several metabolites and the different levels of these metabolites in different individuals with similar rate of tobacco consumption are because of factors like:

- Individual differences in absorption and distribution of nicotine.
- Racial differences
- Genetic factors
- Differences in cotinine elimination.

### Individual Differences

In experiments using radio-labeled nicotine infused intravenously to subjects, considerable individual differences in clearance of nicotine and the percentage of nicotine conversion to cotinine have been demonstrated (Benowitz and Jacob P III, 1994). The excretion of nicotine, cotinine and 3′-hydroxycotinine, measured on the basis of 24 hour urine collection, significantly varies among smokers (Benowitz *et al.*, 1994). Also, the extent of nicotine and cotinine glucronidation is different among individuals (Byrd *et al.*, 1992). Among the individual differences, sex is one important factor which determines the rate of nicotine metabolism. Several studies indicate that male smokers may metabolize nicotine faster than female smokers (Ahijevych, 2000). Daily activities such as consuming a meal also increases nicotine metabolism. An average 42% increase in nicotine clearance, approximately one hour after beginning the meal, may be related to an increase in liver blood flow with the meal. Smokers typically smoke after meals and decreased plasma nicotine caused by increased nicotine clearance with increased hepatic blood flow could contribute to the urge of smoking after meals. The depth and duration of inhalation during smoking and swallowed nicotine-laden saliva intake also influence nicotine metabolism. Nicotine intake is controlled by how intensively a smoker inhales a cigarette—or how deep a "drag" a person takes. Chinese-Americans may take in less nicotine because of their slow metabolism of nicotine and the fact that they need to inhale less deeply to establish a particular level of nicotine in the body. Large individual variability in the kinetics and metabolism of nicotine could, at least partially, explain individual differences in susceptibility to nicotine addiction.

### Racial Differences

Racial/Ethnic differences in nicotine metabolism have been observed in several studies (Pomerleau, 1995). Higher levels of cotinine have been detected in African-Americans (Blacks) as compared to Caucasian (white) smokers resulting in lower smoking rate among the former. African-American women smoked significantly fewer cigarettes as compared to Caucasian women and yet their cotinine level was significantly higher (Perez-Stable *et al.*, 1998). Menthol cigarettes are the predominant choice of African-American smokers. A recently conducted study (Benowitz, 2002) documents that Asian and Latino smokers have the lowest rate of lung cancer, while the Caucasians have higher rates and the African-Americans have the highest rates. Blood analysis showed that it took an average of 152 minutes for half an injection of nicotine to degrade ion in the blood of Chinese-Americans, while nicotine's half-life in Whites and Latinos' was 134 minutes and 122 minutes, respectively. Slow metabolism draws out its effect: White smokers are five times more likely to develop lung cancer than Asian smokers.

### Genetic Factors

Genetic variability is another factor in inter-individual differences in nicotine metabolism (Nakajima *et al.*, 1996). Behavioural genetics research has shown that individual differences in smoking behaviour are substantially heritable. In one investigation, concordance for smoking in 42 pairs of identical twins reared apart was 79% (Shields, 1962), and a meta-analysis of the data from 5 studies, each involving more than 1000 twin pairs, showed an estimated heritability of 60% for the propensity for smoke (Heath and Madden, 1995). Twin studies have also shown that the genetic factor involved in the initiation and cessation of smoking is partially overlapping but mostly independent (Heath and Martin, 1993).

### Differences in Cotinine Elimination

Some *in vitro* studies have identified several different cytochrome P450 isozymes in the C-oxidation of nicotine. CYP2A6 and CYP2D6 have displayed genetic polymorphism suggesting that individuals who lack these enzymes may be poor metabolizers of nicotine. 60 to 80 percent of nicotine is metabolized to cotinine by CYP2A6, which is polymorphically expressed as the wild type and two null alleles CYP2A6*2 and *3. Cotinine formation in human liver microsomes is significantly correlated with CYP2A6 levels leading to the conclusion that CYP2A6 is the principal cytochrome P450 involved in nicotine metabolism. Variations in CYP2A6 are identified as the major reason for inter-individual differences in nicotine kinetics in human liver microsomes. In another study (Fernandez-Salguero, Hoffman, Cholerton *et al.*,1995) smokers homozygous for wild-type active CYP2A6 alleles smoked significantly more cigarettes per day than heterozygous smokers (carriers of one defective CYP2A6 allele) (London, 1999 and Pianezza *et al.*, 1998). While the earlier studies had examined the potential role of CYP2D6 in nicotine metabolism, a recent study reported that CYP2D6 was not important in nicotine metabolism in human liver microsomes. Cotinine formation from nicotine in human liver microsomes is correlated with CYP2A6 levels and coumarin 7-

hydroxylation (Nakajima *et al.*, 1996). The presence of the CYP2A6v1 and CYP2A6v2 alleles significantly decreased the number of cigarettes consumed by the smokers (Pianezza *et al.*, 1998), although this relationship has not been confirmed (London *et al.*, 1999). The frequency of mutated alleles varies considerably among different ethnic populations (Raunio *et al.*, 2001). The frequency of both alleles is low in European populations and very few poor metabolizers have been described in these populations (Oscarson 2001). In addition, CYP2A6 has been shown to metabolically activate pro-carcinogens such as aflatoxin B1 and N-nitrosodiethylamine; thus, the polymorphism of CYP2A6 is important as a factor of cancer susceptibility. These nitrosamines (carcinogens) that are activated by CYP2A6 are found in tobacco smoke.

A homozygous whole deletion allele of CYP2A6 gene has been reported (Nunoya *et al.*, 1999). The whole deletion of CYP2A6 gene could be responsible for the poor metabolism of nicotine to cotinine in humans. A genetic deficiency in nicotine metabolism caused by defective mutations in CYP2A6 may be associated with a lower risk to become tobacco dependent (Pianezza *et al.*, 1998). CYP2A6 has been reported to activate a number of harmful procarcinogens, including tobacco-specific nitrosamines and aflatoxin B1, contained in cigarette smoke (Yamazaki *et al.*, 1992). The individuals who carry a mutation or deletion in CYP2A6 gene may have a decreased risk of tobacco related cancers (Nakajima *et al.*, 2000). Therefore, it has been proposed that CYP2A6 inhibition could be used to reduce the rate of smoking in tobacco dependents and exposure to procarcinogens contained in cigarette smoke or as a part of step-care reduction of smoking, leading to cessation (Sellers 2000). Methoxsalen (8-methoxypsoralen), the drug used in the treatment of psoriasis, has been reported as a potent inhibitor of CYP2A6. However, safety of Methoxsalen during long-term use has not been determined

The link between dopamine release and the addictive properties of nicotine point to dopaminergic genes as logical candidates for genetic effects on smoking behaviour. Lerman *et al* (1999) demonstrated an association between smoking behaviour and allele 9 of a 3′ untranslated region polymorphism in the dopamine transport gene (SLC63A-9) in their case-control study of nonsmokers and current smokers. They found that individuals with an SLC6A3-9 genotype were less likely to be smokers than the individuals without allele 9 and those smokers with SLC6A3-9 genotype had started to smoke later and had been able to quit for longer periods of time than other smokers.

Nicotine metabolism may be affected by some drugs. For example, human hepatocytes for individuals treated in vivo with Phenobarbital show higher-than-normal nicotine oxidation rates on hepatocyte harvest (Williams 1990). On the other hand, no association has been found between the drug histories and the microsomal levels of CYP2A6 protein and CYP2A6 activity in subjects (Nakajima *et al.*, 1996).

Coffee consumption (Kyerematen and Vesell, 1991) and high protein diet (Lee *et al.*, 1989) are reported to influence nicotine metabolism.

The elimination half-life of nicotine in newborns is three to four times that of adults, whereas the half-life of cotinine in newborns is essentially the same as that in adults. Cigarette smoking during pregnancy is associated with adverse pregnancy outcome in the mother and the newborn. In *in vivo* studies, any significant differences in the metabolic profile of nicotine have not been found between pregnant and non-pregnant rabbits (Tutka *et al.*, 2000). *In vivo* human studies have shown that the excretion of nicotine metabolites in the urine of active and passive smokers rises with gestation (Mathai, 1990). The salivary cotine levels are found to be significantly lower in pregnant than non-pregnant women. Nicotine is less rapidly metabolized in pregnant than the non-pregnant women.

## Intake of Nicotine

### *Cigarette Smoking*

Studies indicate that intake from a single filter tipped cigarette is 0.36 to 2.62 mg. Intake was found to be higher in smokers than the nonsmokers. In 22 cigarette smokers, who smoked an average of 36 cigarettes per day, the average daily intake was 37.6 mg (Benowitz, Jacob *et al.*, 1984). The nicotine intake per cigarette averaged 1.06 mg.

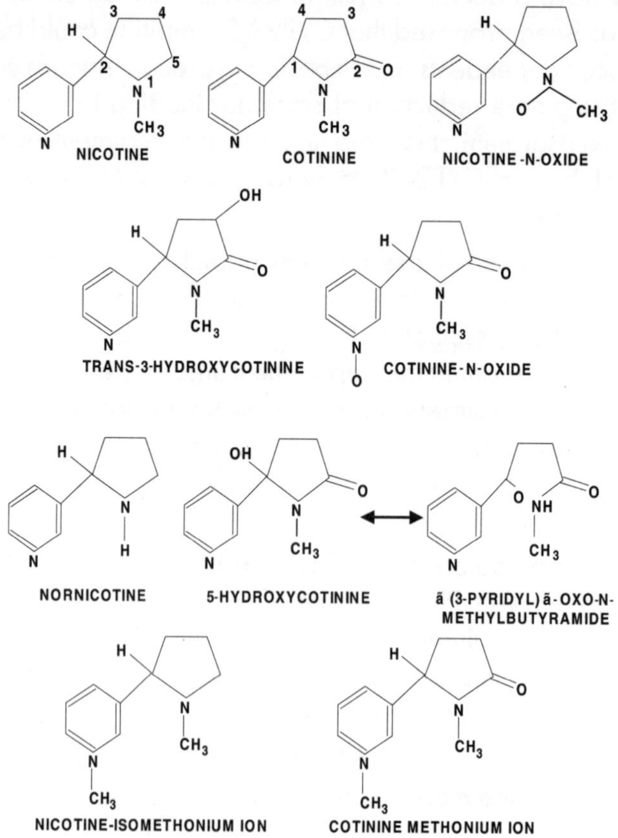

NICOTINE COTININE NICOTINE-N-OXIDE

TRANS-3-HYDROXYCOTININE COTININE-N-OXIDE

NORNICOTINE 5-HYDROXYCOTININE ã (3-PYRIDYL) ã-OXO-N-METHYLBUTYRAMIDE

NICOTINE-ISOMETHONIUM ION COTININE METHONIUM ION

*Figure 6: Nicotine and its metabolites*

## Nicotine and Cotinine Blood Levels During Tobacco Use

### Nicotine Levels

In smokers, plasma nicotine concentrations sampled in the afternoon generally range from 10 to 50 mg/mL. After smoking a cigarette, there is an increase in blood levels from 5 to 30 mg/mL, depending on how the cigarette is smoked (Armitage *et al.*, 1975). The half-life of a drug is useful in predicting its accumulation rate in the body with repetitive doses and also the time course of its decline after cessation of dosing. Assuming a half-life of two hours one would predict nicotine to accumulate over 6 to 8 hours of regular smoking and persist at significant levels even 6 to 8 hours after cessation of smoking. If a smoker smokes until bedtime, significant nicotine level would persist all night. Peaks and troughs follow the use of each cigarette but as the day progresses, trough levels rise and influence of the peak level becomes less important. Thus, nicotine is not a drug to which people are exposed intermittently and that is eliminated rapidly from the body. Smoking represents a multiple dosing situation with considerable accumulation during smoking and with persistent levels for 24 hours of each day.

### Cotinine Levels

Cotinine is present in the blood of smokers in much higher concentrations than nicotine; average levels being 250 to 300 mg/mL (Benowitz, Hall *et al.*, 1983). When smoking is stopped, levels of cotinine decline with a half-life of 20 hours. Fluctuation in cotinine blood concentration is much less in comparison to nicotine because of longer half-life. There is a gradual increase in the cotinine levels during the day, peaking at the end of smoking and persisting in high concentrations overnight.

## Pharmacodynamics of Nicotine

The relationship between nicotine levels in the body and their effect on behavior and physiological function constitutes pharmacodynamics and involves two issues in its understanding: a complex dose-response relationship and level of tolerance that is either preexisting or is produced by administration of nicotine.

### Dose-response

The relationship between nicotine dose and its response (dose-response relationship) is complex and varies with the specific response that is being measured. Nicotine causes ganglionic stimulation in low doses and their blockade in higher doses, following brief stimulation (Comroe, 1960) and this effect pattern is called 'biphasic'. At very low doses, during cigarette smoking, cardiovascular effects seem to be mediated by the CNS either through activation of chemoreceptor afferent pathways or by direct effect on brain stem (Comroe, 1960; Su, 1982). The net result is sympathetic neural discharge with an increase in blood pressure and heart rate. At higher dose, nicotine may act directly on peripheral nervous system, producing ganglionic stimulation and the release of adrenal catecholamines. With high doses or rapid administration, nicotine produces hypotension and slowing of heart rate mediated by peripheral vagal activation or by direct central depressor effect (Henningfield, Miyasato and Jasinki, 1985).

### Biphasic Effects

The initial combination of nicotine with acetylcholine receptor at first stimulates acetylcholine like response, but the fixity of the drug/receptor combination then blocks any further response to acetylcholine (or to more nicotine). The degree of stimulation versus blockade depends upon the amount of nicotine present relative to the number of available acetylcholine receptors. In general, small doses of nicotine produce a predominantly stimulant effect at synapses, larger doses produce a mainly depressant effect, while a lethal dose blocks the nervous transmission altogether. In the complex neural circuits involved in breathing, small doses of nicotine stimulate respiration; large doses depress respiration, while an overdose would cause complete arrest of respiration.

The duration of effect of nicotine at a synapse depends upon its dose. Depending upon factors, such as, the size of the puff, the depth of inhalation and the individual sensitivity of the subject's receptors, a smoker can get either a predominantly inhibitory or a predominantly excitatory effect - or indeed a mixture of both - from one cigarette. The ease with which nicotine can produce rapid, reversible and biphasic effects over a small dose range is another remarkable characteristic, which singles it out from most other drugs.

## Constituents of Tobacco Smoke Other than Nicotine

Of the several thousand compounds isolated from tobacco and tobacco-smoke (Dube and Green, 1982), many are biologically active. Of these thousands of constituents, though, nicotine is the major pharmacological factor; there are many minor alkaloids with qualitative similarity but with lesser potency.

## Other Tobacco Contents

Tobacco smoke is known to be rich in naphthaline and *polycyclic aromatic hydrocarbons* (PAH). In Indian studies, high levels of benzapyrene were reported in *masheri,* snuff and chewing tobacco (Nair *et al.,* 1987 and Bhide *et al.,* 1984). Nitrite content is found to be twice higher in cigarette tobacco as compared to *beedi* (Pakhale *et al.,* 1997). Particulate matter without its alkaloid and water contents is called tar. Tobacco smoke also comprises of some 500 gaseous compounds including nitrogen, oxygen, hydrogen, methane, carbon monoxide, ammonia, hydrogen cyanide and benzene which account for about 95% of the weight of cigarette smoke; the other 5% is accounted for particulate matter. At an alkaline pH, nicotine is detected in gaseous phase also, which seems to add to its absorption. The vapour phase also contains volatile carcinogenic aldehyde, ketones, nitric oxide and volatile nitrates along with additional minor constituents.

### Tar

Tar is a dry particulate matter in tobacco smoke. It is sticky and brown, and stains teeth, fingernails and lung tissue. Role of tar in relation to smoking behaviour is not clear. However, based on the knowledge of taste and aroma constituents of cigarette smoke, it is likely that some chemicals in the tar fraction contribute to tobacco use, if only, by providing distinct sensory stimulation. Therefore, minimal levels of tar are held to be important for the taste characteristics of tobacco smoke.

A number of the isoprenoid compounds that influence the taste and aroma of smoke may be formed by sequential oxidation rearrangement and reduction reactions (Davis, Stevens and Jurd, 1976). Norisoprenoid compounds, which are derived from cyclic carotenoids are important to the aroma of smoke. The taste and aroma of a cigarette can be influenced by the selection of the grade (quality and leaf position on the plant) and type of tobacco use in the blend.

When a smoker lights up a cigarette, the receptors of taste and smell provide the first sensory input, which is generally perceived as pleasurable (Rose *et al.*, 1985). The taste and smell of tobacco smoke are important re-enforcers for tobacco smoking (Jarvik, 1977) — at least, following repeated association with reinforcing effects of nicotine administration. Such behavioural conditioning, sensory cues provided by tar and the flavor additives control the tobacco consuming behaviour of tobacco users.

Many carcinogens, including **Polycyclic Aromatic Hydrocarbons**, N-nitrosamines including TSNAs and aromatic amines have been identified in cigarette tar. Chlorinated hydrocarbon insecticides, N-alkylcarbazols, fluoranthenes, benzofluorones, phenyllindane, pyrenes and cyclo-pentazo-phenanthrene have been detected in sub-fraction of smoke tar. The major carcinogens present in the particulate phase of tobacco smoke are polonium-210, volatie/non-volatile N-nitrosamines and TSNAs. In addition, co-carcinogenic agents such as pyrene, fluoranthene, dichlorostilbene and catechols have been identified in the particulate phase of cigarette smoke. Tar contains the carcinogen benzo (a) pyrene that is known to trigger tumour development (cancer).

### Carbon Monoxide

Mainstream cigarette smoke has carbon monoxide present at concentrations similar to that found in automobile exhaust. It is the dilution of the smoke with room air and the intermittent nature of smoke inhalation that prevents cigarette smoke from being immediately lethal (Burns and David, 1991). Carbon monoxide delivery of cigarette is influenced by the cigarette design and puffing characteristics of smokers. Mainstream delivery of carbon monoxide ranges from 10 to 20 mg per cigarette. The average smoker exhales carbon monoxide of 33 parts per million, which equates to a 5.5% of Carboxyhaemoglobin (COHb). Red blood cells have a 210 to 250 time greater affinity for carbonmonoxide than for oxygen, and fetal haemoglobin binding to carbon monoxide with an even greater affinity. Exhaled carbon monoxide correlates with Carboxyhaemoglobin (COHb) blood levels, and a one pack per day smoker has a reading of 25 to 35 parts per million. A 59 part per million carbonmonoxide level equals a 10% COHb, or a 10% loss oxygen carrying capacity, which may reduce mental awareness and slow reaction time. It has been found that Carboxyhaemoglobin (COHb) level ranges from 3.2 to 14.0 percent in smoker's blood (Steward *et al.*, 1974 and Anderson *et al.*, 1977) with a mean of 8.1 percent and exhaled carbon monoxide of 48 parts per million (Moyer David, 1995). COHb levels gradually decrease in blood after cessation of smoking. Carbon monoxide is eliminated in expired air. The rate of elimination depends on pulmonary blood flow and ventilation. The half-life of COHb is 2 to 4 hours during daytime hours but as COHb is related to the levels of exercise, the half-life may be as long as 8 hours during sleep (Wald *et al.*, 1975). Due to these reasons, many smokers wake up in the morning with substantial levels of COHb despite not smoking overnight (Benowitz *et al.*, 1982). Persons smoking cigarettes with lower nicotine and carbon monoxide yields have only slightly lower levels of COHb when compared with those smoking high yield products (Wald *et al.*, 1981).

### Nitrogen Oxide

It has been shown in animal studies that nitrogen oxide damages lungs and is said to be responsible for causing lung emphysema.

### Hydrogen Cyanide

The lungs contain tiny hair (cilia) that help to clean the lungs by moving foreign substances out. Hydrogen cyanide interferes in working of this lung clearance function and allows poisonous ingredients of tobacco smoke to accumulate inside the lungs.

### Metals

Tobacco smoke contains dangerous metals including arsenic, cadmium and lead. Many of these metals are carcinogenic.

### Radioactive Compounds

Tobacco smoke contains radioactive compounds, which are known to be carcinogenic.

### Acetaldehyde and Other Smoke Contents

Acetaldehyde is a major constituent of tobacco smoke with levels ranging from 0.5 to 1.5 mg per cigarette. Yield over 5.9 mg/cigarette have been reported for large cigars (Hoffmann and Wynder, 1977). Acetaldehyde and acrolein, another important aldehyde in the gas phase of cigarette smoke, activate the sympathetic nervous system (Eagle and Hudgins, 1974). Acetaldehyde, by releasing norepinephrin, results in a pressor effect. Depressor effects occur at high doses of aldehydes in guanethidine-pretreated hypertensive rats. Studies indicate that condensation products of acetaldehyde may be active on endogenous opioid systems. Betacarbolines occur as plant constituents, including minor constituents in tobacco, for example, l-methyl-B-carboline has been identified in tobacco and tobacco smoke. Potential pharmacological effect of aldehydes, have been established, especially with regards to cardio-vascular physiology; however, the evidence is inadequate to determine if these volatile smoke constituents in the doses delivered in tobacco smoke contribute to the behavioral effects of cigarette smoking. Ammonia, a strong chemical found in household cleaners and formaldehyde (used for preserving the organs of dead people in morgues is found in tobacco smoke and damages the lungs.

## REFERENCES


Ahijevych K.: *Nicotine Metabolism Variability and Nicotine Addiction,* Nicotine Conference Programme Index, Ohio State University, 2000.

Anderson W.H., Rivera, C. and Bright, M.: *Carboxyhaemoglobin Blood Levels after Smoking One Cigarette in Relation to Puff Profile,* In: 1975 Symposium Nicotine and Mono-oxide *Proceedings I, University of Kentucky, Lexington, Kentucky,* 130–136, 1977.

Armitage A.K.: *Some Recent Observations Relating to the Absorption of Nicotine from Tobacco Smoke.* In W.L. Dunn, Jr. (eds.) *Smoking Behaviour, Motives and Incentives.* Washington: Winston, 1973.

Armitage A.K., Dollery,C. T., George Housemanet T. H., Lewis, P. J, and Turne, D. M.: Absorption and Metabolism of Nicotine from Cigarettes. *British Medical Journal.* 4: 313 – 316, 1975.

Armitage, A.K., Dollery, C. T., Houseman, T. H., Lewis, P. J., and Turner, D. M.: *Absorption of Nicotine from Small Cigar, Clinical Pharmacology and Therapeutics.* 232 (2): 143 – 151, 1978.

Armitage, A.K., Hall, G. H. and Sellers, M.: Effect of Nicotine on Electro-cortical Activity and Acetylcholine Release from Cat Cerebral Cortex, *British Journal of Pharmacology.* 35: 152–160, 1969.

Baldwin, T. and Schmelz, E.R.: Allocation of ISN from Nitrate to Nicotine: Production and Turnover from a Damage-Induced Mobile *Defence Ecology.* 75: 1703–1713, 1994.

Baldwin, T and Schmelz, E. A.: Immunological in Memory O' in the Induced Accumulation of Nicotine in Wild Tobacco. *Ecology.* 77: 236–246, 1996.

Beckett, A. H., Gorrod, J. W. and Jenner, P.: The Effect of Smoking on Nicotine Metabolism In Vivo in Man. *Journal of Pharmacy and Pharmacology* (suppl.) 23: 62S – 67S, 1971.

Benowitz, N.L. *Human Pharmacology of Nicotine,* In: Capell, H.D. et al (eds) *Research Advances in Alcohol and Drug Problems.* Vol. 9. New York, Plenum Press,1986.

Benowitz, N.L.: Slower Metabolism and Reduced Intake of Nicotine from Cigarette Smoking in Chinese-Americans, *Journal of the National Cancer Institute* Vol. 94, 108–115, 2002.

Benowitz, N.L., Hall, S.M., Herning, N.I., Jacob, P. and Osman, AL: Smokers of Low Yielding Cigarettes Do Not Consume Less Nicotine, *New England Journal of Medicine.* 309(3) 139 –142, 1983.

Benowitz, N.L., Jacob P. III: Daily Intake of Nicotine During Cigarette Smoking. *Clinical Pharmacology and Therapeutics.* 309: 139–142, 1984.

Benowitz N.L. and Jacob P. III: Metabolism of Nicotine to Cotinine Studied by a Dual Stable Isotop Method. Clinical Pharmacology and Therapeutics, 56:483–493, 1994.

Benowitz N.L., Jacob P. III, Fong I., Guota S.: Nicotine Metabolic Profile in Man: Comparison of Cigarette Smoking of Transdermal Nicotine. *Journal of Pharmacology and Experimental Therapeutics*, 68, 296–303, 1994.

Benowitz, N.L., Jacob, P. III, Jones, R.T. and Rosenberg, J.: Inter-individual Variability in the Metabolism and Cardiovascular Effects of Nicotine in Man, *Journal of Pharmacology and Experimental Therapeutics*, 221 (2): 368–372, 1982.

Benowitz, N.L., Kuyt, F. Jacob, P. III, Jones, R.T. and Osman, AL.: Cotinine Disposition and Effects, *Clinical Pharmacology and Therapeutics*, 309: 139–142, 1983.

Benowitz, N. L., Lake, T., Keller, K. H., Lee, B. L.: Prolonged Absorption with Development of Tolerance to Toxic Effects Following Cutaneous Exposure to Nicotine, *Clinical Pharmacology and Therapeutics*. 42 (1): 119–120, 1987.

Bhide S.V. Murdia, U.S. and Nair, J.: Polycyclic Aromatic Hydrocarbon Profiles of Pyrolysed Tobacco Products Commonly Used in India, Cancer Letters, 24:89–90, 1984.

Brunnemann, K.D. and Hoffmann, D. The pH of Tobacco Smoke. *Food and Cosmetic Toxicology*, 12 (1): 115–124, 1974.

Burn David: Physical Fitness and Carbon Monoxide, *Clinics of Chest Medicine*. 633, 1991.

Bush, LP., Grunwald, C. and Davis, D. L.: Influence of Puff Frequency and Puff Volume on the Alkaloid Content of Smoke, *Journal of Agricultural and Food Chemistry*, 20 (3): 676–678, 1972.

Byrd, G.D., Chang, K., Greene J.M. and deBethizy J.D.: Evidence for Urinary Excretion of Glucronide Conjugates of Nicotine, Cotinine and Trans-3′-hydroxycotinine in Smokers, *Drug Metabolism*, 20:19, 1992.

Comroe, J.H.: The Pharmacological Action of Nicotine. Annals of the New York *Academy of Science*, 90 (1): 48–51, 1960.

Creeighton, D.E., Tobacco Smoking Retention, Paper Presented at Conference in Aerosol Physics, *British American Tobacco Co. Ltd., Southampton*, 1973.

Davis, D.L., Steven, K.L. and Jurd, L.: Chemistry of Tobacco Constituents, Oxidation of a-ionone and the Acid Catalyzed Re-arrangement of 5-keto-a-ionone, *Journal of Agriculture and Food Chemistry*, 24(1):187–189, 1976.

Duan, M.J., Yu, L. Savanapridi C. Jacob, P. III and Benowitz, N.L.: Disposition Kinetics and Metabolism of Nicotine-1′-N-oxide in Rabbits, *Drug Metabolism*, 19:667–672, 1993.

Dube, M.F. and Green, C.R.: Methods of Collection of Smoke for Analytical Purposes, *Recent Advances in Tobacco Science*, 8: 42–102, 1982.

Eagle J.L. Jr. and Hudgin P.M.: Dose-dependent Sympathomimetic and Cardio-inhibitory Effects of Acroleitin and Formaldehyde in Anaesthetized Rat, *Toxicology and Applied Pharmacology*, 28:258–266, 1974.

Eudy, L.W., Thome, F.A., Heavner, D.L., Green, C.R. and Ingebrethsen, B.J.: Study on the Vapor Particulate-phase Distribution of Environmental Nicotine by Selected Trapping and Detection Methods. 79th *Tobacco Chemistry Research Conference: Montreal*, 1985.

Faulkner, J.M.: Nicotine Poisoning by Absorption through the Skin, Journal of the American Medical Association, 100 (2): 1664–1665, 1933.

Feyerabend, C., Ings, R.M. and Russel, M.A.H.: Nicotine Pharmacokinetics and its Application to Intake from Smoking. British Journal of Clinical Pharmacology. 19 (2): 239–247, 1985.

Fernandez-Salguero, P., Hoffman, S.M., Cholerton, S., Mohrenweiser, H., Raunio, H., Rautio, A., Pelkonen, O., Huang, JD., Evand, WE. and Idle, J.R.: A Genetic Polymorphism in Coumarin 7-hydroxylation: Sequence of the Human CYP2A Genes and Identification of Variant CYP2A6 Alleles. American Journal of Human Genetics 57: 651– 660, 1995.

Gehlbach, S.H., Williams, W.A., Perry, L.D., Freeman, J.I., Langone, JJ., Petra, L. V. and Van Vunakis, H. (1975) Nicotine Absorption by Workers Harvesting Green Tobacco. Lancet I.: 478–480, 1905.

Geiger, Christopher, G.: The Health and Safety Concerns of Common Insecticides. *Journal of Environmental Health*, 55 (8): 11, 1993.

Gori, G.B., Benowitz, N.L. and Lynch, C.J.: Mouth Versus Deep Airways Absorption of Nicotine in Cigarette Smokers. *Pharmacology, Biochemistry and Behavior*, 25 (6): 1181–1184, 1986.

Gritz E.R.: Smoking Behaviour and Tobacco Abuse, In: Merllo N.K. (eds) *Advances in Substance Abuse*. Vol. I. Greenwich, Connecticut JAI Press, 1980.

Haines, C.F., Mahajan, D.K., Miljkovic, D., Miljkovic, M., and Vessell, ES.: Radioimmunoassay of Plasma Nicotine in Habitual and Naïve Smokers. *Clinical Pharmacology and Therapeutics*. 16:1083 – 1086, 1974.

Haley, N.J. and Hoffmann, D.: Analysis for Nicotine and Cotinine in How to Determine Cigarette Smoker Status. *Clinical Chemistry*. 31 (10): 1598–1600, 1985.

Heath A.C. and Madden P.G.: Genetic Influences on Smoking Behaviouir. In: J.R. Turner, L.R. Cardon, and J.K. Hewitt (Eds), *Behaviour Genetic Approaches in Behavioural Medicine. Plenum:* New York p37–48, 1995.

Heath A.C. and Martin N.: Genetic Models for the Natural History of Smoking: Evidence for a Genetic Influence on Smoking Persistence, *Addictive Behaviour*, 18:19–34, 1993.

Henningfield, J.E., Miyasato, K. and Jansinki, D.R.: Abuse Liability and Pharmacodynamic Characteristics of Intravenous and Inhaled Nicotine. Journal of Pharmacology and Experimental Therapeutics. 234 (1): 1–12, 1985.

Hibberd, A.R., O'Connor, V. and Gorrod, J.W.: Detection of Nicotine, Nicotine-l'N-oxide and Cotinine in Maternal and Fetal Body Fluids. In Gorrod, J. W. (eds.): Biological Oxidation of Nicotine. *Amsterdam. Elseneir/ North Hollan. Biomedical Press*, 1978.

Hibberd, A.R. and Gorrod, J.W. Enzymology of Metabolic Pathway from Nicotine to Cotinine in-vitro. *European Journal of Drug Metabolism and Pharmacokinetics*. 8 (2): 151–162, 1983.

Hoffmann D. and Wynder E.L.: Smoke of Cigarette and Little Cigar: An Analytical Comparison, *Science*, 178:1197–1199, 1977.

Jarvik, M.E.: Biological Factors Underlying the Smoking Habit. In Jarvik, M. E.Cullen, J. W., Gritz, E. R., Vogt, T. M. and West, L. J. (eds.): Research on Smoking Behavior, NIDA Research Monograph 17. U.S. Department of Health and Human Sciences. Alcohol, *Drug Abuse and Mental Health Administration, NIDA. DHEW Publications*, 1977.

Jarvik, M.E., Glick, S.D. and Nakamura, R.K. Inhibition of Cigarette Smoking by Orally Administered Nicotine. *Clinical Pharmacology and Therapeutics*. 11 (4): 574–576, 1970.

Jenner, P., Gorrod, J.W. and Beckett, A.H.: The Absorption of Nicotine- 1′-N-oxide and its Reduction in the Gastro-intestinal Tract in Man. *Xenobiotica* 3 (6): 341–346, 1973.

Jenner P., Gorrod J.W. and Beckett A.H.: Species Variation in Metabolism of R-(+)- and S-(-) Nicotine by Alfa-C- and N-oxidation *in vitro, Xenobiotica,* 3:573–580, 1988.

Kuehl G.E. and Murphy S.E.: N-glucronidation of *Trans*-3′-hydroxycotinine by Human Liver Microsomes. *Chemical research and Toxicology,* 16:1502–1506, 2003.

Kyerematen G.A. and Vesell E.S.: Metabolism of Nicotine, Drug Metabolic Review, 23:3–41, 1991.

Langley, J.N.: On the Reaction of Cells and of Nerve-endings to Certain Poisons, Chiefly as Regard to Reaction of Striated Muscle to Nicotine and to Curari. *Journal of Physiology* (London). 33: 374–413, 1905.

Larson, PS., Haag, H. B. and Silvette, H.: Tobacco: Experimental and Clinical Studies. *Baltimore: Williams and Wilkins,* 1961.

Larson, PS. and Silvette, H.: Tobacco: Experimental and Clinical Studies. Supplement III. *Baltimore: Williams and Wilkins,* 1975.

Lee B.L., Jacob P III, Jarvik M.E. and Benowitz N.L.: Food and Nicotine Metabolism. Pharmacology, Biochemistry and Behaviour, 33:621–625, 1989.

Lerman C., Caporaso N.E, Audrain J., Main D., Bowman E.D., Lockshin B., Boyd N.R. and Shieds P.G. Evidence suggesting the role of Specific Genetic Factors in Cigarette Smoking, *Health Psychology,* 18:14–20, 1999.

London, S.J., Idle J.R., Daly A.K. and Coetzee G.: Genetic Variation of CYP2A6, Smoking, and Risk of Cancer-*Lancet*. 353: 898 – 899. 1999.

Luck, W., Hansen, R., Steldinger, R., and Nau, H.: Nicotine and Cotinine-Two Pharmacologically Active Substances as Parameters for the Strain on Fetuses and Babies of Mother who Smoke, *Journal of Perinatal Medicine,* 10 (52): 107, 1982.

Mathai M., Skinner A., Lawton K. and Weindling A.M.: Maternal Smoking, Urinary Cotinine Levels and birth-weight. Australian and New Zealand Journal of Obstetrics and Gynaecology, 30:33, 1990.

Mazierre, M., Comar, D., Marzano, C. and Berger, G.: Nicotine ′C Synthesis and Distribution Kinetics in Animals. *European Journal of Nuclear Medicine,* 1: 255–258, 1976.

Messina, E. S., Tyndale, R. F. and Sellers, E. M.: A Major Role of CYP2A6 in Nicotine C-oxidation by Human Liver Microsomes, *Journal of Experimental Therapeutics* 282:1608–1614, 1997.

Mishra U.C. and Shaikh G.N.: Determination of Trace Element Concentration of Indian Cigarette Tobacco by Instrumental Neutron Activation Analysis. *Journal of Radioanalytical Chemistry,* 78:385–390, 1983.

Moyer David: Carbon Monoxide. Smokerlyzer Brochure, Bedford Scientific, *Journal of Family Practice.* 690, 1995.

Nakajima M., Yamagischi S., Yamamoto H., Yamamoto T., Kuroiwa Y. and Yukoi T: Deficient Cotinine Formation from Nicotine is Attributed to whole Deletion of CYP2A6 Gene in Humans. *Clinical Pharmacology and Therapeutics,* 67:57–69, 2000.

Nakajima, M., Yamamota, T., Nunoya, K., Yokoi, T., Inoue, K., Funae, Y., Shimada, N., Kamataki, T. and Kuroiwa, Y. Role of Human Cytochrome P450 2A6 in C-oxidation of Nicotine. *Drug Metabolism and Disposal.* 24:1212–1217, 1996.

Nair U.J., Pakhale S.S., Speigelhalden B., Preussmann R. and Bhide S.V. Carcinogenic and Co-carcinogenic Constituents of Masheri, a Pyrolysed Tobacco Product. Indian Journal of Biochemistry and Biophysics, 24:257–259, 1987

Nunoya K.I., Yokoi T., Kimura K., Kainuma T., Satoh K., Kinoshita M. and Kamataki K.: A New CYP2A6 Deletion Responsible for *in vivo* Polymorphic Metabolism of (+)-*cis*-3,5-dimethy-2-(3-pirydyl)Thiazolidin-4-one Hydrochloride in Humans. *Journal of Pharmacology and Experimental Therapeutics*, 289:437-442, 1999.

Oscarson M.: Genetic Polymorphism in the Cytochrome P450 (CYP2A6) Gene: Implications for Interindividual Differences in Nicotine Metabolism, Drug Metabolism Dispos, 29:91–95, 2001.

Pakhale S.S., Dolas, S.S., and Maru, G.B.: Determination of Alkaloids, Nitrate, Nitrite, Moisture and pH in Tobacco Varieties from Different Pats of India. ,*Tobacco Research*, 23:11–18, 1997.

Perez-Stable E.J., Herrera, B. Jacob P. and Benowitz, N. Nicotine Metabolism and Intake in Black and White Smokers, *Journal of the American Medical Association (JAMA)*. 280 (July 8): 152–156, 1998.

Petrakis, N.L., Gruenke, L.D., Beenlen, T.C., Castagnoli, N. and Craig, J.C. Nicotine in Breast Fluid of Non-lactating Women. *Science*. 199 (4326): 303–305, 1978.

Peterson, LA., Trevor, A. and Castagnoli, N. Jr.: Stereochemical Studies on the Cytochrome P-450 Catalyzed Oxidation of (S)-nicotine to (S)-nicotine-D¹É˜, 1987.

Piade, J.J. and Hoffmann, D. Chemical Study on Tobacco Smoke. LXVII Quantitative Determinants of Alkaloids in Tobacco by Liquid Chromatography, Journal of Liquid Chromatography. 3 (10): 1505–1515, 1980.

Pianezza, M.L., Sellers, E.M. and Tyndale, R.F.: Genetically Variable CYP2 influences Smoking Behaviour. Clinical Pharmacology and Therapeutics. 63: 71, 1998.

Pianezza ML, Dellers EM. and Tyndale R.F.: Nicotine Metabolism Defect Reduces Smoking, Nature, 393:750, 1998.

Pomerleau, O. F.: Individual Differences in Sensitivity of Nicotine: Implications in Genetic Research on Nicotine Dependence, Behavioural Genetics. 25: 161–177, 1995.

Rathkamp, G., Tso, T.C. and Hoffmann, D.: Chemical Studies on Tobacco Smoke. XX: Smoke Analysis of Cigarettes Made from Bright Tobacco Differing in Variety and Stalk Positions. *Bietrage zur Tobakforschung*, 7(3):179–189, 1973.

Raunio H, Rautio A, Gullsten H. and Pelkonen O.: Polymorphism of CYP2A6 and its Practical Consequences. British Journal of Clinical Pharmacology, 52:357–363, 2001.

Rose JE, Tashkin DP., Ertle A, Zinser MC. and Lafer R.: Sensory Blockade of Smoking Satisfaction. *Pharmacology, Biochemistry and Behaviour*,23(2): 289–293, 1985.

Russell, MAH. Tobacco Smoking and Nicotine Dependence. In: Gibbins, R., Israel, Y., Kalant, H., Popham, RE., Schmidt, W. and Smart, RC. (eds.) *Recent Advances in Alcohol and Drug problems*, John Wiley and Sons, New York, 1976.

Russell, M.A.H.: Smoking Addiction: In Swartz, J. L. (eds.) Progress in Smoking Cessation. New York: *American Cancer Society/WHO*, 1978

Russell, MAH. and Feyerabend, C.: Cigarette Smoking: A Dependence on High Nicotine boli. *Drug Metabolism Reviews.* 8 (11): 29–57, 1978.

Russell, MAH. and Feyerabend, C.: Smoking as Dependence Disorder. In Ramstrom, LM. (eds.) The Smoking Epidemic: Proceedings of the Fourth World Conference on Smoking and Health. Stockholm: *Almqqvist and Wiksell* International, 1980.

Russell, M.A.H., Feyerabend, C. and Cole, P.V.: Plasma Nicotine Levels After Cigarette Smoking and Chewing Nicotine Gum. *British Medical Journal.* 1: 1043 –1046, 1976.

Russell, MAH., Jarvis, MJ., Devitt, G. and Feyerabend, C.: Nicotine Intake by Snuff Users. *British Medical Journal.* 283 (6295): 814–817, 1981.

Russell, MAH., Raw, M. and Jarvis, M.J.: Clinical Use of Nicotine Chewing Gum. *British Medical Journal.* 280 (623): 1599–1602, 1980.

Sasson, I.M., Haley, N.J., Hoffman, D., Wynder, E.L., Hellberg, D. and Nilsson, S.: Cigarette Smoking and Neoplasia of Uterine Cervix: Smoke Constituents in Cervical Mucous (letter). *New England Journal of Medicine.* 312 (5): 315–316, 1985.

Schmeltz, I. And Hoffmann, D.: Nicotine Containing Compounds in Tobacco and Tobacco Smoke. *Chemical Review.* 77 (3): 295–311, 1977.

Sellers, E,M., Kaplan H.L. and Tyndale, R.F.: Initiation of Cytochrome P4502A6 Increases Nicotine's Bioavailability and Decreases Smoking. *Clinical Pharmacology and Therapeutics*, 68:35–43, 2000.

Shields J.: Monozygotic Twins Brought-up Apart and Brought-up Together. *Oxford University Press*: London, 1962.

Spector R. and Goldberg M.J.: Active Transport of Nicotine by the Isolated Choroids Plexus *in vitro. Journal of Neurochemistry*, 38:594–596, 1982.

Steward, R.T., Berret, E.D., Platte, L.R., Stewart, E.B., Kalbfleisch, J.H., Van, Yserloo, B. and Rimm, A.A.: Carboxyhemoglobin Levels in American Blood Donors. *Journal of the American Medical Association.* 229 (9): 1187–1195, 1974.

Su, C.: Actions of Nicotine and Smoking on Circulation, *Pharmacology and Therapeutics*, 17 (1): 129–141, 1982.

Travell, J.: Absorption of Nicotine from Various Sites, *Annals of the New York Academy of Science.* 90 (1): 13–30, 1960.

Turner, DM., Armitage, A.K., Briant, R. H. and Dollery, C.T. Metabolism of Nicotine by the Isolated Perfused Dog's lung. *Xenobiotica.* 5 (9): 539–551, 1975.

Turner, J.A., Sillet, R.W., Taylor, D.M. and McNicol, M.W.: The Effects of Supplementary Nicotine in Regular Cigarette Smokers. *Post-graduate Medical Journal.* 53: 683 – 686, 1977.

Tutka P., Dempsey D. Benowitz N.L. and Kroetz D.: Metabolism of nicotine in Pregnant and Non-pregnant Rabbits. Clinical Pharmacology and Therapeutics, 67:32, 2000.

Tutka P., Mosiewicz J and Wielosz M.: Pharmacokinetics and Metabolism of Nicotine. *Pharmacological Reports*, 57:143–153, 2005.

Wald, N., Howard, S. and Smith, PG.: Use of Carboxyhemoglobin Levels to Predict the Diseases Associated with Cigarette Smoking. *Thorax.* 30: 133–140, 1975 .

Wald, N.J., Idle, M., Boreham, J., Bailey, A.: Carbon Monoxide in Breath in Relation to Smoking and Caboxyhemoglobin Level. *Thorax*. 36 (5): 366–436, 1981.

Westman E.C.: Does Smokeless Tobacco Cause Hypertension? *South Medical Journal*, 88:716–720, 1995.

Williams D.E., Ding XX. and Coon M.J.: Rabbit Nasal Cytochrome P450 Nma has High Activity as a Nicotine Oxidase. *Biochemistry and Biophysics Research*, 166:945–952, 1990.

Yamazaki H., Inoue K., Hashimoto M. and Shimada T.: Roles of CYP2A6 and CYP2B6 in Nicotine C-oxidation by Human Liver Microsomes. *Archives of Toxicology*, 73:65–70, 1999.

Yamazaki H., Inui Y, Yun CH., Guengerich FP. and Shimada T.: Cytochrome P4502E1 and 2A6 Enzymes as Major Catalystsfor Metabolic Activation of N-nitrosodialkyl-amines and Tobacco Related Nitrosamines in Human Liver Microsomes. *Carcinogenesis*, 123:1789–1794, 1992.

Zevin S., Gourlay S.G. and Benowitz N.L.: Clinical Pharmacology of Nicotine. *Clinical Dermatology*, 16:557–564, 1998.

Zevin S., and Benowitz N.L.: Drug Interaction with Tobacco Smoking: An Update, *Clinical Pharmacology*, 36:425–438, 1999.

CHAPTER

# 5 Addiction Model: Tobacco Use as Drug Dependence

*"Cigarette smoking is probably the most addictive and dependence producing object-specific self-administered gratification known to man."*

— Russell MAH, 1976

Substance abuse involves the use of a substance despite social, interpersonal, or other problems caused by the use of the substance while dependence is a more severe disorder entailing signs of physical or psychological tolerance. Dependence refers to compulsive drug use that is derived by strong and often irresistible urge that persist despite a desire to quit or even repeated attempts to quit. From behavioural point of view, addiction or dependence to a drug can be defined as repeated self-administration of a drug or substance despite of adverse medical and social consequences and attempts to abstain from it. At the cost of social and occupational commitments, an addict's daily activities centre on obtaining and consuming the drug. Addictive behaviour like human behaviour in general is the outcome of genetic and biochemical characteristics, past learning experiences, motivational states, psycho-social antecedents and cultural context in which it unfolds (Sutker, 1977). Initial decision to use a drug is generally influenced by genetic, psycho-social and environmental factors that initiate smoking in an individual. Therefore, substance dependence or addiction is a primary brain disease, determined genetically, expressed biochemically, and has psycho-social consequences. These consequences can and do occur in all aspects of the addict's life, influencing the social, vocational, legal, family, spiritual, psychological and physical spheres. The disease is characterized by its chronic, progressive, relapsing, and lethal nature. There are four cardinal features generally seen in drug addiction:

- Loss of *control* over the use of drug
- *Continuous* use despite of adverse consequences.
- *Compulsive* use.
- *Craving* when the drug is withheld.

Often present in the definitions of dependence or addiction are two characteristics: the *compulsion* to use a drug leading to its excessive and uncontrolled consumption and appearance of *withdrawal symptoms* when the drug is withheld after a period of its continuous consumption. Other characteristics noticed are that the addicts use *more* of the substance than intended, or use it for a *longer period of time* than intended. There is a *persistent desire* to use, or unsuccessful efforts to cut down or control use. They spend *more time or resources* to obtain the substance and take longer time in recovering from its use. Two factors that modulate behaviour – re-enforcement and neuroadaptation – contribute to addictive process. Psycho-active effects are achieved with drug-reinforced behaviour. "*Reinforcement*" refers to the quality of being able to get users to do something repeatedly, such as to consume the substance repeatedly. Neuroadaptations in the brain cells result from repeated exposure to a drug of abuse. These adaptations contribute to produce the complex behaviours that define an addictive state.

International Classification of Diseases (1992), 10th Revision (ICD-10) by World Health Organization (WHO) defines drug dependence as "a state psychic and sometimes also physical, resulting from the interaction between a living organism and a drug, characterized by behavioural and other responses that always include a compulsion to take the drug on a continuous or periodic basis in order to experience its psychic effects, and sometimes to avoid discomfort of its absence..." Tolerance may or may not be present (Cohen, Pickworth and Henningfield, 1991). According to all these parameters, nicotine is an addictive substance and nicotine addiction has been classified as a disease by the WHO's International Classification of Diseases (ICD) 10th Revision.

Based on the WHO criteria for drug dependence the US Surgeon General has concluded that tobacco delivered nicotine is addictive and the Food and Drug Administration (FDA) has declared nicotine as an addictive drug on 12th July, 1996[1].

***Table 1: Diagnostic criteria for substance dependence* and examples of their application to nicotine dependence (Hughes 1993)**. A maladaptive pattern of substance abuse leading to clinically significant impairment or distress, as manifested by three (or more) of the following, occurring at any time in the same 12 month period:***

| *Criteria* | *Examples* |
|---|---|
| *Tolerance, as defined by either*<br>A need for markedly increased amounts of the substance to achieve intoxication or desired effect. | Most smokers escalate use to one packet per day or more by age 25. |

*Contd...*

[1] Anonymous. FDA can't regulate nicotine as addictive drug.

| | |
|---|---|
| Markedly diminished effect with continued use of the same amount of the substance. | Absence of nausea, dizziness, etc. |
| *Withdrawal as manifested by either* | |
| The characteristic withdrawal syndrome for the substance. The substance is taken to relieve or avoid withdrawal symptoms. | Known nicotine withdrawal symptoms are experienced by a dependent smoker. Many smokers light up immediately after being in a smoke-free area. |
| The substance is often taken in large amounts or over a longer period than intended. | Most smokers do not intend to smoke 5 year later, but in fact, over 70% continue to use. |
| *There is persistent desire or unsuccessful effort to cut down substance use* | 77% of the smokers have tried to stop, 55% of these have not been able to stop despite repeated attempts and only 5%–10% of self-quitters are successful. |
| A great deal of time is spent in activities necessary to obtain the substance, use the substance or recover from its effects. | Leaving worksite to smoke. |
| Important social, occupational or recreational activities are given up or reduced because of substance use. | Not taking a job due to on-job smoking rest`rictions. |
| The substance use is continued despite knowledge of having a persistent or recurrent physical or psychological problem that is likely to have been caused or exacerbated by the substance. | Many smokers have heart disease, chronic obstructive pulmonary disease or ulcers and continue to smoke. |

* *Diagnostic and Statistical Manual (4th Edition) American Psychiatric Association, 1994.*
** *Courtesy: American Psychiatric Association, Practice Guidelines for the Treatment of Psychiatric Disorders, 2000 Washington DC.*

American Psychiatric Association's internationally used Diagnostic and Statistical Manual for Mental Disorders (1994), 4th Edition (DSM-IV) outlines the criteria for substance dependence and includes nicotine dependence and nicotine withdrawal as disorders. Nicotine abuse is not included because clinically significant psychosocial problems from tobacco use are rare (Hughes, 1994).Nicotine intoxication is also not included as it is very rare. Table 1 illustrates how the generic DSM IV criteria for substance dependence apply to nicotine dependence. The applicability and reliability of DSM diagnosis of nicotine dependence appears high (Hughes, 1993). The Diagnostic and Statistical Manual of Mental Disorders, 4th Edition (DSM-IV) 1994 classifies nicotine addiction as Nicotine Use Disorder. The criteria for diagnosis include any three of the following within a 1-year time span:

- *Tolerance* to nicotine with decreased effect and increasing dose to obtain same effect.

- *Withdrawal* symptoms.
- Smoking *more than the usual.*
- *Persistent desire to smoke* despite efforts to decrease intake.
- *Extensive time spent* smoking or purchasing tobacco.
- *Postponing* work, social and recreational events in order to smoke.
- *Continuing* to smoke despite health hazards.

***Table 2: Items and scoring for Fagerstrom test for nicotine dependence****

| *Question* | *Answer* | *Point* |
|---|---|---|
| 1. How soon after you wake up do you smoke your first cigarette? | Within 5 minutes | 3 |
| | Within 6–30 minutes | 2 |
| | Within 30–60 minutes | 1 |
| | After 60 minutes | 0 |
| 2. Do you find it difficult to refrain from smoking in places where it is forbidden, e.g. in library, in the cinema hall, etc? | Yes | 1 |
| | No | 0 |
| 3. Which cigarette would you hate most to give up? | The first one in the morning | 1 |
| | All others | 0 |
| 4. How many cigarettes per day do you smoke? | 10 or less | 0 |
| | 11–20 | 1 |
| | 21–30 | 2 |
| | 31-or more | 3 |
| 5. Do you smoke more frequently during the first hours of waking than during rest of the day? | Yes | 1 |
| | No | 2 |
| 6. Do you smoke if you are so ill that you are in bed most of the day? | Yes | 1 |
| | No | 0 |

**Courtesy: American Psychiatric Association, Practice Guidelines for the Treatment of Psychiatric Disorders, 2000, Washington DC.*

The American Psychiatric Association (APA) and the World Health Organization (WHO) have refined their definitions of drug dependence they have issued criteria for specific behavioural and psychological identifiers that can be used as diagnostic criteria. The various sets of criteria change slightly as succeeding versions of the diagnostic categories are issued, reflecting growth in scientific understanding of addiction and in societal comprehension of its impact. One comprehensive definition of addiction comes from a report issued to the Royal Society of Health and Welfare Canada. In this report, addiction or dependence on a drug is described as a strongly established pattern of behaviour characterized by (1) the repeated self-administration of a drug in amounts which reliably produce reinforcing psycho-active effects and (2) great difficulty in achieving voluntary long-term cessation of use, even when the user is strongly motivated to stop[2]. Therefore, tobacco use is not just a random or capricious activity of human beings that simply occurs at will or pleasure of those who use it. It is a repetitive, stereotypic and compulsive behaviour characteristic of drug dependence. This seemingly irrational behaviour is strongly driven by the pharmacological actions of nicotine on the brain and that cigarette and smokeless tobacco products are extraordinarily effective at maximizing the addictive effects of nicotine. The activity of lighting, smoking and extinguishing cigarette including puffing and inhaling also become regular in smokers over time. Most smokers do not continue to smoke out of choice but because they are addicted to nicotine. A majority of smokers have tried to quit or at least would like to quit, 65 percent of smokers had made at least one serious attempt to quit and another 21 percent expressed their desire to get rid of this problem if there were an easy way to do so (US DHHS, 1986). Number of puffs, depth of inhalations, and many other variables and constituents of smoke such as nicotine, tar, and carbon monoxide (CO) affect the intake of tobacco smoke. The process of producing cigarette smoke constituents is a complex one (Figure 1) (US DHHS, 1981). This complexity emphasizes the importance of the use of careful measurement to ensure accurate characterization of cigarette smoking. The measurement determines the intensity and severity of cigarette smoking.

A widely used measure of nicotine dependence is the Fagerstrom Tolerance Questionnaire or the more recent version—the Fagerstrom Test for Nicotine Dependence (Table 2). Scores of greater than seven on the scales indicate nicotine dependence.

Once the body has accustomed to functioning with a level of nicotine in the blood, it seeks to maintain this level and smokers feel the need to continue self-administering the drug. Its quick absorption and distribution in the body and its psychopharmacology has helped move definitions of tobacco use from the outdated concept of "habit" to the current concept of "nicotine dependence." Nicotine's action on brain and body, and consequently the mechanism of action which causes addiction, is the subject matter to be discussed in this chapter.

---

[2] Royal Society of Health and Welfare, Canada, 1989.

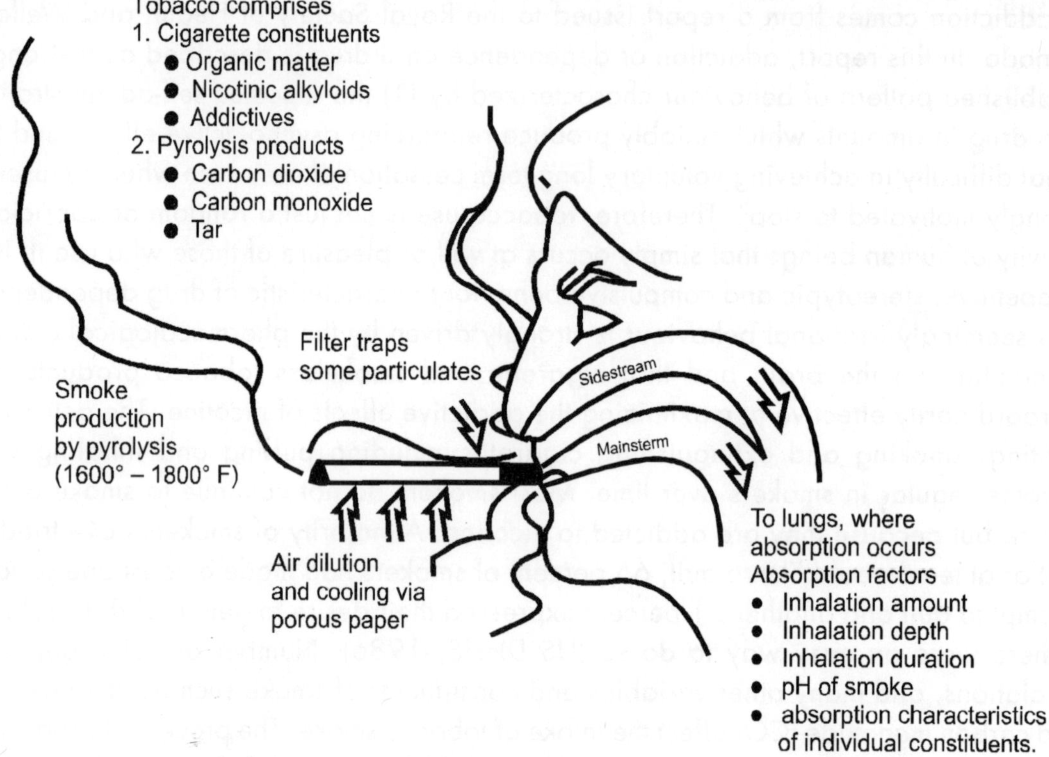


***Figure 1: Production and fate of cigarette smoke constituents***

*NOTE: Description of complexity of process by which nicotine is extracted from cigarette. Amount of nicotine ultimately absorbed is as much a function of smoker behaviour as of cigarette characteristics.*

**Source:** *Henningfield, 1984.*

Tobacco dependence or addiction is presently a problem of many millions world-wide who indulge in tobacco smoking, chewing, snuffing or taking it inside their body in various other forms. Vulnerability to tobacco dependence is almost universal, based on the effects of nicotine on the brain and the body.

Tobacco dependence has been a complex and challenging phenomenon to describe aetiologically, psychologically and behaviourally. Tobacco-intake behaviour and its remarkable intractability to change is addiction to nicotine (Himbury and West, 1985) with wider ramifications. Addictive properties of tobacco are similar to those of other dependence producing drugs (Hughes *et al.,* 1994) such as heroin and cocaine. Although the psychoactive effect of nicotine is less dramatic than that of heroin or cocaine, the strength of addiction is as powerful or more powerful.

## Nicotine in Tobacco

Nicotine is one of the 4000 chemicals found in tobacco smoke and about 3000 in smokeless tobacco[3]. It is a naturally occurring pale yellow to dark brown liquid with slightly fishy odour when warm, derived from the tobacco plant, was first isolated from tobacco leaves by Posselt and Reimanbasic in 1828 (Jain and Mukherjee, 2003) and since then it has been studied extensively and shown to have a number of complex and sometimes unpredictable effects on the brain causing chemical and biological changes in the brain and the body.

Nicotine, an alkaloid (1-methyl–2–[3-pyrodyl] pyrrolidine), is conveyed in the body through the lungs, skin, and mucous membranes. Pulmonary absorption, which is the most favoured and perhaps commonest, occurs in a matter of seconds.

Cigarette smoke containing nicotine is absorbed mainly through the alveolar surface of the lungs. Acidic pH of cigarette smoke allows nicotine in the smoke to be ionized and thus can not be absorbed completely through the mucous membrane of the mouth while more alkaline smoke of cigars which is non-ionized is absorbed through the mucous membrane of the mouth. From the lungs, chemicals in the smoke are absorbed into body's systems and carried quickly to different parts of the body. Oral snuffs and other smokeless tobacco products are absorbed more gradually (Benowitz, Porchet and Sheiner, 1988). The extent of tobacco exposure to lung alveoli depends upon the length and the number of puffs of a cigarette, the intensity and depth of inhalation, the mixture of air and smoke, and the amount of available smoke. The amount of nicotine intake from one cigarette varies widely, in accordance with the smoker's latitude for adjusting the dose level. Nicotine intake ranges from 10 mg/day to 80 mg/day, or 0.4 mg-1.6 mg/cigarette (Benowitz and Jacob, 1984).

Nicotine, the primary pharmacological factor in tobacco, influences and reinforces all tobacco-use behaviour. The vulnerability to smoking behaviour is also familial and cultural and is heightened by the tobacco's powerful reinforcing effects and by the nature of the tobacco products, which are designed in many cases to be optimally addictive (Hoffmann and Hoffmann, 1997). Development of tobacco smoking behaviour depends upon a complex interplay of these multiple factors. The factors which initiate the process of tobacco intake may be quite different from those which contribute to its continuation. User becomes pharmacologically involved and progresses along a continuum from occasional smoking or taking for fun to regular smoking and using to dependence. After absorption, nicotine travels rapidly to the brain, in a matter of seconds (Figure 2), therefore, the psycho-active rewards associated with smoking occur quickly

---

[3] Report on Tobacco Control in India, Ministry of Health and Family Welfare, Government of India, Centre for Disease Control and Prevention, USA and World Health Organization, 2004.

and these rewards are highly reinforced. A drug is most reinforcing if the psycho-active effect quickly follows the administration of the drug.

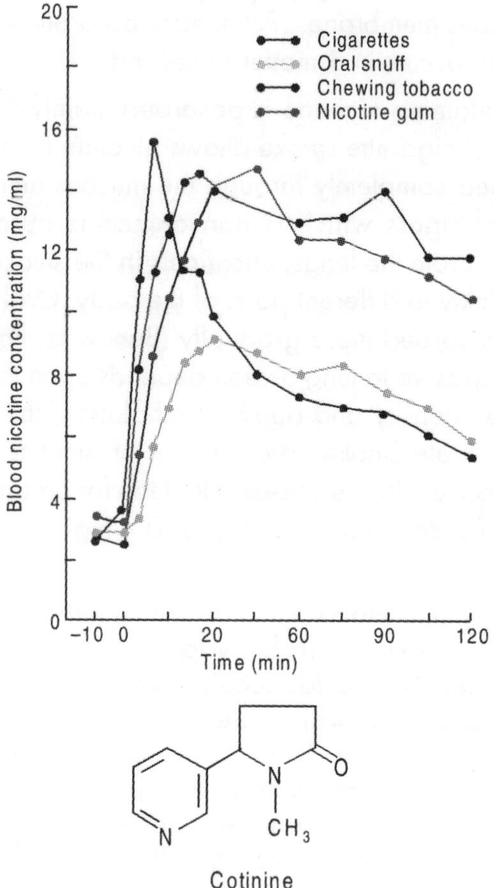


*Figure 2: Nicotine ingestion and plasma concentration*

***Source:*** *Sinauor Associates, Inc., Feldman Fundamentals of Neuro Psyco-pharmacology.*

Nicotine binds to the receptors in the brain where it influences the cerebral metabolism. Nicotine is then distributed throughout the body, mostly to skeletal muscles. As already mentioned, nicotine is a potent addictive substance as powerful as "hard drugs," it acts as a gateway drug for other addictive substances. Effects of nicotine include changes in respiration, blood pressure, constriction of arteries, and increased alertness. Many of these effects are produced through its action on both the peripheral and central nervous system.

Nicotine generates dependence by producing centrally mediated reinforcing effects, by regulating elements such as body weight and mood in ways that are perceived as useful or desirable by tobacco user and by leading to a physical dependence such that abstinence may result in adverse symptoms. In a cigarette smoker, following initiation of smoking there is a gradual increase in cigarette intake over time until he/she achieves the level that remains stable, day after day, during the smoker's life (Schuman, 1977). The initial cigarette of the day is smoked soon after waking (Fagerstrom, 1978) and in which smoking throughout the day is regulated from day to day (Griffiths and Henningfield, 1982).

If nicotine were not absorbed quickly from the lungs, people would not take it in the form of smoke; if it were not taken up into the brain, it would not exert its *psycho-pharmacological* effects; if it were not rapidly metabolized and excreted, it would probably not be taken in such often-repeated doses.

## Mechanism of Action

Nicotine has structural similarity to a body neuro-transmitter acetylcholine (Ach) which conveys information from one neuron to another. When a nerve is stimulated, the excitation is initially propagated along the nerve fibre in the form of electrical impulse. At the nerve ending, acetylcholine is released from the synaptic vesicle into the synaptic cleft and stimulates acetylcholine receptors in the next neuron; electrical changes occur which initiate a further electrical impulse in the next neuron. Each time synaptic contact is made in this way, the neurotransmitter is used as the messenger to pass on the information carried in the nerves. This way messages are carried from the body to the brain, from the brain to the body and between different parts of the brain and spinal cord.

Acetylcholine is an important neurotransmitter involved in systems concerned with mental and physical arousal, learning and memory, and several aspects of emotion. There are also other receptors for acetylcholine in the body, apart from the ones at synapses. They are also found at the junction of nerve and muscles and nerves and certain glands. Acetylcholine-receptors respond only to acetylcholine in order to pass on the nerve message correctly. These receptors do not respond to other chemicals or neurotransmitters present in the vicinity. Acetylcholine-receptor recognizes the acetylcholine molecule by the position of two electrical charges, one positive and one negative, located at certain sites of the molecule (Figures 3 and 4).

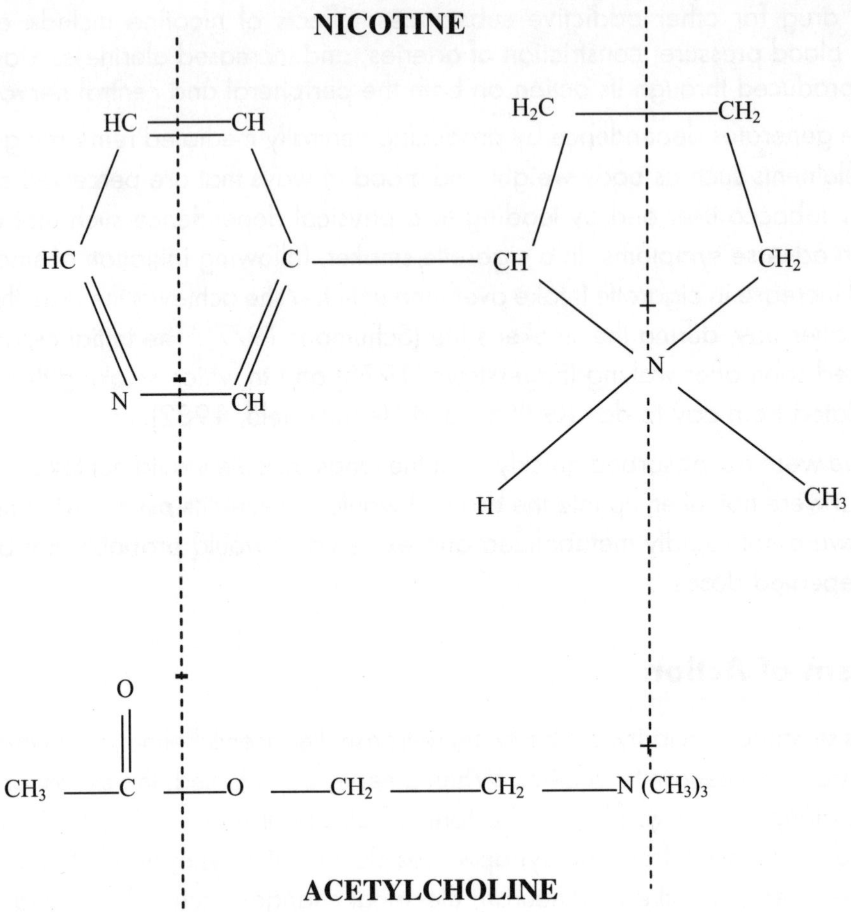


*Figure 3: The structure of nicotine and acetylcholine*

The positive and negative charges are the same distance apart in the two molecules.
***Source:*** *Ashton and Stepney,* 1982.

The distance between these two charges is always the same and corresponds with two equally spaced and oppositely charged sites on the receptor. The acetylcholine molecule is attracted to the acetylcholine-receptor and then fits snugly into it by virtue of their mutually satisfying configuration. Other molecules without the electrical and spatial characteristics of acetylcholine simply pass the receptor by.

In the nicotine molecule the positive charge on the ammonium head and the negative charge on pyridine ring are just the same distance apart as they are in the acetylcholine molecule. This structural similarity makes nicotine molecule to interact with acetylcholine receptors.

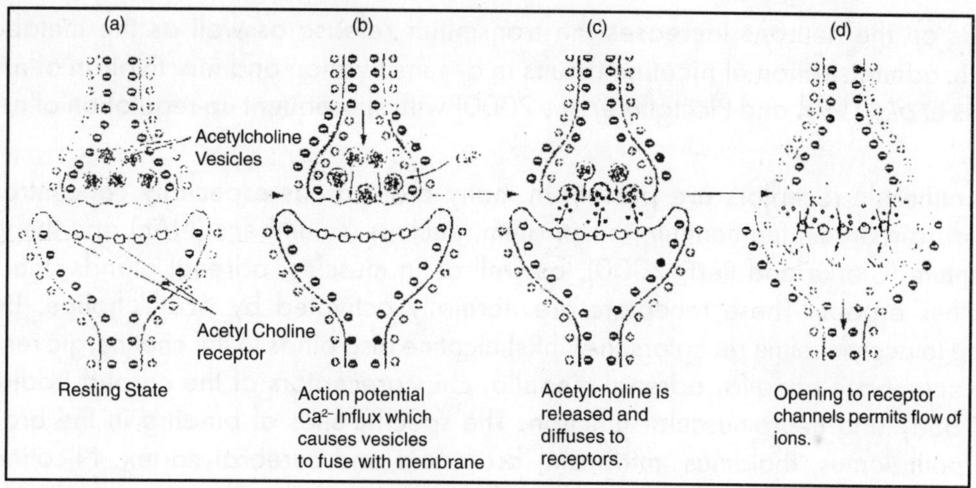


**Figure 4: Cell-cell communication at the synapse**

(a) *Mediated by neuro-transmitters such as acetyl-choline, produced from choline by cholineacetyltransferase. The arrival of action potential the synaptic knob.*

(b) *Opens $Ca^2+$ channels in presynaptic membrane. Influx of $Ca^2+$ induces the fusion of acetylcholine containing vesicles with the plasma membrane and release of acetylcholine into synaptic cleft.*

(c) *Binding of acetylcholine to receptors in the postsynaptic membrane opens Na+ channels.*

(d) *The influx of Na+ depolarizes the postsynaptic membrane, generating a new action potential. O (7) nicotine locks this ionchannel in the IopenO conformation.*

**Source:** *Kelvin B (2000) Nicotine: Chemistry of Drugs and Poisons. Chemistry 377, Spring.*

Acetylcholine receptors throughout the body are traditionally classified as nicotine receptors (those that respond to nicotine) and muscarine receptors (those that respond to muscarine). The ability of nicotine to combine with acetylcholine-receptors means that it can exert actions like acetylcholine at all synapses where nicotine acetylcholine-receptors (nAChRs) are present and can trigger impulses down postsynaptic nerve fibres, resulting in effects which otherwise occur only when acetylcholine is released following stimulation of the pre-synaptic nerves. Synapses involving acetylcholine are very widespread in the body, affecting systems ranging from the cardiovascular to the psychological and also interacting with other transmitter systems showing that nicotine has multifarious actions. Electrical excitation of a nerve produces not just one impulse but a whole train of impulses. This multiplicity imposes the requirement at the synapse that the combination of transmitter with the receptor must be quickly reversed between each impulse, leaving the receptor free to combine with the next pack of acetylcholine released.

Nicotine binds to the acetylcholine receptors (nAChRs) in the brain where it influences the cerebral metabolism by stimulating these receptors. The stimulation of presynaptic nAChRs on the neurons increases the transmitter release as well as the metabolism. Chronic administration of nicotine results in desensitization and inactivation of nAChRs (Collins *et al.*, 1994 and Picciotto *et al.*, 2000) with subsequent up-regulation of nAChRs sites.

Cholinergic receptors are present in many brain areas especially concentrated in the midbrain areas, tegmentum, the striatum, nucleus accumbens (NAc) and the ventral tegmentum (Clarke and Pert, 2000), as well as in muscles, adrenal glands, the heart, and other organs. These receptors are normally activated by acetylcholine. Besides binding to acetylcholine receptors (nAChRs) nicotine also binds to the cholinergic receptors in the autonomic ganglia, adrenal medulla, chemoreceptors of the carotid bodies and aortic body and neuromuscular junction. The specific sites of binding in the brain are the hypothalamus, thalamus, midbrain, brainstem and cerebral cortex. Nicotine also binds to the receptors in nigrostriatal and mesolimbic dopaminergic neurons. As and when dopaminergic receptors are stimulated they release acetylcholine, norepinephrine, dopamine, serotonin, vasopressin, growth hormone and ACTH. Nicotine is one of the most potent stimulants of the midbrain dopamine reward pathway (Epping-Jordan *et al.*, 1998; Picciotto *et al.*, 1998 and Pidoplichko VI *et al.*, 1997). Nicotine acts on locus ceruleus regulating vigilance, arousal, concentration and stress reactions making the tobacco users more alert. Because of the interaction between nicotine and neuronal high-affinity nicotine high affinity acetylcholine receptors nicotine affects learning, memory and other functions.

Nicotine also alters the function of some of the neurotransmitters implicated in the pathogenesis of some of the major psychiatric disorders. These include dopamine, norepinephrine, serotonin (5-HT), glutamate alfa-aminobutyric acid (GABA) and endogenous opioid peptides (George *et al.*, 2000; McGhee *et al.*, 1995). These effects could be presynaptic, preterminal, or cell body nicotine receptors, rather than mediated through neurotransmission wherein presynaptically released acetylcholine acts on postsynaptic, junctional nAChRs to cause neuronal firing (Wonnacot *et al.*, 1990).

## Biological Theories of Nicotine Dependence

### *1. Dopamine and Reward Pathways*

Nicotine plays a vital role in maintaining the tobacco smoking habit and as a result many habitual smokers become dependent on it. Nicotine addiction, like other drug addictions, is fundamentally a neurobiologically mediated brain disorder characterized by cellular and molecular reinforcing effects which lead to dependence. A drug is considered to be most reinforcing if the psyco-active effect quickly follows the administration of the drug. The drug-addicted brain is structurally and functionally different from non-addicted brain, and changes that occur are an important part of addiction itself (Bigelow, Rand and

Gross, 1986 and Ferry and Burchette, 1994). Nicotine addiction is related to the effects of nicotine on dopaminergic and noradrenergic systems of the brain—the mesolimbic system and locus ceruleus respectively (Figure 5). The neurobiological processes that determine nicotine addiction are similar to those that determine addiction to drugs such as heroin or cocaine.

Nicotine is a powerful reinforcing agent in both animals and humans. Behaviour studies in animals do indicate that nicotine reinforces self-administration, place preference and increases locomotion. The effects of nicotine on test reinforcement and behavioural sensitization are primarily mediated through the mesolimbic dopamine system. It activates the brain's mesolimbic dopamine system, particularly in nucleus accumbens, important in the development of dependence or addiction. The mesolimbocortical dopamine system consists of neurons with cell bodies localized in ventral tegmental area (VTA) and the axons projecting to the nucleus accumbens (NAc) and the medial prefrontal cortex (PFC), being referred to as mesolimbic and mesocortical projections respectively. Nicotine receptors concentrated in the VTA and NAc activate the mesolimbic dopamine system, responsible for reinforcing behaviour like stimulant and dependence producing properties of nicotine. Nicotine increases "burst activity", that is rapid sequential electrochemical spikes, as measured electrophysiologically in the ventral tegmental area (VTA) of the brain. Ventral tegmental area (VTA) is significant in nicotine's physiologic impact on motivation, learning and cognition. These bursts trigger a massive release of dopamine, as high as six times the baseline level. The consequent changes in the electrochemical brain activity are seen in attention and reward systems; thus nicotine mirrors the reward response of the mesolimbic dopamine system. In this way nicotine is similar to other dependence producing drugs such as amphetamines, cocaine, opiates and alcohol (Imperato, 1986). The VTA and its projections to NAc are involved in reward and mediate reinforcing actions of the drug abuse (Nestler, 1992).

Thus, the key brain chemical involved in mediating the desire to consume drug is the neurotransmitter dopamine. In the brain, nicotine stimulates the release of the dopamine in the pleasure circuit. This stimulation relates to the dopaminergic system of brain that include the mesolimbic, nucleus accumbens (NAc) and nigrostriatal system. Nicotine increases the extracellular level of dopamine in direct receptor mediated action on nerve terminals. Chronic administration of nicotine can result in increased density of nicotine acetylcholine receptors (nAChRs) in the brain, which occurs before measurable tolerance is developed. nAChRs are associated with the reinforcing properties of nicotine because of their mediation of nicotine induced effects in the brain's reward system. Chronic exposure to nicotine results in changes in at least one subtype of nicotine acetylcholine receptors (Perry, Devila-Garcia and Stockmeir, 1999).

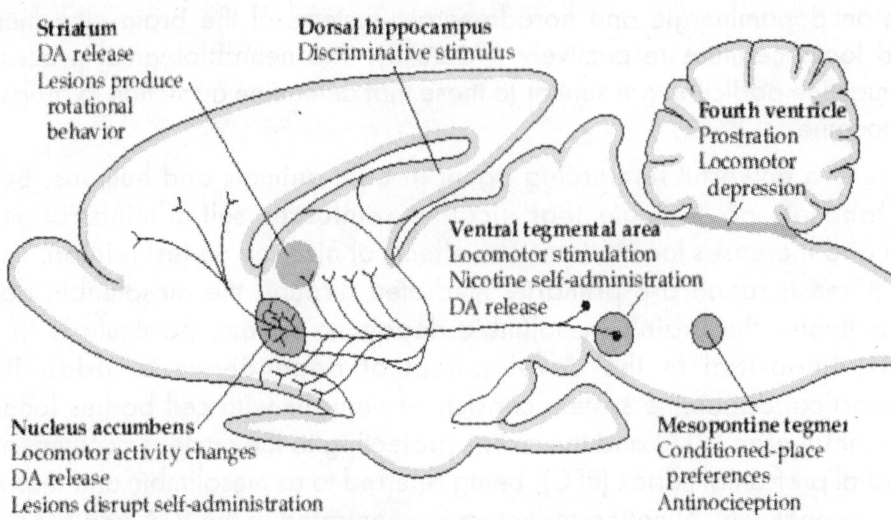


*Figure: 5 Brain regions and pathways in the behavioural and neurochemical effects of nicotine brain regions and pathways of nicotine*

Local injection of nicotine or nicotine agonist into the VTA can result in increased locomotion (Mifsud *et al.*, 1989; and Shoab *et al.*, 1994). The strongest effects of nicotine appear to be on dopamine cell bodies of the VTA. Injection of nicotine agonist locally into the dopamine terminal fields of NAc stimulates dopamine release (Risinger and Oakes, 1995) or locomotor activity (Cox, Goldstein and Nelson, 1984) indicating that nicotine receptors on the dopamine terminals are involved in mediating the actions of nicotine. Lesions of mesolimbic dopamine neurons attenuate nicotine self-administration in rats (Leikola-Pelho and Jackson, 1992). It also attenuates the locomotor stimulant effect of the systematically administered nicotine (Museo and Wise, 1994). Researchers have discovered using the microanalysis method which allows minute quantities of neurotransmitter to be measured in precise brain area that nicotine causes an increase in release of dopamine in the nucleus accumbens (NAc). Such a release also occurs with other drugs of abuse such as heroin and cocaine, and is thought to underline the pleasurable sensation experienced by many smokers.

Cravings are thought to occur as a result of sensitized responses. The decline in dopamine levels that result from nicotine deprivation between cigarettes or following smoking cessation may play a part in the developments of cravings.

## 2. Other Biological Theories Related to Addiction to Nicotine

Nicotine provides its central effects through nAChRs. The cholinergic receptors are relatively large consisting of several components called subunits (alfa2-alfa10 and beta2-beta10) which play central role in autonomic transmission. Different combinations of these subunits make different types of receptors which vary in terms of affinity and localization within the brain. One of these subunits, the beta subunit plays an important role in nicotine addiction. The alfa4-beta2 subunit combination has greater sensitivity to nicotine. Researchers have produced a new strain of mice devoid of gene that produces beta subunit – known as "knock out mice" (Picciotto *et al.*, 1998). These knock out mice were found not to self-administer nicotine unlike others who had intact beta subunit. Beta-subunit plays a critical role in mediating the pleasurable effects of nicotine.

Repeated tobacco smoke inhalation generates nicotine boli delivered into the brain superimposed on a relatively stable nicotine plasma level maintained throughout the smoking day. This basal level will keep some of the nAChRs desensitized while remaining nAChRs are available for activation by nicotine boli, if appropriate concentrations are achieved. This explains how smokers manipulate their plasma nicotine profile to achieve balance desensitization versus activation. That is why the first cigarette of the day is most satisfying, as the overnight abstinence allows a substantial recovery from nAChRs desensitization. This further suggests that when a smoker is asleep, plasma level of nicotine is decreased and nicotine receptors can gradually recover their active functional state (up regulation) and this might contribute to the development of withdrawal symptoms and craving.

Moreover it is well established that the number of [3H] nicotine binding sites (nAChRs) are increased in the brain of smokers examined post-mortem (Benwell, Balfour and Anderson, 1988 and Breese *et al.*, 1997) and in the brain of rodents given nicotine for few days (Wonnacott, 1990). The alfa4-beta2 nAChR is more prone to inactivation than alfa3-beta2 nAChR (Kuryatov *et al.*, 2000).

The interaction between nicotine and GABAergic system has recently been discovered. Electrophysiological studies demonstrate that nicotine agonists stimulate the release of GABA from rodent brain tissue and this release was $Ca^{2+}$ dependent (Lu *et al.*, 1998 and Zhu and Chiappinelli, 1999). Actions of nicotine on ventral tegmental GABAergic interneuron, which modulate the mesolimbic dopamine excitability, have been studied (Yin and French, 2000). Using extra-cellular recording techniques in rat brain slices, nicotine was found to increase the firing rate of dopamine and non-dopamine neurons while former was more vigorous. These results suggest that nicotine stimulates the firing rate of dopaminergic neurons of VTA and GABAergic neurons which may be an important target for the effects of nicotine on central nervous system.

Acute nicotine administration stimulates the release of noradrenalin (NA) in the different parts of the brain, and nicotine acts primarily at locus ceruleus level (Fu *et al.*, 1998). Moreover, it is also found that in the hippocampus, maximum desensitization of nicotine stimulated NA occurs as early as 40 minutes and persists for at least 100 minutes; therefore, desensitization becomes the dominant process (Fu, Matta, Valentine *et al.*, 1998).

Tobacco smoking and chronic nicotine administration decreases the concentration of 5-HT because smoking is associated with selective increase in the density of 5-$HT_{1A}$ receptors in this area. There is evidence that hippocampus receives serotonergic innervation from the median raphe nucleus. Supression of 5-HT release in this part of hippocampus brings about anxiolytic response to nicotine when given locally by microinjection into the dorsal hippocampus (Quagazzal *et al.*, 1999). The effects of nicotine on 5-HT are difficult to dissociate from those on dopamine neurons. Increased exposure to stressful stimuli is likely to increase the desire to smoke as reported by smokers (Pomerleau and Pomerleau, 1987). The effects of nicotine withdrawal on dopamine release in the brain may be exacerbated by exposure to stressful stimuli and may underlie the role of stress as a factor in tobacco smoking, as well as the role of nicotine on reducing the effects by acting on 5-HT neurons within the hippocampus. Currently, there is little evidence of involvement of serotonergic system in positive reinforcing effects of nicotine, but there is some evidence that this system might be involved in the negative reinforcing effects of nicotine withdrawal. However, smoking results in increased platelet serotonin receptor density, which increases binding of fibrinogen receptors (Markowitz, Tolbert and Winders, 1999).

A recent study suggests that cotinine stimulates nicotine receptors to evoke the release of dopamine (DA) in a calcium-dependent manner from super fused rat striatal slices (Dwoskin *et al.*, 1999).

Nicotine's electrophysiological effects on the brain are relatively lateralized and localized and that it affects the central nervous system at large. During stressful or high-arousal conditions, nicotine appears to reduce right-hemisphere processing more than the left-hemisphere processing. Nicotine appears to activate left hemisphere more than the right in the highly engaging vigilance tasks (Hasenfratz and Batting, 1992). The laterality of nicotine's effects is thus believed to vary by situation as well as to be affected by a variety of behaviours and personality traits.

Nicotine administration to animals and humans produces altered spontaneous electroencephalogram (EEG) —there are signs of electroencephalographic activation such as increased beta power, decreased alfa and theta power, and increased alfa frequency, evoked brain electrical potentials, and local cerebral glucose metabolism, increased adrenal hormone release (including adrenocorticotropic hormone, beta-endorphin, beta-lipotropin, growth hormone, vasopressin, and neurophysin), increased heart rate, and caused changes in skeletal muscle tension (Pickworth: Herning and Henningfield, 1989). Most of these effects are related to the dose of nicotine, and tolerance develops to differing degree across effects.

Specific elements of the striatopallidal and extended amygdale systems may mediate the acute reinforcing action of nicotine (Koob, 1999). Chronic use results in dysregulation of brain's reward system, characterized by decreased reward function. Withdrawal raises threshold for reward. Decrease in dopamine and serotonin neurotransmission in the nucleus accumbens (NAc) and increase in corticotrophin-related factor (brain-stress neurotransmitter) could mediate such changes. These factors may help explain the compulsive seeking and self-administration of nicotine. In experimental animals, nicotine is shown to increase the release of stress-induced serotonin through the stimulation of nicotine acetylcholine receptors (Takahashi, Takada and Nagai, 1998).

Positron Tomographic (PET) studies reveal that cigarette smoking causes a marked decrease in the levels of an important enzyme, monoamine oxidase (MAO), responsible for breakdown of dopamine. The decrease in its two forms— MAO-A and MAO-B, results in increased dopamine levels. Although nicotine causes increased brain dopamine, nicotine itself does not alter MAO levels. It affects dopamine through other mechanisms which point towards the possibility of another component of cigarette smoke other than nicotine may be inhibiting the MAO. There may be multiple ways by which smoking alters the neurotransmitter dopamine to ultimately produce feeling of pleasure and reward (Cao *et al.*, 1993; Brioni *et al.*, 1993 and Volkow *et al.*, 1999).

CYP2A6 is an enzyme responsible for the majority of inactivation of nicotine in humans; it is also responsible for activating tobacco related procarcinogens such as the nitrosamines. A common genetic defect in nicotine metabolism decreases smoking. Genetic variation in CYP2A6 gene may protect individuals from becoming nicotine-dependent smokers. Mimicking this gene defect by inhibiting CYP2A6 one can decrease nicotine metabolism (Tyndale *et al.*, 1999). Cigarette smoking like other behaviours shows evidence of heterogeneity. Dopamine transporter (DAT) gene (SLC6A3) encodes protein that regulates the synthetic levels of dopamine in the brain and leads to addictive behaviour (Vandenbergh *et al.*, 2002). It is expected that recent advances in molecular biology, including the completion of draft sequence of the human genome may help in identifying gene markers that predict a heightened risk of using tobacco to increase our understanding of nicotine dependence (Hall *et al.*, 2002).

## Principal Studies

### *1. Learning and Memory*

Nicotine enhances cognition and improves learning or performance (Clarke and Fibiger 1987). In recent studies, nicotine has been shown to produce a sort of place performance in rats and mice (Rose *et al.*, 2001 and Berlin and Antenelli, 2001). The self-administration of nicotine has also been demonstrated in rats (Corrigall and Coen 1989 and Costall *et al.*, 1989) and mice (Levin, 1992). Nicotine and nicotine agonists improve performance in a variety of cognitive tasks by animals with basal forebrain lesion (Levin *et al.*, 1992). Chronic nicotine intake affects attention and working memory in rodents. Nicotine enhances acquisition of spatial radial maze and water maze tasks in normal animals. Rats treated with chronic nicotine for a week and then stopped it also showed enhanced acquisition of tasks as compared to the controls (Singer, Wallace and Hall, 1982).

### 2. *Tolerance and Dependence*

Animal studies include studies of withdrawal signs upon cessation of chronic nicotine administration (Hildebrand *et al.,* 1997) and studies of onset and persistence of nicotine self-administration (Donny *et al.,* 2000). Wonnacott (1990) suggests that chronic exposure to nicotine increases high affinity binding of nicotinic agonists to brain tissue and induces chronic tolerance to many of drug's behavioural and physiological effects. The increase in receptor number (up regulation) has been interpreted as compensation for agonist induced desensitization of nAChRs and this proposed desensitization has been proposed as a mechanism to chronic tolerance to nicotine (Robinson, Marks and Collins, 1996). The effects of acute and chronic nicotine administration on locomotor activity have been studied. Nicotine administration in experimentally naïve rats can depress locomotor activity, an effect to which acute and chronic tolerance can develop. In a conditioned taste aversion paradigm, rat learns to avoid consuming distinctly flavoured solutions that have previously paired with nicotine solutions. In rats exposed to test apparatus, nicotine produces moderate increase in activity and with repeated exposure to the drug, sensitization occurs. Effects of selective dopaminergic drugs in nicotine tolerance have also been studied and the result suggests that tolerance to nicotine may be mediated through dopaminergic system (Jain Varma and Mohan, 2001).

Nicotine affects much more than brain functions related to concentration, alertness, arousal etc. Nicotine's half life of 2–4 hours keeps nicotine present and active for 6–8 hours in a typical tobacco user. Nicotine acts on sympathetic nervous system, resulting in constriction of some blood vessels, an increased heart rate, a moderate increase in blood pressure and an increase in myocardial contractility. Nicotine increases heart's workload while constricting coronary blood vessels, a condition that presages ischaemic events. Chronic exposure to nicotine results in the development of tolerance to nicotine's cardiovascular effects, but such tolerance is never sufficiently complete, thus allowing cardiovascular damage to occur even with the development of tolerance.

Nicotine has a demonstrable effect on performance of cognitive tasks. Nicotine agonists can also facilitate performance. Nicotine influences working memory, though not necessarily other types of memory. Unlike other effects of nicotine, memory improvement does not exhibit any signs of tolerance. Nicotine facilitates synaptic activity in the hippocampus of the brain, long known as an important structure associated with memory functions. Nicotine interacts with several neurotransmitter systems that constitute the neural basis of cognition. Nicotine induces the release of various neurotransmitters, including acetylcholine, dopamine, serotonin, norepinephrine and glutamate, and may have some association with other systems, including the aminobutyric acid, opioid and histaminergic systems.

## Nicotine Addiction and Withdrawal

Withdrawal is an important component of the addiction process. Cessation of tobacco consumption after long-term use, like with other drugs of abuse, usually results in withdrawal symptoms (Hughes and Hatsukami, 1986). Decrease in exposure to nicotine, whether from total abstinence or merely cutting back on tobacco consumption, results in a constellation of symptoms that vary considerably among individuals but usually involve marked effects and can be unpleasant and distressing. The DSM-IV criteria for nicotine withdrawal are listed in table 3. In addition to these symptoms, craving for tobacco, a desire for sweets, increased coughing, and impaired performance on vigilance tasks may occur (Hughes, Huggins and Hatsukami 1990 and Hughes and Hatsukami, 1992). Withdrawal symptoms begin within a few hours and peak 24–48 hours after cessation (Hughes and Hatsukami, 1992). In most cases, these symptoms begin within 12 hours of cessation of smoking, peak within a few hours, and persist for several weeks (Hughes, 1994). Individual experiences most severe symptoms during first three days of abstinence. Symptoms and effects of nicotine abstinence peak within 1–2 weeks and persist for as long as 3–4 weeks. More than 40% smokers, who quit smoking, report experiencing withdrawal symptoms for more than 4 weeks. Most symptoms last an average of 4 weeks, but hunger and craving can last 6 months or more (Hughes and Hatsukami, 1992). Nicotine withdrawal symptoms are due, in large part, to nicotine deprivation. Cessation of smoking can cause slowing on EEG, decreases in cortisol and catecholamine levels, sleep EEG changes and a decline in metabolic rate (Hughes, Huggins and Hatsukami, 1990).

Symptoms typically include: Nicotine craving, anxiety, irritability, impatience, difficulty in concentrating, headache, dizziness, insomnia or other sleep disturbances, digestive disturbances, hunger, depressed mood, heart palpitation, sweating, tremours, restlessness.

*Table 3: The characteristic withdrawal*

A. Daily use of nicotine for at least several weeks.

B. Abrupt cessation or reduction of nicotine use, followed within 24 hours by four or more of:

1. Dysphoric or depressed mood
2. Insomnia
3. Irritability, frustration or anger
4. Anxiety
5. Difficulty concentrating
6. Restlessness
7. Decreased heart rate
8. Increased appetite or weight gain

C. The above symptoms cause clinically sufficient distress or impairment in social, occupational or other important areas of functioning.

D. The symptoms are not due to a general medical condition and are not better accounted for by another mental disorder.

** As identified by the Diagnostic and Statistical Manual (DSM-IV)*

It is typical for symptoms to change over the course of time, with symptoms replacing others that were less prominent at the onset of the abstinence. Overall, tobacco abstinence in nicotine-dependent individuals entails experiencing a substantial number of withdrawal symptoms, some of which have the potential to adversely affect occupational and social functioning (Sommese and Patterson, 1995). Some tobacco users routinely achieve some cognitive and affective stabilization or enhancement through exposure to nicotine (Gilbert, 1995); these effects diminish as tobacco exposure is reduced. It may take at least several weeks for some former user of tobacco to attain cognitive and affective stasis in the absence of nicotine. Therefore, a tobacco user who attempts to quit without substantial nicotine replacement is likely not only to experience abstinence symptoms but also to lose stabilizing and enhancing effects of nicotine. Additionally, evidence indicates that nicotine-dependent smokers metabolize certain other substances, including caffeine and alcohol, differently for a period of time after initial cessation (Swanson, Lee and Hopp, 1994). The toxicity from other substances adds to the potential for temporarily impaired cognitive, affective and performance related functions. Withdrawal symptoms due to tobacco abstinence increase occupational accident risk (Waters, Jarvis and Sutton, 1998). Regular smokers experience deterioration in mood and performance within a few hours of abstinence (Snyder, Davis and Henningfiels, 1989). Findings of 'No Smoking Day' data indicate the increase in the number of accidents on this day (West and Russell, 1985). Nicotine deprived smokers experience decreased efficiency in reaction time and overall vigilance. Nicotine administration can reverse performance deficit in nicotine-deprived, tobacco-dependent smokers (Parrott and Craig, 1992).

Symptoms of nicotine toxicity, otherwise known as acute nicotine poisoning, include nausea, vomiting, salivation, pallor, abdominal pain, diarrhea, and cold sweat.

## Common Features Between Nicotine and Other Drugs of Abuse

Nicotine addiction, like other drug addictions, is fundamentally a neurobiologically-mediated brain disorder. The drug addicted brain is structurally and functionally different from the non-addicted brain, and these changes are an important part of the addiction itself. Nicotine addiction is related to the effects of nicotine on dopaminergic and noradrenergic systems in the brain – the mesolimbic system and locus ceruleus, respectively.

The effect of nicotine is faster than that of heroin. A common feature that nicotine shares with non-psychostimulant drugs such as narcotic analgesic, delta-9-hydrocannabinol and ethanol, is the ability of stimulating dopamine transmission preferentially in the shell of nucleus accumbens by activating dopamine neurons that project to this area (Picciotto, 1998). Psychostimulant drugs such as amphetamines, cocaine and phencyclidine preferentially stimulate dopamine transmission in the shell, but reduce the firing activity of dopamine neurons as a result of an interference with the dopamine reuptake carrier, leading to accumulation of dopamine extracellularly and stimulation of dopamine autoreceptors. Nicotine dependence resembles nonpsychostimulant drugs with regards to its dopamine stimulating property upon an endogenous tone on u-opioid receptors and 5-HT$^3$-receptors.

Nicotine addiction, like addiction to other drugs of abuse, is likely to be the result of molecular changes in the brain area that mediate reinforcement. Nicotine withdrawal has been shown to result in changes in firing pattern of VTA neurons, implying that adaptation takes place in mesolimbic dopamine neurons following chronic treatment (Rasmussen and Czachura, 1995). Many drugs of abuse such as cocaine, morphine and ethanol alter the mRNA levels, protein or activity of tyrosine hydroxylase (TH) in the mesolimbic dopamine system. Like acute cocaine administration, acute administration of nicotine increases TH activity in NAc (Smith, Mitchell, and Joseph, 1991). In addition, chronic administration of nicotine can increase TH, mRNA levels and activity in locus ceruleus. That has been reported following chronic morphine treatment (Guitart *et al.*, 1990). These changes in activity and levels of the rate-limited biosynthetic enzyme for catecholamines are likely to be common markers for the development of dependence for these drugs of abuse.

Self-administration of either nicotine or cocaine results in increased expression of chronic fos-related antigens (fras) in the NAc, the prefrontal cortex and the medial caudate (Merlo-Pich *et al.*, 1997). The common biochemical response to nicotine or cocaine suggests that the similar mechanisms may be involved in the development of dependence to these different drugs of abuse. Repeated exposure to nicotine induces adaptive changes such as tolerance, and sensitization, in the level of dopamine in the shell and in the core of the nucleus accumbens that resemble those of other drugs of abuse.

Activation of the mesolimbic system, resulting in a surge of dopamine in the nucleus accumbens (NAc) – thought to induce positive mood effects (i.e. feeling of pleasure or elation) that become associated with nicotine administration. The rapid action of inhaled nicotine on this 'reward' pathway provides immediate positive reinforcement. The smoker is motivated to repeat the behaviour, leading to compulsive use of the drug. Chronic nicotine administration produces tolerance (as evidenced by changes in the sensitivity and abundance of nicotine receptors) so that a certain level of nicotine in the brain becomes necessary to maintain normal function and smokers need to smoke more to achieve the same effects. At this stage, it is no more a matter of personal choice to abstain from tobacco than to reverse metastatizing lung cells. After several weeks of nicotine exposure physical dependence on nicotine develops the cellular and neurological adaptations that produce tolerance also lead to physical dependence. In fact, compared to non-smokers, the cigarette smoker has an elevated pulse, elevated circulating catecholamines, lower bodyweight, and increased receptor binding sites (Benwell, Balfour and Anderson, 1988). Such increases in brain receptors may affect the smoker's subsequent risk for neuropsychiatric disorders.

Like other addictions, nicotine dependence results in compulsive use of the drug, tolerance to its effects, a characteristic withdrawal syndrome, and inability to control use despite negative consequences. However, nicotine dependence has several unique features.

## Biphasic Action

Nicotine's action at the synapse is one of the reasons for the biphasic effects of nicotine. The initial combination of nicotine with the acetylcholine receptor at first stimulates an acetylcholine-like response, but the fixity of drug/receptor combination then blocks any further response. The degree of stimulation versus block depends on the amount of nicotine present relative to the number of available acetylcholine receptors in general, small doses of nicotine produce a predominantly stimulant effect, at synapse larger doses produce a mainly depressant effect, while the effect of lethal dose is to block nervous transmission altogether. For example, in the complex neural circuit involved in breathing, small doses of nicotine stimulate respiration; larger doses of nicotine depress respiration, while a nicotine overdose causes complete arrest of respiration. This is the reason, nicotine's cardio-vascular and neurotransmitter effects do not follow a positive linear dose-response pattern. A high dose of nicotine, therefore, is not necessarily proportionally more toxic than a low dose, and a low dose can be associated with adverse effects. The intensity of nicotine's effects depends upon the rate of delivery. This is why the rapid delivery of nicotine through cigarettes is desirable to smokers, because it results in higher arterial levels of nicotine (Benowitz, 1998). Nicotine administration elicits "biphasic response" in humans and laboratory animals. In the human body, low doses of nicotine produce an arousal response, with heightened vigilance and attention. Smokers can adjust the speed with which nicotine is delivered to the brain and thus can adjust the psychological effects. The extent of the dose interacts with the rate of delivery and the preexisting baseline condition to determine the overall magnitude and direction of the nicotine's effects. A cigarette smoker controls the dose and delivery rate of nicotine with each puff; consequently, it is not sufficient merely to count puffs when determining nicotine exposure. Rather the volume of each puff, the depth to which smoke is inhaled, and the rate and intensity of puffing are all aspects of smoking topography that must be analysed in order to accurately characterize the way nicotine is taken into the body through cigarette smoke.

Nicotine penetrates the nerve tissue and briefly concentrates into the brain cells. So nicotine is able to combine with acetylcholine receptors and stimulate acetylcholine as a neurotransmitter, it blocks acetylcholine and briefly concentrates in the nerve cells. Combination of these three features provides basic mechanism by which nicotine exerts its widespread effects.

Psychoactive effects of nicotine are also related to its absorption and titration, which depend to a great extent on the nature of the delivery system. Smokers vary nicotine levels, and presumably also vary the psychoactive impact of nicotine, by varying the intensity and rapidity of their inhalation of tobacco smoke (Russell, Jarvis and Iyer, 1980).

## Characteristics of Cigarette Smoking Behaviour

The process of cigarette smoking involves a complex series of events. Even the act of taking a single puff is complex. Typically, a smoker puffs a volume of smoke into the mouth, where it is held for a short period of time (McBride *et al.*, 1984). The post-puff inhalation is generally longer and larger in volume than normal inspiration. After a variable period of breath holding, the smoker exhales, usually through the mouth. The duration and volume of puffing are generally highly correlated although they vary somewhat from smoker to smoker (Adam *et al.*, 1983). Peak smoke flow rate has been reported to be moderately correlated with puff duration (Gritz, Rose and Jarvik, 1983). Puff per cigarette and puff duration has been found to be inversely related (Lichtenstein and Anlonuccio, 1981).

Carbon monoxide (CO) intake (measured either from expired air or blood sample) also tends to be positively related to measures of smoking behaviour, including total puff volume (Gust and Pickens, 1982) and mean puff volume (Zacny *et al.*, 1987). These findings illustrate that specific aspects of smoking behaviour can affect absorption of smoke constituents.

**Puffing and Inhaling Pattern**

During smoking of a single cigarette, the duration of each puff tends to decrease and time duration between two puffs tends to increase (Graham *et al.*, 1963). The nicotine concentration of smoke increases as the cigarette is smoked (Kozlowski, 1981).

## Dose Related Determinants of Tobacco Intake

Cigarette smoking is a complex but orderly behaviour. The behaviour characteristics include:

***Self-administration*** determines the amount of tobacco smoked and the time when dose is required.

Unlike most other forms of drug-delivery, the control and measurement of ***cigarette dose level*** *is complex*. In other drugs such as opioids and alcohol precise amount of constituents can be measured. But CO, tar and nicotine can vary in level in tobacco smoke. The total smoke dose is positively related to the number of puffs taken per cigarette.

***Smoke concentration delivered*** to the lungs can be changed by diluting with air. One way to study the possible effects of smoke dilution is to use ventilated cigarette holders. This can help quit smoking when the smoker gradually reduces the level of dependence to nicotine by using holders of gradually increasing ventilation level.

If cigarette is shorter in ***length***, people smoke more cigarettes (Jarvik *et al.*, 1978), length also determines how people smoke each cigarette. Smokers shorten their intervals between puffs and spend greater proportion of their time puffing on a smaller cigarette, smoker takes relatively more puffs and leave shorter butts. Puff duration and puff volume are inversely proportional to the length of tobacco rod even for the first puff of the cigarette (Nemeth, Coselett, and Griffiths, 1984). Smokers often switch to lower tar/nicotine yielding cigarette brands in order to reduce their exposure to toxins and to reduce their level of nicotine dependence. The number of cigarettes smoked per day is only slightly increased when lower nicotine yield cigarette brands to reduce their exposure to tobacco constituents and to gradually reduce their dependence.

Rate of renal nicotine ***excretion*** is partially determined by the acidity of urine, lower pH value (higher acidity) increase the rate of excretion. There is a direct relationship between rate of nicotine excretion and cigarette smoking suggesting that the alkaline diets may be useful for the persons trying to decrease their cigarette smoking (Grunberg and Kozlowski, 1986).

***The drugs that block the effects of nicotine*** on the nervous system are nicotine antagonists:

(i) Those drugs which do not readily enter the brain but are active in the peripheral nervous system, they are ganglion blockers, such as – Pentolinium, Hexamethonium.

(ii) Those drugs which do enter the brain and thus work in both peripheral and central nervous system (Taylor, 1985) such as mecamylamine.

Smoking is also affected by the ***chemicals*** which act on respiratory tract and not on the nervous system. The region of the respiratory tract just below the larynx is assumed to be a site of some cigarette smoke related sensations (Cain, 1980). This site corresponds to the region 2 cm. below the narrow opening of the larynx where particles entering the trachea change direction (Chan and Schreck, 1980).

***Tar and volatile gases*** present in the cigarette smoke contribute to the taste, olfactory and trachea-bronchial sensations elicited by cigarette smoke.

Besides its causal role in lung cancer and other diseases, tar may function to mask the harshness and irritation of nicotine (Herskovic, Rose and Jarvik, 1986). Consistent with this hypothesis, nicotine aerosol delivering devices of nicotine similar to those in mainstream cigarette smoke are rated as extremely harsh and irritating by cigarette smokers (Russell 1986). Similarly, some gaseous components of smoke, such as acrolein and formaldehyde, are irritating and could also contribute to the trachea-bronchial sensations elicited by smoke (Lundberg *et al.,* 1983).

Natural history and course of tobacco use make it evident that tobacco is often used in combination of other substances. The initiation function on many levels, influencing the effects of tobacco use on health risks, medical treatment and metabolism of other substances. Drugs whose effects can be altered by nicotine include theophylline, caffine, tacrine, imipramine, haloperidol, pentazocine, propranolol, flecanide, estradiole, heparine, insulin, s-blockers, benzodiazepines, ethanol, and opioids (Zevin and Benowitz, 1999).

Nicotine serves as a major reinforcer both in humans and animals. It is a complex behavioural phenomenon comprising effects on several neural systems. Actions of nicotine on dopaminergic system increase dopaminergic activity and release, leading to nicotine induced reinforcement. Action of nicotine on many systems, including brain-stem, cholinergic, GABAergic, noradrenergic, and serotonergic nuclei, may also help to mediate nicotine effects related to nicotine addiction. The use of molecular genetic techniques along with beavioural analysis will help us in further understanding of nicotine addiction.

## REFERENCES


Adams L, Lee C, Rawbone R. and Guz A.: Patterns of smoking: Measurement and Variability in Asymptomatic Smokers, *Clinical Science* 65(4):383–392, 1983.

American Psychiatric Association, *Diagnostic and Statistical Manual of Mental Disorders* (fourth edition) Wasington DC American Psychiatric Association, 1994.

Ashton H. and Stepney R.: *Smoking: Psychology and Pharmacology*, Tavistock Publications, London, 1982.

Benowitz N.L.: ) Cardiovascular Toxicity of Nicotine: Pharmacokinetic and Pharmacodynamic Considerations. In: Benowitz NL., ed. *Nicotine Safety and toxicology.* Oxford University Press: New York NY, 19–27, 1998.

Benowitz N.L. and Jacob P. III.: Daily Intake of Nicotine During Cigarette Smoking. Clinical Pharmacology and Therapeutics, 35: 499–504, 1984.

Benowitz N.L., Porchet H., and Sheiner L.: Nicotine Absorption and Cardiovascular Effects with Smokeless Tobacco Use: Comparison with Cigarette and Nicotine Gum. *Clinical Pharmacology and Therapeutics*, 44, 23–28, 1988.

Benwell M.M., Blafour D.J. and Anderson J.M.: Evidence that Tobacco Smoke Increases the Density of (–)-[$^3$H] Nicotine Binding Sites in Human Brain. *Journal of Neurochemistry*, 50:1243–1247, 1988.

Berlin I and Antenelli RM: Monoamine Oxidase and Tobacco Smoking. *International Journal of Neuropsychopharmacology*, 4:33–42, 2001.

Bigelow GE., Rand CS., and Gross J.: Smoking Cessation and Response Among Cardiac patients. In: *Relapse and Recovery in Drug Abuse. NIDA Research Monograph* 72, Rockville, Maryland US Department of Health Human Services, 167:71, 1986.

Breese CR, Marks MJ: Logel J, Adam CF, Sullivan B, and Collin A.C.: Effect of Smoking History on [3H] Nicotine Binding in Human Post-mortem Brain. *Journal of Pharmacology and Experimental Therapeutics*. 282:7–13, 1997.

Brioni JD, O'Neill A: Kim DJB, and Decker M.W.: Nicotine Receptor Agonists' Exhibit Anxiolytic Like Effects on the Elevated Plus Maze Test. *European Journal of Pharmacology*, 238:1–8, 1993.

Cain W.S.: Sensory Attributes of Cigarette Smoking, In: Gori GB, Bock F (Eds) Banbury Report 3: *A Safe Cigarette*? Cold Spring Harbour Laboratory, New York, 239–249, 1980.

Cao W., Burkholder T., Wilkins I. and Collins A.C.: A Genetic Comparison of Behavioural Actions of Ethanol and Nicotine in the Mirrored Chamber. *Pharmacology, Biochemistry and Behaviour*, 54:803–809, 1993.

Chan TL. and Schreck R.M.: Effect of the Laryngeal Jet on Particle Deposition in Human Trachea and Upper Bronchial Airways, *Journal of Aerosol Science* 11(5/6): 447–459, 1980.

Clarke PBS and Fibiger H.C.: Apparent Absence of Nicotine–Induced Conditioned Place Preference in Rats. *Psychopharmacology*, 92(1): 84–88, 1987.

Clarke PBS and Pert A.: Autoradiographic Evidences for Nicotine Receptors in Nigrostriatal and Mesolombic Dopaminergic Neurons. *Brain Research*, 348:355–358, 2000.

Cohen C., Pickworth W. B. and Henningfield J.E.: Cigarette Smoking and Addiction, *Clinical Chest Medicine*, 12:701–710, 1991.

Collins A.C., Luo Y. and Marks M.J.: Sensitivity to Nicotine and Brain Nicotine Receptors are Altered by Chronic Nicotine and Mecmylamine Infusion. *Journal of Pharmacology and Experimental Therapeutics*, 271:125–133, 1994.

Corrigal W.A. and Coen K.M.: Nicotine Maintains Robust Self-administration in Rats in A Limited Access Schedulr. *Psychopharmacology*, 99: 473–479, 1989.

Costall B., Kelly ME, Nylor N.J. and Onaivi E.S.: The Action of Nicotine and Cocaine in A Mouse Model of Anxiety. *Pharmacology, Biochemistry and Behaviour*, 33:197–203, 1989.

Cox BM, Goldstein A. and Nelson W.T.: Nicotine Self-administration in Rats. *British Journal of Pharmacplogy*, 83:49–55, 1984.

Donny E.C., Caggiula A.R., Rowett P.P., Ghurib M.A., Maldovan V. and Booth S.: Differential Effects of Reference-contingent and Response Independent Nicotine in Rats. *European Journal of Pharmacology*.402:321–240, 2000.

Dwoskin L.P., Teng L., Buxton S.T. and Crooks P.A.: (S)-(-)- Cotinine the Major Nicotine Metabolite of Nicotine, Stimulates Nicotine Receptors to Evoke [3h] Dopamine Release From Rat Striatal Slices in A Calcium Dependent Manner. *Journal of Pharmacology and Experimental Therapeutics*, 288–905–911, 1999.

Epping-jordan M.P., Watkin S.S., Koob G.F. and Markou A.: A Dramatic Decrease in Brain Reward Function During Nicotine Withdrawal, *Nature*, 393:76–79, 1998.

Fagerstrom K.O.: Measuring Physical Dependence to Tobacco Smoking with Reference to Individualization of Treatment. *Addictive Behaviour*, 3(3/4): 235–241, 1978.

Ferry L.H., and Burchette R.J.: Efficacy of Bupropion for Smoking Cessation in Nondepressed Smokers. *Journal of Addictive Disorders*, 13:9a, 1994.

FU Y., Matta S.G., James T.J. and Sharp B.M.: Nicotine Induced Nrepinephrine Release in Rat Amygdale and Hippocampus Is Mediated Through Brain-stem Cholinergic Receptors. *Journal of Pharmacology and Experimental Therapeutics*.284:1188–1196, 1998.

FU Y., Matta S.G., Valentine J.D. and Sharp B.M.: Desensitization and Resensitization of Epinephrine Release in The Rat Hippocampus with Repeated Nicotine Administration. *Neurosciences*, 241:147–150, 1998.

George T.P., Vernico C.D., Picciotto MR and Roth RH. Nicotine Modulation of Mesofrontal Dopamine Neurons: Pharmacologic and Neuroanatomic Characterization. *Journal of Pharmacology and Experimental Therapeutics*, 295:58–66, 2000.

Gilbert D.G.: *Smoking: Individual Differences, Psychopathology, and Emotion*, *Taylor and Francis*, Washington DC, 1995.

Graham S., Crouch S., Levin M.L. and Bock F.G.: Variations in Amounts of Tobacco Tar Reprieved From Selected Models of Smoking Behaviour Simulated by Smoking Machine. *Cancer Research*, 23:1025–1030, 1963.

Griffths R.R. and Henningfield J.E.: Experimental Analysis of Human Cigarette Smoking. *Behaviour Federation Proceedings*, 40(2): 234–240, 1982.

Gritz Er, Rose J.E. and Jarvik M.E.: Regulation of Tobacco Smoke Intake with Paced Cigarette Presentation. *Pharmacology, Biochemistry and Behaviour*, 18(3):457–462, 1983.

Grunberg N.E. and Kozlowski L.T.: Alkaline Therapy as an Adjunct to Smoking Cessation Programmes. *International Journal of Biosocial Research*. 8(1): 43–52, 1986.

Guitart X., Hayward M., Niserbaum L.K., Beitner-johnson D.B., Haycock J.W. and Nestler E.J.: Identification of Marppp-58, A Morphine and Cyclic Amp Regulated Phosphoprotein of 58kda, As Tyroxine Hydroxylase: Evidence for Regulation of Its Expression by Chronic Morphine in Rat Locus Ceruleus. *Journal of Neurosciences*, 10:2649–2659, 1990.

Gust S.W. and Pickens R.W.: Does Cigarette Nicotine Yieldaffect Puff Volume? *Clinical Pharmacology and Therapeutics*, 3214):418–422, 1982.

Hall W., Madden P. and Lynskey M.: The Genetics of Tobacco Use: Findings and Policy Implications. *Tobacco Control*, 11:119–124, 2002.

Hasenfratz M. and Battig K.: Action Profiles of Smoking and Caffeine: Stroop Effect, Eeg and Peripheral Physiology. *Pharmacology, Biochemistry and Behaviour*, 42: 155–161, 1992.

Henningfield J.E.: Behavioural Pharmacology of Cigarette Smoking. In: Thompson T, Dews PB, Berret J.E. (Eds) Advances in Behavioural Pharmacology, Vol. 4. Academic Press: Orlando, 1984.

Herskovic, J.E., Rose J.E. and Jarvik M.E.: Cigarette Desirability and Nicotine Preference in Smokers. *Pharmacology, Biochemistry and Behaviour*.24 (2):171–175, 1986.

Hildebrand BE., Nomokos GG., Bondjers C., Nisell M. and Svensson T.H.: Behavioural Manifestations of Nicotine Abstinence in Rat: Peripheral Versus Central Mechanisms. *Psychopharmacology*, 129:348–356, 1997.

Himbury S. and West R.: Smoking Habit After Laryngectomy. *British Medical Journal*, 291:514–515, 1985.

Hoffman D. and Hoffman I.: The Changing Cigarette 1950–1995. *Journal of Toxicology and Environmental Health*, 50: 307–364, 1997.

Hughes J.R.: Nicotine Withdrawal, Dependence and Abuse in Dsm IV Sourcebook Vol. I Edited by Widiger TA, Frances AJ, Pincus HA, First MB, Ross R, Davis W. *American Psychiatric Association*, Washington Dc Pp109–116, 1994.

Hughes J.R.: Non-nicotine Therapies for Smoking Cessation. *Journal of Drug Development*, 6: 197–203, 1994.

Hughes J.R.: Smoking as a Drug Dependence: A Reply to Robinson and Pritchard. Psychopharmacology, 113:282–283, 1993.

Hughes JR. and Hatsukami D.K.: Signs and Symptoms of Tobacco Withdrawal. *Archives of General Psychiatry*, 43: 289–294, 1986.

Hughes J.R. and Hatsukami D.K.: The Nicotine Withdrawal Syndrome: A Brief Review and Update. International Journal of Smoking Cessation, 1:21–26, 1992.

Hughes J.R., Higgins ST and Hatsukami D.K.: Effects of Abstinence From Tobacco. In: Kpzlowski LT, Annis HM and Cappell HD, Eds. *Research Advances in Alcohol and Drug Problems*. Plenum Publishing Corporation, New York, 1990.

Hughes Jr, Higgins and Bickel W.K.: Nicotine Withdrawal Versus Other Drug Withdrawal Syndromes: Similarities and Differences. *Addiction*, 89: 1461–1470, 1994.

Imperato A., Mulas A. and D.I. Chiara G.: Nicotine Preferentially Stimulates Dopamine Release in The Limbic System of Freely Moving Rats. European *Journal of Pharmacology*, 132:337–338, 1986.

Jain R. and Mukherjee K.: Biological Basis of Nicotine Addiction. *Indian Journal of Phsarmacology*, 35:281–289, 2003.

Jain R., Varma S. and Mohan D.: Effects of Selective Dopaminergic Drugs in Nicotine Tolerant Rats. *Drug and Alcohol Dependence*, 63:72, 2001.

Jarvik Me, Popeh P, Schneider NG, Baer Weiss V, Gritz E.R.: Can Cigarette Size and Nicotine Content can Influence Smoking and Puffing Rates? *Psychopharmacology* 58(3):303–306, 1978.

Koob G.f.: The Role of The Striatopallidal and Extended Amygdala Systems in Drug Addiction. *Annals of New York Academy of Science*, 877: 445–460, 1999.

Kozlowski L.T. Tar and Nicotine Delivery of Cigarettes: What a Difference a Puff Makes. *Journal of the American Medical Association*. 245(2):158–159, 1981.

Kuryatov A., Olabe F., Choi C. and Lindstrom J.: Acetylcholone Receptor Extracellular Dopamine Determines Sensivity to Nicotine Induced Inactivation. *European Journal of Pharmacology*, 393:11–21, 2000

Leikola-pelho Tand Jackson D.M.: Prefrential Stimulation of Locomotor Activity by Ventral Tegmentum Microinjections of (–) Nicotine. *Pharmacology and Toxicology*, 70:P50–52, 1992.

Levin ED., Briggs SJ., Christopher Wc. and Rose J.E. Persistence of Chronic Nicotine Induced Cognitive Facilitation. *Behavioural and Neural Biology*, 58:152–156, 1992.

Levin E.D.: Nicotine Systems and Cognitive Functions. *Psychopharmacology*, 108:417–431, 1992.

Lichtenstein E. and Antonuccio D.O.: Dimensions of Smoking Behaviour. *Addictive Behaviour*, 6(4):365–367, 1981.

Lundberg J.M., Mastling C.R., Saria A., Folkers K., and Rosell S.: Cigarette Smoking Induces Airway Oedema Due Ton Activation of Capsaicin-sensitive Vagal Afferent and Substance P. Release. *Neurosciences* 10(4):1361–1368, 1983.

Lu Y., Grady S., Marks MJ., Picciotto M., Chaneux J.P., and Collins A.Cc.: Pharmacological Characteristiucs of Nicotine Receptor-stimulated Gaba Release From Mouse Brain Synaptosomes. *Journal of Pharmacology and Experimental Therapeutics*, 67:331–337, 1998.

Markovitz JH., Tolbert L. and Winders S.E.: Increased Serotonin Receptor Density and Platelet Gphb/Iiia Activation Among Smokers. *Arteriosclerosis, Thrombosis and Vascular Biology*, 19: 262–266, 1999.

Mcbride M.J., Gyatt A.R., Kirkham A.J.T., Gumming G.: Assessment of Smoking Behaviour and Ventilation of Cigarettes of Different Nicotine Yields. *Clinical Sciences*, 67(6):619–631, 1984.

Mcghee D.S., Heath M.J., Gelber S., and Devay R.: Nicotinic Enhancement of Fast Excitatory Synaptic Transmission in CNS by Presynaptic Receptors. *Science*, 269:1692–1696, 1995.

Merlo–Pich E, Paglius SR., Tessari M, Talaboy Ayer D., Hooft Van Huijsduijnen R and Chiamulera C.: Common Neural Substances for the Addictive Properties of Nicotine and Cocaine. *Science*, 275:83–86, 1997.

Mifsud J.C., Hemandez L and Hoebel B.G. Nicptine Infusion Into The Nucleus Accumbens Increases Synaptic Dopamine as Measured in Vivo Microdialysis. *Brain Research*, 478:365–367, 1989.

Museo E. and Wise R.A.: Place Preference Cionditioning with Ventral Tegmental Injections in Cysticine. Life Sciences, 55:1179–1186, 1994.

Nemeth-coslette R and Griffths R.: Determinants of Puff Duration. *Pharmacology, Biochemistry and Behaviour*, 21(6), 903–912, 1984.

Nestler E.: Molecular Mechanisms of Drug Addictions. *Journal of Neurosciences*, 12:2439–2450, 1992.

Parrott A.C. and Craig D.: Cigarette Smoking and Nicotine Gum: Effect on Four Visual Attention Tasks. *Neuropsychobiology*, 25: 34–43, 1992.

Perry DC, Davila-garcia Miand Stockmeir C.A.: Increased Nicotine Receptors in Brains from Smokers: Membrane Binding and Autoradiography Studies. *Journal of Pharmacology and Experimental Therapeutrics*, 289: 1545–1552, 1999.

Picciotto M.R.: Common Aspects of the Action of Nicotine and other Drugs of Abuse. *Drug and Alcohol Dependence*, 51:165–172, 1998.

Picciotto M.R., Caldarone B.J., King S.L. and Zacharion V.: Nicotine Receptors in The Brain: Links Between Molecular Biology and Behaviour. *Neuropsychopharmacology*, 22:451–456, 2000.

Picciotto M.R., Zoli M., Rimondini R., Lena C., Marubio L.M. and Pich E.M.: Acetylcholine Receptors Containing The Beta 2 Subunit Are Involved in The Reinforcing Properties of Nicotine. *Nature*, 391:173–177, 1998.

Pickworth W.B., Herning R.I. and Henningfield J.E.: Spontaneousd E.E.G. Changes During Tobacco Abstinence and Nicotine Substitution, *Journal of Pharmacology and Experimental Therapeutics*, 251:976–982, 1989.

Pidoplichko VI., Debiasi M., Williams J.T. and Dani J.A.: Nicotine Activates and Desensitizes Midbrain Dopamine Neurons. *Nature*, 390:401–404, 1997.

Pomerleau CS and Pomerleau O.F.: The Effect of Psychological Stressor on Cigarette Smoking and Subsequent Behavioural and Physiological Responses. *Psychophysiology*, 24:278–285, 1987.

Quagazzal A.M., Kenny P.J. and File S.E.: Modulation of Behaviours on Trials 1 and 2 in The Elevated Plus Maze Test of Anxiety After Systemic and Hippocampal Administration of Nicotine, *Psychopharmacology*, 144:54–60, 1999.

Rasmussen K. and Czachura J.F.: Nicotine Withdrawal Leads to Increased Firing Rates of Midbrain Dopamine Neurons. *Neuroreporter*, 380:347–351, 1995.

Risinger F.O. and Oakes P.A.: Nicotine Induced Place Preference and Conditioned Place Aversion in Mice. *Pharmacology, Biochemistry and Behaviour*, 51:457–461, 1995.

Robinson S.F. and Marks M.J. and Collins A.C.: Inbred Mouse Strains Vary in Oral Self-selection of Nicotine. *Psychopharmacology*, 124:332–339, 1996.

Rose JE, Behm FM, Ramsey C and Ritchie JC Jr: Pkatelet Monoamine Oxidase, Smoking Cessation and Tobacco Withdrawal Symptoms. *Nicotine, Tobacco Research*, 3:383–390, 2001.

Russell, M.A.H.: Tobacco Smoking and Nicotine Dependence. In: R.J. Bibbins *Et Al* (Eds) Research Advances in Alcohol and Drug Problems (Vol. 3) Wiley and Sons: New York, 1976.

Russell M.A.H.: Tobacco Smoking and Nicotine Dependence. Proceedings of the World Congress, Cambridge: Massachusetts Institute of *Study of Smoking Behaviour and Policy*. Pp 90–107, 1986.

Russell M.A., Jarvis M. and Iyer R.: Relation of Nicotine Yield of Cigarettes to Blood Nicotine Concentrations in Smokers. *British Medical Journal*, 280: 972–976, 1980.

Schuman L.M.: Patterns of Smoking Behaviour. in Jarvik ME, Cullen J.W., Grit ER, Vogt T.M., and West L.J. (Eds) Research on Smoking Behaviour, Nida Research Monograph 17. UD Department of Health Education and Welfare. Public Health Service, *Alcohol, Drug-abuse and Mental Health Administration* Nida, Dhew, Publication No. (Adh) 78–81,581 Pp36–66, 1977.

Shoab M., Stolerman I.P. and Kumar R.C. Nicotine Induced Place Preference Following Prior Nicotine Exposure in Rats. *Psychopharmacology*, 113:445–452, 1994.

Singer M, Wallace M and Hall R.: Effect of Dopaminergic Nucleus Accumbens Lesions on Acquisition of Schedule Induced Self Injection of Nicotine in The Rat. *Pharmacology, Biochemistry and Behaviour*, 17:579–581, 1982.

Smith KM, Mitchell SN and Joseph M.H.: Effects of Chronic and Subchronic Nicotine on Tyrosine Hydroxylase Activity in Non-adrenergic and Dopaminergic Neurons in The Rat Brain. *Journal of Neurochemistry*, 57:1750–1756, 1991.

Snyder FR, Davis Fc and Henningfield J.E. The Tobacco Withdrawal Syndrome: Performance Decrements Assessed on a Computerized Test Battery. *Drug and Alcohol Dependence*, 23:259–266, 1989.

Sommese T. and Patterson J.C. Acute Effects of Cigarette Smoking withdrawal: A Review of The Literature. *Aviation, Space and Environmental Medicine*, 66: 164–167, 1995.

Sutker Patricia: Drugs and Psychopathology: Research Issues 19. *National Institute of Drug Abuse Research* Maryland, 1977.

Swanson JA, Lee JW and Hopp J.W.: Caffein and Nicotine: A Review of Their Joint use and Possible Interactive Effects in Tobacco Withdrawal. *Addictive Behaviour*, 19: 229–256, 1994.

Takahashi H, Takada Y and Nagai N. Nicotine Increases Stress-induced Serotonin Release by Stimulating Nicotine Acetylcholine Receptor in Rat Stratum. *Synapse*, 28: 212–219, 1998.

Tylor P.: Cholionergic Agonists. In: Gillman AG, Goodman LS, Rall TW and Murad F (Eds) Goodman and Gillman's *The Pharmacological Basis of Therapeutics*. 7th Edition, Pp100–107, 1985.

Tyndale R.F., Pianezza M.L. and Sellers E.M.: A Common Genetic Defect in Nicotine Metabolism Decreases Risk for Dependence and Lowers Cigarette Consumption. *Nicotine and Tobacco Research* (Suppl. 2):63–67 and 69–70, 1999.

United States Department of Health and Human Services: The Health Consequences of Smoking: The Changing Cigarette. A Report of The Surgeon General. US Department of Health and Human Services, Public Health Service. Dhew Publication No (Phs) 81–50156, 1981.

United States Department of Health and Human Services: The Health Consequences of Using Smokeless Tobacco. *A Report of Advisory Committee of Surgeon General*. US Department of Health and Human Services, Public Health Service. National Institute of Health (Nih) Publication No 86–2874, 1986.

Vandenbergh D.J., Bennett C.J., Grant D., Strasser A.A., O'connor Rand Stauffer R.L.: Smoking Status and Human Dopamine Transporter Variable Number of Tandem Reports (VNTR) Polymorphism: Failure to Replicate and Finding That Never Smokers May Be Different. *Nicotine and Tobacco Research*, 4:333–340, 2002.

Volikow N.D., Fowler J.S., Ding Y.S., Wang G.J. and Gatley S.J.: Imaging the Neurochemistry of Nicotine Actions: Studies with Positron Emission Tomography. *Nicotine and Tobacco Research*, 1 (Suppl. 2): 127–132 and 139–140, 1999.

Waters A.J., Jarvis M.J. and Sutton S.R.: Nicotine Withdrawal and Accident Rates. *Nature*, 394: 137, 1998.

West R.J. and Russell M.A.H.: Effects of Withdrawal From Long-term Nicotine Gum Use. *Psychological Medicine*, 15:891–893, 1985.

Wonnacott S.: The Paradox of Nicotine Acvetylcholine Receptor Upregulation by Nicotine. *Trends in Pharmacological Science*, 11:216–219, 1990.

Wonnacott S. Drasdo A., Sandeerson R. and Rowell P.: Presynaptic Nicotine Receptors and Modulation of Transmission Release. In: Block G, Marsh J Editors. *The Biology of Nicotine Dependence*. Wiley: Chichester, 1990.

World Health Organization. *International Classification of Diseases and Health Related Problems* 10[th] Revision, Volume 1) Geneva, Who, 1992.

Yin R. and French E.D.: A Comparison of Effects of Nicotine on Dopamine and Norepinephrine Neurons in The Rat Ventral Tegmental Area: in Vitro Electrophysiological Study. *Brain Research Bulletin*. 51:507–514, 2000.

Zacny JP., Stitzer MC., Brown F.Z., Yingling J.Ee., Griffths R.R.: Human Cigarette Smoking: Effects of Puffs and Inhalation Parameterson Smoke Exposure. *Journal of Pharmacology and Experimental Therapeutics*, 240(2):554–564, 1987.

Zevin S. and Benowitz N.L.: Drug Interactions with Tobacco Smoking: an Update. *Clinical Pharmacokinetics*, 36: 425–438: 1999.

Zhu PJ and Chiappinelli V.A.: Nicotine modulates Evoked GAB Argec Transmission in the Brain. *Journal of Neurophysiology*. 82:304, 1999.

CHAPTER

# 6 People at Risk: Initiation and Maintenance of Tobacco Use

*Adolescents who begin smoking at a younger age are more likely to become regular smokers and less likely to quit smoking.*

— Breslau and Peterson, 1996 and Escobedo *et al.*, 1993.

The process of initiation of tobacco use in an individual is multi-factorial, linked to environmental and personal factors (Aghi *et al.*, 2001) which determine how and why a person has the first taste of tobacco, continues to use it and becomes regular user and dependent without even realizing that he got addicted to it. This process is the complex interplay of positive and negative factors which diminish or enhance the initiation and continuation of tobacco use. The long-term tobacco dependence has resulted primarily from the initiation of tobacco use during adolescence. The earlier the onset of tobacco smoking more severe the addiction is likely to be (Breslau and Peterson, 1996). Tobacco use primarily begins in early adolescence, typically by age 16, with almost all first use occurring by the time one attains the age of 18 years (Townsend, Riderick and Cooper, 1994). Youth risk behaviour survey reported cigarette, smokeless tobacco, and cigar use among 42.7% of US students in grade 9–12 and an increase in current cigarette smoking from 27.5% in 1991 to 36.45 in 1997. [1] It is expected that 75% of daily teenaged smokers will continue to smoke throughout adult life (Johnson *et al.*, 1992). Although some try their first cigarette as children, the majority of smokers start smoking in their teens. In most countries, where smoking is long established, few people start smoking after the age of 18 – 21 years[2]; however, in some countries such as China, prevalence is low during adolescence and increases during early adulthood (WHO, 1992). In India where tobacco is consumed in

---

1 Centres for Disease Control (CDC), 1998.

2 International Union against Cancer – A manual on tobacco and young people for the industrialized world. Geneva: UICC, 1990.

different forms, 50% of those who use smokeless tobacco tend to start before 10 years of age and 80% of the users start within first 20 years of their life (Gupta, 1996). These data predict that tobacco use will be a long-term addiction for many adolescents who start using it now. By age 17, 50% smokers have tried to quit and failed, two-third regret even having started smoking and 40% smokers want some form of treatment to get rid of smoking behaviour[3]. The median cessation age for those who started smoking as adolescents has been found to be 33 years and 37 years respectively for males and females. Thus, 50% of males may smoke for 16 years and 50% females for 20 years, based on a median age of smoking initiation of 16 to 17 years (Pierce and Gilpin, 1996). These data are the indicators of the severity of smoking initiation and maintenance in adolescence and the formidable challenges that the therapeutic and preventive interventions present. In a study, in 1996, it was estimated that unless current trends changed, some 30-40% of the 2.3 billion children and teenagers in the world would become smokers in early adult life (Peto *et al.*, 1996) and 250 million of these future smokers will be killed by tobacco smoking[4].

Initiation of tobacco smoking is complex (Conrad, Flay and Hill, 1992) with multiple factors which contribute in the onset of this behaviour. The psycho-social factors influencing the initiation of tobacco use vary from developed world to the developing nations, region to region and culture to culture. While there are numerous other factors that affect the initiation of smoking behaviour, genetics and nicotine metabolism could be other important contributory factors.

## Risk Factors for Smoking Initiation

Factors influencing the predilection for tobacco smoking can be classified as:

1. Biological:
   - i. Developmental and demographic such as age and gender
   - ii. Genetic and biochemical
2. Psychological
3. Social and Environmental

### 1. Biological

*(i) Developmental and Demographic factors*

*Developmental* aspects of adolescence include (a) establishing independence and autonomy, (b) forming a coherent self-identity and (c) adjusting to psycho-social changes associated with physical maturation (Franzkowiak, 1987). Smoking can become a way for adolescents to instantly become independent and mature while fitting in with peers who smoke (O'Neill *et al.*, 1983, Stone and Kristeller, 1992); therefore, among various socio-demographic factors influencing initiation of tobacco use, *age* is an important factor.

---

3 Center for Disease Control (CDC), 1994.

4 Tobacco Control fact sheet: Youth and Cigarette Smoking, 2004.

Initiation and prevalence of tobacco use among adolescents typically rise with increasing *age* (Botvin *et al.*, 1992 and Camp *et al.*, 1993). Adolescents who begin smoking at a younger age are more likely to become regular smokers (Escobedo *et al.*, 1993) and less likely to quit smoking (Breslau and Peterson, 1996).

*Gender*: Countries with Western cultural orientation such as England, New Zealand, and the United States have a higher prevalence of cigarette smoking among females (Aghi *et al.*, 1999; McNeill *et al.*, 1988; and Oakley, Brannen and Dodd, 1992) as compared to Eastern ones. In the Eastern countries such as China, Japan, Sri Lanka, and India, there is higher smoking prevalence among males (Ogawa *et al.*, 1988; Mendis, 1990; Gupta, 1996 and Zhu *et al.*, 1996). Studies reveal that Vietnamese boys have higher risk of current smoking than Vietnamese girls of these *ethnic/racial* groups (Wiecha, 1996). African-Americans have significantly lower levels of initiation and current smoking than Caucasians and Hispanics (Bachman *et al.*, 1991). In African-American smokers mechanism of smoking differs from that for Caucasians; in Caucasian adolescents smoking serves more of a social function because they are more strongly influenced by peer smoking (Headen *et al.*, 1991).

Women smokers consume fewer cigarettes than men do; prefer filter tipped, low tar and low nicotine brands; do not smoke 'roll your own cigarette'; inhale less deeply; and leave more cigarette un-smoked than men (Nicolaid-Bouman *et al.*, 1993). Since smoking-related diseases are quantitatively related to the dose of cigarette smoke measured in terms of packs of cigarettes per day, this further reduces the overall risk of smoking related diseases in women.

*(ii) Genetic and biochemical factors*

Individual differences in smoking behaviour are substantially heritable (Sabol *et al.*, 1999). The earliest studies found that genetic identity increases the similarity of the smoking pattern. In their study, Friberg and associates (1959) found 74% of identical twins and 50% of non-identical twins having the same smoking status. Subsequent studies confirmed these findings that the concordance rate in identical twins reared apart was as high as 79% (Shields, 1962), and a meta-analysis of the data from five studies, each involving more than 1,000 twin pairs, showed an estimated heritability of 60% for the propensity to smoke (Heath and Madden, 1995). Twin studies have also shown that one's predilection for starting and/or quitting smoking are independent genes (Hamer, 2000) but partially overlapping (Heath and Martin 1993). The risk factors that may be related to inheritance are (a) vulnerability to nicotine addiction secondary to nicotine receptor genes, and (b) genes to determine personality.

*Personality traits* such as anxiety, depression, irritability, impulsivity (neuroticism) which are generally linked with nicotine intake, are said to be associated with serotonin. Gene for serotonin transport in nicotine users has been examined. Although each person has only 1 type of serotonin transporter (compared with the at least 12 different kinds of serotonin receptors found in humans), there appeared to be 2 different forms of the gene, a long version and short version, and the long version makes twice as much transporter as the short version. As a result, people who have the long version of this gene transport serotonin twice as much as people with the short version. There is mild correlation between the short version and neuroticism, but a strong correlation between the combination of both the short and long and high neuroticism score and difficulty quitting smoking.

The reinforcing properties of nicotine are in part due to activation of the mesolimbic dopamine reward system and release of dopamine in nucleus accumbens, the brain's pleasure and reward centre (Carr *et al.*, 1992). Cigarette smoking also contains substances that inhibit brain mono-amine oxidase B, which is responsible for degradation of dopamine (Fowler *et al.*, 1996). The link between dopamine release and the addictive properties of nicotine point to dopaminergic genes as logical candidates for genetic effects on smoking behaviour. Genetic variations influence the function of dopamine receptors and liver enzymes that metabolize nicotine. Consequently, certain individuals incur elevated risk for nicotine addiction. Variations in the effects of nicotine could be mediated by polymorphism in the dopamine receptor gene resulting in greater or lesser reward and vulnerability to drug-addiction (Noble *et al.*, 1991 and Noble *et al.*, 1994). In a recent molecular genetic study, in individuals with (Al and A2) and Taq IB (B1 and B2) of the $D^2$ dopamine receptor gene were more likely to have smoked 100 or more cigarettes in their lifetime and to have had an earlier onset of smoking and fewer attempts at quitting. Individuals lacking fully functional CYP2A6, a genetically variable enzyme of the cytochrome P450 system, were significantly protected from tobacco dependence because of impaired nicotine metabolism (Pianezza *et al.*, 1998). These findings suggest that some component of nicotine dependence and its consequences are heritable. Lerman *et al.*, (1999) demonstrated an association between smoking behaviour and allele 9 of a 3′ un-translated region polymorphism in the dopamine transporter gene (SLC63A3-9) in their case control study of nonsmokers and current smokers. Individuals with SLC6A3-9 genotype were less likely to be smokers than individuals without allele 9 and that smokers with SLC6A3-9 genotype had started to smoke later and had been able to quit for longer periods of time than other smokers.

There is involvement of multiple genetic and environmental risk factors in the pathway of nicotine dependence (Kendler *et al.*, 1991). However, a recent study suggests that genetic factors explained much of the variation in the use of tobacco in adolescents (Maes *et al.*, 1999). Heritability for both lifetime and current initiation of tobacco use were approximately 80%, dizygotic correlates reaching approximately half the monozygotic correlates.

Relevance of nicotine metabolism in development of nicotine-addiction can not be underestimated since metabolism influences an individual's exposure to nicotine. Individual variations in nicotine metabolism play a role in person's level of smoking, as well as transition from initiation to maintenance of smoking behaviour pattern. Slower nicotine metabolism permits longer exposure to nicotine and therefore, may yield fewer cigarettes smoked per day. Slower metabolism in naïve smokers may potentially reduce the likelihood of their becoming regular smokers, which is related to more aversive symptoms from nicotine exposure. Persons with faster nicotine metabolism may smoke more cigarettes per day to maintain nicotine levels and be more likely to develop and maintain a smoking pattern.

Various studies illustrate differences in individual metabolism variability in the natural environment (Pomerleau, 1995 and Seaton and Vesell, 1993). These studies have identified higher cotinine levels in African-American compared with Caucasian smokers, resulting in lower smoking rates among African-Americans. It is also observed that men metabolized nicotine faster than women. That is why women require fewer cigarettes than men. African-American women smoke significantly fewer cigarettes per day than do the Caucasian women, and yet their average cotinine level is found to be significantly higher.

Higher levels of cotinine in African-American smokers compared with Caucasians may also be related to the findings of a recent study of nicotine and cotinine clearance in African-American and Caucasian smokers assessed with dual-labeled nicotine and cotinine infusions. While clearance of nicotine is similar for both African-Americans and Caucasians, the clearance of cotinine is found to be significantly slower in African-Americans (Ahijevycoh, 2000).

Variability in nicotine metabolism related to differences in nicotine absorption and distribution, difference in depth and duration of inhalation during smoking and differences in cotinine elimination, play an important role in smoking initiation and maintenance. Plasma nicotine half-life in "chippers" (persons who smoke fewer cigarettes intermittently) is found to be similar to the nicotine half-life in regular smokers. This provides information about nicotine levels in persons with smoking patterns that may resemble youth in smoking initiation. The chippers' lower smoking rate does not yield increased nicotine levels as a result of diminished nicotine disposition or clearance. Other biological measures of smoke constituent exposure in youth in initiation phase are lacking.

Individual differences in sensitivity to nicotine address the range of responses to a specified drug dose. Sensitivity has been described in relation to the initial experiences with smoking and individuals subsequently becoming smokers or nonsmokers. Smokers classified as "more dependent" recalled significantly more pleasurable sensations with initial smoking experiences than less dependent smokers. The ratio of pleasurable to unpleasant sensations was significantly higher in more dependent versus less dependent smokers. Those who become smokers are more sensitive to reinforcing properties of nicotine and are undeterred by the negative effects. In addition, examination of first-dose sensitivity to nicotine in mice indicates that those more reactive initially develop greater tolerance and become more willing to self-administer.

### 2. Psychological

*(i) Personality variables*

There have been attempts to identify the specific personality characteristics in smokers which could differentiate them from others. Eysenk *et al* (1960) in their attempt found a positive correlation between smoking and extraversion; they observed that the average extraversion score increased as smoking became heavier. Smokers have been found to be more extrovert than non-smokers in various UK, US and Australian studies in school students and in adult population as well as in both the sexes. An association between smoking and lower emotional stability may exist amongst certain age groups or particular populations, but the existence of any more general link between smoking and emotionality is not proven. Risk taking behaviour is positively associated with smoking in both sexes with more impulsivity in boys. Eysenk and Eaves (1980) reported smokers to be high on the personality dimension psychoticism which reflects emotional coldness, egocentricity and hostility. Personality traits that predispose to smoking are depression/anxiety and impulsivity/novelty seeking. There is a strong relationship between depression and anxiety traits and smoking. Hamer (2000) used a scale that measured negative effects such as depression, anxiety, irritability, and impulsivity and were able to score subjects on the extent to which they had these character traits, referred to collectively as neuroticism. On the neuroticism score, the current smokers scored higher on the free-floating and phobic anxiety (Haines *et al.*, 1980) it was also found that the current smokers had higher neuroticism scores compared with either ex-smokers or nonsmokers (Coger *et al.*, 1996).

*(ii) Cognitive*

Possible factors contributing to initiation and development of nicotine dependence are the perceived beneficial effects of nicotine. Many smokers report that smoking improves their concentration. It is well documented that nicotine deprivation impairs attention and cognitive abilities and that nicotine and smoking can reverse such deficits (Heishman *et al.*, 1994, Levin *et al.*, 1998). It is not known, however, whether these performance enhancing effects of nicotine are present in adolescents, and if so, whether they play a role in the initiation of cigarette smoking in their age group.

The psycho-social factors influencing the initiation of tobacco use vary from developed world to the developing one.

### 3. Social and Environmental

Parental and peer influence plays an important role in initiation and maintenance of tobacco use as a risk factor in adolescents. Other factors influencing the tobacco use initiation are family structure, peer pressure, self-image, curiosity, stress, boredom, self-assertiveness and rebelliousness (Landrive *et al.*, 1994).

*(i) Parental influence*

Parents are the first influence and are particularly important for the young children. Children whose parents smoke are twice as likely to become smokers as those whose parents do not smoke (Eiser *et al.*, 1989). Some studies have found significant relationship between parental smoking and smoking in adolescents (Banks *et al.*, 1978). Bauman and co-workers (1990) found that smoking among adolescents is more strongly related to whether a parent has ever smoked than to whether a parent currently smokes. Perceived parental opinion is also a major factor, parental disapproval of smoking makes a child less likely to initiate smoking (Aaro *et al.*, 1981).The strength of relationship whether a parent has ever smoked and children smoking was strong as the relationship between adolescents smoking and their friends smoking. This finding suggests that parental influence on children's smoking is more likely attributable to other processes than a modeling. Parents who have smoked during their life-time are more likely to express their opposition clearly and explicitly to their children smoking than are parents who have never smoked.

First grade children, whose parents smoke, perceive it as an acceptable habit more often than do children whose parents do not smoke (Evans *et al.*, 1978). Female adolescents are more likely to be smokers if both the parents are smokers. There is a strong correlation between mother smoking and female youth becoming a smoker (Elkind, 1985; Gottlieb, 1982 and Nolte *et al.*, 1983).

The popular interpretation is that smoker parents serve as models for the behaviour of their children. However, there are many ways parental smoking could influence adolescents' smoking behaviour. Being raised in a home where parents smoke exposes a young person to a good deal of cigarette smoking; such exposure may accustom a young person to the presence of smoke. Parents who smoke may also facilitate their children's smoking simply by giving children early access to cigarettes. Finally, parents who smoke may be less likely to oppose their children's smoking, once peer influence prompts children to experiment, children are also more likely to smoke if their older siblings are smoking (Severson and Lichtenstein, 1986).

*(ii) Family structure*

Family structure plays significant role in initiation of tobacco use. Intact and two parent families are protective against smoking (Covey and Tam, 1990). Higher levels of parental and socio-economic variables such as education, and social class have been inversely related to tobacco use among adolescents (Miller and Hunter, 1990). Prevalence of smoking is more common in families which are with lower socio-economic educational strata of the society. The children and adolescents hailing from the families which are deprived and marginalized are at a greater risk for smoking initiation.

*(iii) Peer influence*

Friends are the greatest influence in youth smoking. It is not necessarily peer-pressure but peer-bonding that acts making peer tobacco use consistently related to adolescent tobacco use initiation (Biglan *et al.*, 1995 and Spear and Akers, 1988). The onset of smoking has been related to having a close friend who smokes (Gritz 1982 and Krohn *et al.*, 1980). Female adolescents with best friend who smokes are nine times more likely to be smokers (USDHHS, 1987). In fact, smoking is usually a shared activity with important socializing functions for female youth (McGraw *et al.*, 1991). Same sex friends are influential in the smoking behaviour of female adolescents. Young people smoke because they want to belong to a particular group (Michell, 1997). Others may lack the skills to refuse a cigarette offered by a friend or someone they would like to be their friend (De Vries, 1988). The single most direct influence on smoking among adolescents is how many of their five best friends smoke (Biglan and Lichtenstein, 1984). Peer smoking also predicts continued smoking among young people who have already begun to smoke (Ary and Biglan, 1988). Adolescents who begin and continue smoking receive social reinforcement from peers.

*(iv) Role model*

Film stars, pop stars and fashion models make smoking seem attractive (Bandura, 1977) to the adolescents.

*(v) Advertising and promotion*

It is estimated that the tobacco companies have to recruit about 4,000 new smokers daily to just to maintain their current market size. About 1,100 smokers die every day from smoking related illnesses, and more than 3,000 quit smoking every day (USDHHS, 1990) in the United States. Recruiting younger people to smoke is vital to profit maintenance. Marketing to young people is not just a matter of ensuring future sales but also a significant source of profit for the tobacco companies. In the USA alone, $900 billion to $1540 billion worth of cigarettes are sold annually to people less than 18 years of age (Difranza and Tye, 1990). Advertising is an effective weapon to influence the decision of youth to initiate smoking (Hastings, Aitken, and Mackintosh, 1991). This includes poster and print advertisements, sports and art sponsorship, brand-stretching and portrayal of cigarette brands, and smoking in films and television programmes. 12-13 years old boys whose television sports include motor-racing are twice as likely to become regular smokers as their peers who do not watch it (Charlton, While and Kelly, 1997). Advertising bans have been found to be very effective in reducing cigarette smoking prevalence in youth (Bjartveit, 1990). Young smokers smoke the most heavily advertised brand (Chapman and Fitzgerald, 1982). The packaging of these brands is regarded by the young people as important in portraying an image and making a fashion statement (Deppe, 1996). In the year 2003, Indian Government banned advertising of cigarette and other tobacco products through an Act[5].

*(vi) Socio-economic factors*

There is an almost universal social class gradient of higher smoking rate in lower income groups. The social class gradient is reflected in differences in smoking prevalence by occupation. For example, in Canada in 1998 there was a decline in smoking intensity among all workers except 'blue-collar occupations' (Gaudette and Richardson, 1998). Between 1987 and 1990 in the US, occupational prevalence was 57.8% for roofers and 57.6% for crane and tower operators, and between 1985 and 1992, 40% of the men employed as handlers/labourers in transportation/material movers were smokers.

---

[5] The Cigarette and Other Tobacco Products (production, advertisement, and regulation of trade and commerce, production, supply and distribution) Act, 2003.

Adolescents from low socio-economic background are more likely to become smokers than the middle-class counterparts (Brunswick, 1984 and Eckert, 1983). This difference in smoking pattern may reflect divergent beliefs and attitudes about tobacco use based on socio-economic status (Graham, 1976). Attitudes and beliefs regarding tobacco are more easily influenced by advertising than others. However in an Indian study conducted in the metropolitan city of Bombay (Mumbai) it was found that children from higher income groups attending public schools have a higher smoking prevalence rate compared to the children attending municipal Indian-language schools (Jayant, Notani, Gulati and Gadre, 1991). This elucidates that those children from higher income groups are more likely to use tobacco compared to their middle class counterparts.

However, in the lower strata of Indian society *beedi* smoking is more prevalent for the reasons of low price, easy availability and convenient use. *Price* is a major factor in adult smokers (Townsend, Roderick and Cooper, 1994). Research in Canada and the USA (Biener *et al.*, 1998) shows that a decrease in youth smoking followed an increase in the real price of cigarettes.

### *(vii) Availability*

Availability is often assumed to be very important in youth smoking; however, it is probably not the strongest influence. However, it is morally wrong to sell cigarettes to children and that is the reason most of the countries have legislation forbidding sale of cigarettes to children and within 100 meters of the schools. In the UK, a National Parents' Group lobbied for tighter legislation governing prevention of cigarette sales to minors and for increased penalties for those who broke the law.

### *(viii) Personal factors*

There are certain personal factors which are consistently associated with tobacco use such as knowledge, attitude and beliefs, self esteem, and locus of control. These factors are very close to young people since many of these are related to personal appearance, status in the group, self-esteem and so on. Their belief that smoking makes them control their weight, calms their nerves, gives them confidence, provides them adult appearance and fills them with fun, enjoyment and sociability (Charlton and Blair, 1989).

### *(ix) Knowledge, attitudes and beliefs*

Knowledge about detrimental health effects of tobacco use has been found to be preventive in some studies (Prokhorov and Alexandrov, 1992). Adolescents who smoke are generally less knowledgeable about the health risks involved, do not believe that smoking will affect them personally or consider that short-term benefits outweigh any health risks. However, knowledge alone is not sufficient to prevent smoking among adolescents, since many misinterpret the risks involved. In China, 61% of the adult smokers in 1996 believed that cigarette did them "little" or no harm (World Bank, 1999). Smokers in higher-income countries are generally aware of their increased risk of disease, but that they judge the size of these risks to be smaller and less established than do nonsmokers. Evidences from various countries show that smokers may have a distorted perception of the health risks compared with other health risks. Most smoking starts early in life, and children and teenagers may know less about health effects of smoking than do adults. Younger people underestimate the risk of becoming addicted to nicotine, and therefore grossly underestimate the future costs from tobacco use. Even teenagers who have been told about the risks of tobacco use may have a limited capacity to use the information wisely (Aghi, Asma, Chng and Rose, 2001).

Positive attitude towards tobacco use and tobacco users tend to be related to an increased likelihood of tobacco use (Spear and Akers, 1988). Beliefs about smoking also predict initiation of smoking (Gilchrist, Schinke, Nurius, 1989). Adolescent smokers demonstrate less knowledge about the negative consequences of smoking, discount the addictive properties of tobacco and negate the risks of experimental smoking as compared to their nonsmoking counterparts. Although most female teenagers believe that long-term smoking is a health hazard, their own smoking is believed to be unrelated to the chronic smoking habits of the adults (Silvis and Perry, 1987).

In some low income groups there is a prevalent belief among pregnant teenagers that cigarette smoking decreases the pain and length of labour. This belief serves as an incentive for young females to smoke (Lawson, 1994); such enticement may be particularly significant for pregnant adolescents who fear losing control during childbirth.

### *(x) Self-esteem*

The process of individuation and identity formation is inherent to adolescence. The sense of self evolves with the interactions at school with the peers and the parents at home and considers options for the future. One's self-esteem plays an important role in initiation of tobacco smoking among adolescents. Adolescents who smoke possess low self-esteem and low expectations for future achievements (Johnston, O'Malley and Bachman, 1987). Young people with low perceptions of their academic achievement and behaviour are at increased risk of becoming smokers, and the girls who are unhappy about their appearance often take up smoking because they believe that smoking makes them more attractive (Minagawa; While and Charlton, 1993). In fact, they may regard smoking as a means of coping with stress, anxiety and depression associated with lack of self-confidence. In traditional Indian society with graded inequality, low castes, always subjected to every kind of deprivation and discrimination, were more vulnerable to indulgence in intoxicants including tobacco consumption. Use of narcotics and alcohol was significantly higher in these communities (Briggs, 1920) with excessive tobacco smoking.

### *(xi) Self-image*

It is likely that some adolescents smoke cigarettes just to enhance their low self-esteem by improving their external image i.e. by appearing mature, or 'cool'. Role models who smoke are frequently seen as tough, sociable and sexually attractive. Adolescents who believe that smoking bestows these attributes may use smoking as a powerful mechanism for self-enhancement. These young people may experiment with smoking to try to adopt a perceived positive social image and thereby improving the way others, particularly peers view them. If peers respond favourably to this strategy, these new smokers continue to smoke, since the behaviour has proved functional for them in creating an acceptable self-image.

*(xii) Advertising*

Advertising portrays smoking as a means of attaining maturity, adulthood and being sophisticated, sociable and sexually attractive. To a great extent, media is responsible in promoting an image of female attractiveness that equates being thin with desirability, evidence shows that weight control and dieting are the major pre-occupations among adolescent girls. For these girls, smoking serves as an appetite suppressant to cope with weight gain. A male shown smoking in an advertisement is depicted as tough, masculine and manlier for easy imitation.

Rates of smoking observed among people living in institutions are considerably higher than for those with similar illnesses living at home. The highest rates were also observed for those homeless who were sleeping rough. Environment plays very important role in smoking initiation.

## Stages of Tobacco Smoke Initiation

A young smoker who initiates smoking goes through a series of stages (Charlton *et al.*, 2004). Each stage is influenced by different factors. These stages are not a one-way process; rather, the stages are fluid and may reverse and restart several times (McNeil, 1991). These stages are as follows:

1. *Pre-contemplation:* The adolescent is not thinking about smoking, but receives messages about it. At this stage, parental and siblings' smoking, advertising, films, television and role models all exert influence.
2. *Contemplation*: The adolescent receives images or peer influence, builds up to a point where curiosity takes over and the young person considers trying a cigarette. Friends' behaviour is now added to the pre-contemplation influences.
3. *Initiation:* Most young people try smoking, but the majority do not become regular smokers. At this stage, friends are the strongest influence.
4. *Experimentation*: This stage involves repeated attempts to smoke. Young people may become addicted to nicotine after smoking a very small number of cigarettes and it is not uncommon that many experimenters become regular smokers.
5. *Regular Smoking*: It may involve a new set of influences. Personal factors such as beliefs about the benefits of smoking, self-efficacy, self-perception and coping join earlier influences. Societal factors such as price and availability, and interpersonal factors such as school policy, provide a background.
6. *Maintenance:* All these factors contribute in maintenance; however, addiction to nicotine is the most important factor.

7. *Quitting:* It occurs when the relative importance of these factors changes. A new non-smoking partner, steep increase in the price of cigarettes, decrease in spending money, and beginning work where smoking is not permitted can all trigger a decision to stop smoking.

**Characteristics of Nicotine Use in Adolescents**

As we have discussed earlier, the onset of and the first self-generated efforts to control tobacco addiction occurs most typically during adolescence. (Flay *et al.*, 1998). Three important clinical phases precede tobacco dependence: *trial, occasional use,* and *daily use.* No formal criteria have been adopted to define adolescent nicotine dependence (Moolchan *et al.*, 2000). Establishing the prevalence of tobacco dependence in youth would help anticipate the specific level of need for smoking cessation programmes.

**Maintenance of Tobacco Use**

Individuals vary in their vulnerability to dependence on nicotine and other drugs as they vary in their vulnerability to other medical disorders. Some people show a high degree of resistance to the disorder despite multiple exposures to the causative agent, whereas others very quickly become dependent or otherwise sick. Once a person starts smoking, there is a likelihood that the person continues to smoke because of the complex interplay of individual and psycho-social factors. Continued smoking is often the result of an individual's physiological addiction to nicotine and psychological and social factors. There are several biological, psychological and social factors which favour initiation of tobacco use during adolescence and late childhood. These factors need to be kept in mind before planning any preventive or therapeutic strategies.

## Factors Responsible for Maintenance of Tobacco Smoking

1. Physiological
2. Cognitive
2. Psychosocial
   (i) Stress
   (ii) Body-weight
4. Psychiatric illnesses.

### *1. Physiological*

*Dependence:* Cigarette and other forms of tobacco use are addictive and that nicotine is the drug in tobacco that leads to addiction, is well documented[6]. A substance is said to be addictive if the discontinuation of its use produces cravings and other withdrawal reactions, if a period of deprivation of substance produces higher than usual compensatory consumption, and if consummatory behaviour functions to regulate blood levels of the substance (McMorrow and Fox, 1983). Cigarette smoking and other forms of tobacco use meet all these criteria. Smokers who are deprived of cigarettes experience diverse unpleasant sensations, including headache, irritability and anxiety (Hughes and Hatsukami, 1986).

They tend to compensate for the periods of deprivation by increasing consumption when cigarettes become available, and such compensatory activity regulates the nicotine level in their blood stream.

Evidence indicates that smokeless tobacco use produces the same effects (Biglan, LaChance and Benowitz, 1992).

Nicotine's dependence producing properties are responsible for its reinforcing effects. Once a person has begun to use tobacco habitually, his attempts to stop produce symptoms of withdrawal.

The aversive events can be reduced or terminated by resuming smoking or chewing tobacco. Termination of these events constitutes negative reinforcement. A tobacco user experiences numerous trials each day when the aversive effects of nicotine withdrawal are terminated by consuming tobacco. A person who tries to quit but fails, experiences longer and more substantial aversive events, which are then reinforced by giving in to the usages. In unsuccessful effects to quit, most tobacco users inadvertently shape powerful aversive reactions to nicotine withdrawal (Lewin, Biglan and Inman, 1986).

Nicotine withdrawal symptoms include nausea, headache, constipation, diarrhea, increased appetite, drowsiness, fatigue, and insomnia, inability to concentrate, irritability, hostility, anxiety and craving for tobacco. Nicotine dependence is recognized as a mental disorder due to psychoactive substance abuse, according to the Diagnostic and Statistical Manual of Mental Disorders, 4th Edition (DSM-IV, 1994), the American Psychiatric Association.

## 2. *Cognitive*

A prominent component of nicotine withdrawal syndrome is impaired cognitive performance; re-administration of nicotine provides rapid relief, thus providing a potentially powerful source of reinforcement for continued tobacco usage. It has even been suggested that nicotine does not really produce dependence but that instead people self-administer cigarettes primarily to provide cognitive benefit (Warburton, 1989); however, the presence or lack of therapeutic efficacy is not a criterion for the determination of addictive liability. Furthermore, the only conditions under which reliable cognitive benefits of nicotine administration have been documented are in persons who are cognitively impaired during nicotine withdrawal or possibly by Alzheimer's disease.

In nonsmokers, nicotine administration can increase finger-tipping rate and slightly (but significantly) attenuate the deterioration in attention that occurs during protracted testing.

---

[6] US Department of Health and Human Services. Nicotine Addiction. A Report of the Surgeon General, US Government Printing Office, Washington DC.

### 3. Psycho-social

*(i) Stress*

People often smoke in response to negative life experiences which indicate low self-esteem. People also smoke to control their emotions, particularly to suppress their anger. Women more often than men use smoking as a mechanism to attain and maintain ideal body-weight. The factors that contribute to women's maintenance of smoking are the stresses they are continuously exposed.

*(ii) Body-weight*

One of the most common reasons females give for maintaining smoking behaviour and relapsing upon cessation is their belief that tobacco helps control their appetite and body weight. Relationship between smoking and body weight, body image and dietary behaviour is widely studied (Gritz and Crane, 1991; Croft *et al.*, 1992; Page *et al.*, 1993) and there is substantial literature that documents the robust effect of nicotine exposure to reduce body weight and prevent developmental weight gain in animals and humans (Klesges *et al.*, 1989). A significant number of adolescent girls report smoking for weight management (Weekley *et al.*, 1992). Women's concern about weight may encourage smoking initiation, be a barrier to smoking cessation, and increase relapse rates among women who stop smoking (French *et al.*, 1992). Studies reveal that nearly 40% female cigarette smokers endorse smoking as a method to control their appetite and weight versus only 12% of male smokers (Camp *et al.*, 1993). Female weight control smokers report higher dietary restraint and more eating disorder symptoms suggesting a greater tendency toward chronic dietary and restrained eating behaviour. In addition, restrained eaters endorse the use of smoking for weight-control purposes significantly more than do unrestrained eaters (Ogden and Fox, 1994). This relationship is a consequence of cigarette smoking and not simply a correlate (Eisen *et al.*, 1993).

Several mechanisms have been postulated to account for the appetite and weight-suppressing effects of cigarettes (Kresges *et al.*, 1989). Those that appear specific to nicotine include a selective decrease in appetite for sweet carbohydrates, increased metabolic rate, and decreased appetite through serotonergic mechanisms. The slowly releasing form of nicotine provided by the transdermal medications does not provide the weight attenuating effect of either continued smoking or nicotine polacrilex use (Fagerstrom, Schneider and Lunell, 1993). The more pronounced catecholamine-releasing effects of faster forms of nicotine delivery (Benowitz, 1990) might account for cigarettes appearing to be particularly efficacious anorectants, polacrilex less so, and transdermal systems without such an effect.

### Psycho-social Factors in Indian Society to Maintain Tobacco Consumption

The traditional Indian society is a hierarchical society wherein the caste of an individual determines his social status and the way he should deal with the members of other caste groups. Each caste being a social unit in it is governed by precise rules regarding the acceptance or rejection of food or drink or tobacco smoke from a member of other caste on purity-pollution basis.

*Hookah* smoking is quite common in rural India (especially in North India) which is shared among the members of one's caste. Tobacco consumption in such a way acquires a whole range of symbolic connotations. Louis Dumont, when referring to the notion of purity and pollution, avers that sharing the *hookah* pipe among individuals depends upon the caste and the age of the participant in *hookah* smoking ritual (Dumont L, 1999). The inclusionary aspect of tobacco use may be most clearly depicted through the exclusionary aspect exemplified in a statement of "*hookah-paani band*" (suspension of sharing of water and tobacco smoke) i.e. barring someone from sharing social life with other equals. In most cases, this implies designating a person – and his family – as an outcaste by refusing to share *hookah* with him or accepting or giving him water.

Inclusion or exclusion of the individuals or castes, communities or classes from shared consumption be it smoking, drinking or eating together, acts to maintain equality or inequality. Tobacco has been a consumption good consistently associated with this kind of symbolic value in Indian society.

### 4. Psychiatric Illnesses

Studies reveal that there has been a strong association between tobacco use and psychiatric disorders. Nicotine administration and withdrawal have diverse effects on brain and endocrine function that may be of functional significance in the aetiology of psychiatric and neurological disorders such as affective Disorders, Alzheimer's and Parkinson's diseases, Tourette' Syndrome, and maintenance of cognitive functions (Jarvik, 1991 and Newhouse and Hughes, 1991). In Parkinson's disease, nicotine provides a weak protective effect (Newhouse and Hughes, 1991) with some evidence that nicotine is an effective treatment for the disorder, or even that the protective effect is specific to nicotine. Smoking appears to be positively associated with Alzheimer's disease development but there is no conclusive evidence. Studies suggest that nicotine administration might be of benefit to Alzheimer's patients (Sahakian, Jones, Levy, Gray and Warburton, 1989).

Smoking in psychiatric patients is found to be much higher than in the general population. Prevalence of cigarette smoking is higher among psychiatric patients such as Schizophrenia, Mania, Personality disorders, and Depression, Panic Disorder etc. In Schizophrenics smoking prevalence is as high as 88%. An association between tobacco smoking with depression and anxiety has also been demonstrated in adolescents. Adolescents who initiate smoking report more symptoms of depression than adolescents who do not smoke (Kandel and Davies, 1982). Smoking is found to be associated with an increased rate of major depression and substance abuse. Adolescents with depression and anxiety symptoms show high risk of smoking initiation than asymptomatic adolescents. There is a strong evidence for association between child and adolescent psychopathology and tobacco use in conditions such as Conduct problems, Attention Deficit Hyperactivity Disorder etc. (Tobacco use and psychiatric illnesses have been discussed in details in another chapter).

*Depression:* Depressed smokers are less likely to quit smoking. Smoking with a history of depression has a greater risk of relapse after cessation attempt. Smoking cessation causes more intense depressed mood in smokers with history of depression and these symptoms are related to low success rates for cessation. Depressed adolescents are more likely than non-depressed adolescents to report daily smoking in future (Kandel and Davies, 1986). There is an association between heavy smoking and depression.

Several social, personal and biological factors lead an adolescent to initiate smoking and smoking may continue if factors favourable to maintain smoking behaviour are operative in smoker's life. These factors are necessarily not the same factors which make the individual to initiate smoking. For any therapeutic and preventive intervention these factors need to be carefully addressed.

## REFERENCES

Aaro L.E, Hauknes A., Berglund, E. L: Smoking Among Norwegian School Children 1975–1980: The influence of the Social Environment. *Scandinavian Journal of Psychology*, 22:297–309, 1981.

Aghi M, Asma S., Vaithinathan R. and Chng C.Y.: Initiation and Maintenance of Tobacco use. Paper presented at the *Kobe International Conference on Women and Tobacco*. Kobe Japan, 1999.

Aghi M., Asma S., Chng C.Y. and Vaithinathan R.: Initiation and Maintenance of Tobacco Use. *Women and the Tobacco Epidemic: Challenges for the 21st Century*. WHO Publication, 2001.

Ahijevych K.: Nicotine Metabolism Variability and Nicotine Addiction. *Nicotine Conference Programme Index*, Ohio Sate University, 2000.

American Psychiatric Association, Diagnostic and Statistical Manual of Mental Disorders: DSM-IV, 4th Ed.: 1994) Washington: *American Psychiatric Association*.

Ary DV and Biglan A.: Longitudinal changes in Adolescent Cigarette Smoking Behaviour: Onset and Cessation. *Journal of Behavioural Medicine*. 15(5): 413–422, 1988.

Bachman JG, Wallacs J.M. Jr and O'Malley PM: Racial/ethnic Differences in Smoking, and Illicit drug-use Among American High School Seniors. *American Journal of Public Health*, 81: 372–377, 1991

Bandura A.: *Social Learning Theory*, Eaglewood Cliffs, Prentice Hall, 1977.

Banks MH, Bewley BR, Bland JM, Dean J.R. and Pollard V.: Long-term Study of Smoking by Secondary School Children. *Archieves of Disorders of Children*. 53(1): 12–19, 1978.

Bauman K.E., Foshee V.A., Linzer M.A., and Koch G.G.: Effect of Parental Smoking Classification on the Association Between Parental and Adolescent Smoking. *Addiction Behaviour*, 15(5): 413–422, 1990.

Benowitz N.L: Pharmacokinetic Considerations in Understanding Nicotine Dependence. In: *The Biology of Nicotine Dependence*. Ciba Foundation Symposium. Wiley: Chichester, 186–209, 1990.

Biener J.R. Aseltine R., Cohen B. and Anderka M.: Reactions of Adult and Teenaged Smokers to the Massachusetts Tobacco Tax. *American Journal of Public Health*, 88:1389–1391, 1998.

Biglan, A., LaChance P.S. and Benowitz N.L.: Experimental Analysis of the Effects of Smokeless Tobacco Dependence. *Oregon Research Triangle*, 1992.

Biglan A. and Lichtensteine: A Behaviour-analytic Approach to Smoking Acquisition: Some Recent Findings. *Journal of Applied Social Psychology*, 14(3): 207–223, 1984.

Biglan A., Duncan T.E., Ary D.V.: Peer and Parents Influences on Adolescent Tobacco Use. *Journal of Behavioural Medicine*, 18: 315–330, 1995.

Bjartveit K.: Fifteen Years of Comprehensive Legislation: Results and Conclusions. *Proceedings of the 7th World Conference on Tobacco and Health*, Perth Australia, 1990.

Botvin G.J., Baker E., Goldberg C.J.: Predictors of smoking Prevalence Among New York, Latino Youth. *Addictive Behaviour*, 17: 97–103, 1992.

Breslau N. and Peterson E.L.: Smoking Cessation in Young Adults: Age at Initiation of Cigarette Smoking and other Suspected Influences. *American Journal of Public Health*, 86(2): 214–220, 1996.

Briggs G.W.: *The Chamars: The Religious and Social Life of India*. Association Press, Calcutta, 1920.

Brunswick A., Messeri: Gender Differences in the Process Leading to Cigarette Smoking. *Journal of Psychology and Oncology*, 2: 49–69, 1984.

Camp D.E., Klesges R.C., Relyea G.: The Relationship between Body-weight Concerns and Adolescent Smoking. *Health Psychology*, 12(1): 24–32, 1993.

Carr L.A., Basham J.K., York B.K. and Rowell P.P.: Inhibition of Uptake of 1-methyl-4-Phenylpyridinium Ion and Dopamine in Striatal Synaptosomes by Tobacco Smoke Components. *European Journal of Pharmacology*, 215:285–287, 1992.

Chapman S, and Fitzgerald B.: Brand Preference and Advertising Recall in Adolescent Smokers: Some Implications for Health Promotion. *American Journal of Public Health*, 72:491–494, 1982.

Charlton A. and Blair V: Predicting the Onset of Smoking in Boys and Girls. *Social Science and Medicine*, 29: 813–818, 1989.

Charlton A., Cheryl Moyer, Prakash Gupta and David Hill: *Tobacco Control Fact-sheets: Youth and Cigarette Smoking*. World Bank, 2004.

Charlton A., While D. and Kelly S: Boys' Smoking and Cigarette-brand-sponsored Motor-racing. *Lancet*, 350:1474, 1997.

Coger R.W., Moe KL, Serafetinides E.A.: Attention Deficit Disorder in Adults and Nicotine Dependence: Psychobiological Factors in Resistance to Recovery? *Journal of Psychoactive Drugs*, 28:229–240, 1996.

Conrad K.M. Flay BR and Hill D.: Why Children Start Smoking Cigarettes: Predictors of Onset. *British Journal of Addiction*, 87: 1711–1724, 1992.

Covey L.S. and Tam D.: Depressive Mood, The Single Parent Home, and Adolescent Cigarette Smoking. *American Journal of Public Health*, 80: 1330–1333, 1990.

Croft J.B., Strogatz D.S., James S.A., Keenan L.A., Ammerman A.S., Malarcher AM and Haines P.S.: Socio-economic and Behavioural Correlates of Body-mass Index in Black Adults: The Pitt County Study. *American Journal of Public Health.* 82(6): 821–826, 1992.

Deppe B.: An Explanation of the Social Image of Smoking Held By Adolescent Girls. Msc Thesis. Department of Public Health and Health Promotion. *School of Epidemiology and Health Sciences,* Faculty of Medicine, University of Manchester, Uk, 1996.

De Vries H., Dijkstra M, and Kuhlman P: Self-efficacy: The Third Factor Besides Attitude and Subjective Norm As A Predictor of Behavioural Intentions. *Health Education Research,* 3: 273–282, 1988.

Difranza JR, Tye JB: Who Profits From Tobacco Sale to Children? *Journal of American Medical Association* (Jama), 263(20), 2784–2787, 1990.

Dumont L.: *Homo Hierarchicus*: The Caste-system and Its Implications, Oxford University Press, New Delhi, 1999.

Eckert P: 1983) Beyond the Statistics of Adolescent Smoking. *American Journal of Public Health,* 73: 4439–4441.

Eisen S.A., Lyons M.J., Goldberg J., True W.R.: The Impact of Cigarette and Alcohol Consumption on Weight and Obesity: An Analysis of 1911 Monozygotic Male Twin Pairs. *Archives of Internal Medicine,* 153:2457–2463, 1993.

Eiser J.R., Morgan M., Gammage P. and Gray E.: Adolescent Smoking: Attitude, Norms and Parental Influence. *British Journal of Social Psychology,* 28:193–202, 1989.

Elkind A.K.: (1985) The Social Definition of Women's Smoking Behaviour. *Social Sciences and Medicine,* 20, 1269–1278.

Escobedo L.G., Marcus S.E. and Holzman D.: Sports Participation, Age At Smoking Initiation, and Risk of Smoking Among Us High School Students. *Journal of American Medical Association* (Jama), 269: 1391–1395, 1993.

Evans R.I., Rozelle R.M., Mittlemark M.B., Hansen W.B., Bane A.T. and Havis J.: Deterring the Onset of Smoking in Children: Knowledge of Immediate Physiological Effects and Coping with Peer Pressure, and Parent Modeling. *Journal of Applied Social Psychology.* 8: 126–135, 1978.

Eysenk H.J., Tarrant M., Wolf M. and England L.: Smoking and Personality. *British Medical Journal,* 1:1456–1460, 1960.

Eysenk H.J. and Eaves L.J.: The Causes and Effects of Smoking. *Maurice Temple Smith*: London. 1980.

Fagerstrom K.O., Schneider N.G. and Lunell E.: Effectiveness of Nicotine Patch and Nicotine Gum As Individual Versus Combined Treatments for Tobacco Withdrawal Symptoms. *Psychopharmacology,* 111:271–277, 1993.

Flay BP, Hu FB and Richardson J: Psychosocial Predicators of Different Stages of Smoking Among High School Students. *Preventive Medicine,* 27 (5): Part 3a9–A18, 1998.

Fowler J.S., Volkow N.D., Wang G.J., Pappas N., Logan J., MacGregor R., Alexoff D., Shea C., Schyler D., Wolf A.P., Warner D., Nenulkova I. and Cilento R.: Inhibition of Mono-amine Oxidase B in the brain of smokers. *Nature,* 379:733–736, 1996.

Franzkowiak P: Risk Taking and Adolescent Development: The Functions of Smoking and Alcohol Consumption in Adolescents and Its Consequences for Prevention. *Health Promotion*, 2:51–61, 1987.

French S.A., Jeffery R.W., Pirie L., and McBridge C.M.: Do Weight Concerns Hinder Smoking Cessation Efforts? *Addiction Behaviour*. 17: 219–226, 1992.

Friberg l, Kaij L, Dencker S and Jonson E: Smoking Habit of Monozygotic and Dizygitic Twins. *British Medical Journal*, 1:1090–1092, 1959.

Gaudette, LA and Richardson A: Which Workers Smoke? Health Reporter, 10(3): 35–45, 1998.

Gilchrist L.D., Schinke S.P. and Nurius P.: Reducing Onset of Habitual Smoking Among Women. *Preventive Medicine*, 18: 235–248, 1989.

Gottlieb NH: The Effects of Peer and Parental Smoking and Age on the Smoking Careers of College Women. A Sex Related Phenomenon. *Social Sciences and Medicine*, 16:595–600, 1982.

Graham H.: Smoking in Pregnancy. The Attitudes of Expectant Mothers. *Social Sciences and Medicine*, 10: 399–405, 1976.

Gritz E.R.: The Female Smoker: Research and Intervention Targets. In: Jw Cullen and Lr Martin, (Eds), *Psychological Aspects of Cancer*. New York: Raven, 39–49, 1982.

Gritz E.R., and Crane L.A.: Use of Diet Pills and Amphetamines to Lose Weight Among Smoking and Non-smoking High School Seniors. *Health Psychology*, 10(5): 330–335, 1991.

Gupta P.C.: Survey of Socio-demographic Characteristics of Tobacco Use Among 99598 Individuals in Bombay, India Using Hand Held Computers. *Tobacco Control*, 5(2): 114–121, 1996.

Hamer D.H.: Genes, Personality and Smoking Cessation. *International Journal of Neuropsychopharmacology*, 3 (Suppl. 1):S58. Abstract S 36.2, 2000.

Hastings G, Aitken PP and Mackintosh A.M.: From the Billboard to the Playground. *Glasgow Centre for Social Marketing*. University of Strathclyde, 1991.

Haines A.P., Imeson J.D. and Meade T. W: Psychoneurotic Profile of Smokers and Nonsmokers. British Medical Journal, 1:1422, 1980.

Headen S.W., Bauman K.E., and Deane G.D.: Are the Correlates of Cigarette Smoking Initiation Are Different for Black and White Adolescents? *American Journal of Public Health*, 81: 8548, 1991.

Heath A.C., and Madden P.G.: Genetic Influence on Smoking Behaviour. In: J.R. Turner, L.R. Cardon and J.K. Hewitt (Eds) *Behaviour Genetic Approaches in Behavioural Medicine* (Pp 37–48), Plenum, New York, 1995.

Heath A.C. and Martin N.: Genetic Models for the Natural History of Smoking: Evidence for A Genetic Influence on Smoking Persistence. *Addictive Behaviour*, 18:19–34, 1993.

Heishman S.J., Tylor R.C., Henningfield J.E.: Nicotine and Smoking: A Review of Effects on Human Preference. *Experimental Clinical Psychopharmacology*, 2:345–395, 1994.

Hughes JR, Hatsukami D: Signs and Symptoms of Tobacco Withdrawal. *Archieves of General Psychiatry*, 43: 289–294, 1986.

Jarvik ME: Beneficial Effects of Nicotine. *British Journal of Addiction*, 86:571–575, 1991.

Jayant K., Notani P.N., Gulati S.S. and Gadre V.V.: Tobacco Usage in School Children in Bombay, India. A Study of Knowledge, Attitude and Practice. *Indian Journal of Cancer*, 28(3): 139–147, 1991.

Johnston L., Bachman J, and O'Malley P.: *Monitoring the Future:* Questionnaire Response From the Nation's High School Seniors. University of Michigan, *Institute for Social Research*, 1992.

Johnston L.D., O'Malley P.M. and Bachman J.G.: National Trends in Drug-use and Related Factors Among American High School Students and Young Adolescents, 1975–1986. *Us Government Printing Office*: Washington Dc, Department of Health and Human Services No. Adm-87–1535, 1987.

Kandel D.B. and Davies M.: Epidemiology of Depressive Mood and Adolescence: An Empirical Study. *Archives of General Psychiatry*, 39:1205–1212, 1982.

Kandel DB, and Davies M: Adult Sequelae of Adolescent Depressive Symptoms. *Archives of General Psychiatry*, 43(3): 255–262, 1986.

Kendler K.S., Neale M.C., Sullivan P. Gardener C.O. and Precott C.A.: A Population Based Twin Study in Women of Smoking Initiation and Nicotine Dependence. *Psychological Medicine*, 29:299–308, 1991.

Klesges R.C., Meyers A.W., Klesges L.M. and LaVasque M.E.: Smoking, Body Weight and Effects on Smoking Behaviour: A Comprehensive Review of Literature, *Psychological Bulletin*, 106:553–555, 1989.

Krohn M.D., Massey J., Skinner W.F. and Laner R.M.: Social Bonding Theory and Adolescent Cigarette Smoking. A Longitudinal Analysis. *Journal of Health Society and Behaviour*, 24: 337–349, 1980.

Landrine H., Richardson J., Klonoff E., and Flay B.: Cultural Diversity in the Predictors of Adolescent Smoking: The Relative Influence of Peeras. *Journal of Behavioural Medicine*, 17: 331–347, 1994.

Lawson E.J.: The Role of Smoking in the Lives of Low Income Pregnant Adolescents: A Field Study. *Adolescence*, 29: 61–79, 1994.

Lerman C., Caporaso N.E., Audrain J., Main D., Bowman E.D., Lockshin B., Boyd N.R. and Shields P.G.: Evidence Suggesting the Role of Specific Genetic Factors in Cigarette Smoking. *Health Psychology*, 18:14–20, 1999.

Levin E.D., Conner C.K., Sparrow E. and Silva D.: Trans-dermal Nicotine Effects on Attention. *Psychopharmacology*, 140:135–147, 1998.

Lewin L.M., Biglan A. and Inman D: Operant Conditioning of Emg Activity Using Cigarette Puffs As A Reinforcer. *Addictive Behaviour*, 11(2): 197–200, 1986.

Maes HH, Woodars CE and Murrelle L: Tobacco, Alcohol and Drug Use in Eight to Sixteen Year Old Twins: The Virginia Twin Study of Adolescent Behaviour Development. *Journal of Study of Alcohol*, 60:293–305, 1999.

McGraw S.A., Smith KW, Schensul J.J. and Carrillo E.: Socio-cultural Factors Associated with Smoking By Puerto Rican Adolescents in Boston. *Social Sciences and Medicine*, 33, 1355–1364, 1991.

McMorrow M.J., and Foxx R.M.: Nicotine's role in Smoking: An Analysis of Nicotine Regulation. *Psychological Bulletin*, 93(2): 302–327, 1983.

McNeill AD: The Development of Dependence on Smoking Among Children. *British Journal of Addiction*, 86:589–592, 1991.

McNeill A.D., Jarvis M.J., and Stapleton J.A.: Prospective Study of Factors Predicting Uptake of Smoking in Adolescents. *Journal of Epidemiology and Community Health*, 43:72–78, 1988.

Mendis S.: Tobacco Use in A Cohort of Children in Sri Lanka. *British Journal of Addiction*. 85: 397–398, 1990.

Michell L.: Loud, Sad or Bad Young People's Perception of Peer Group and Smoking. *Health Education Research*, 12:1–14, 1997.

Miller W.J. and Hunter L.: The Relationship Between Socio-economic Status and Household Smoking Patterns in Canada. *American Journal of Health Promotion*, 5: 36–43, 1990.

Minagawa K., While D. and Chrlton A.: Smoking and Self-perception Among Secondary School Students. *Tobacco Control*, 2:215–221, 1993.

Moolchan E.T., Ernst M. and Henningfield J.E.: A Review of Tobacco Smoking in Adolescents: Treatment Implications. *Journal of American Academy of Child and Adolescent Psychiatry*, 39:682–693, 2000.

Newhouse P.A. and Hughes J.R.: The Role of Nicotine and Nicotinic Mechanism in Neuro-psychiatric Disease. *British Journal of Addiction*, 86:521–526, 1991.

Nicolaides-Bouman, Wald N, Forey B and Lee P: *International Smoking Statistics*. Wolfson Institute of Preventive Medicine, Oxford University Press, London, 1993.

Noble E., Blum K, Ritchie T, Montgomery A and Sheridan P: Allelic Association of the D[2] Dopamine Receptor Gene with Receptor Binding Characteristics in Alcoholism *Achieves of General Psychiatry*, 48: 648–654, 1991.

Noble E., St Joer ST and Ritchie T: D[2] Dopamine Receptor Gene and Cigarette Smoking: A Reward Gene. *Medical Hypotheses*, 42:257–260, 1994.

Nolte A.F., Smith BJ and O'Rourke T: The Relative Importance of Parental Attitude and Behaviour Upon Youth Smoking. *Journal of Science and Health*, 53:256–271, 1983.

Oakley A., Branner J and Dodd K: Young People, Gender and Smoking in the United Kingdom. *Health Promotion Institute*, 7: 75–88, 1992.

Ogawa H., Tominaga S, and Gellort G.: Smoking Among Junior High School Students in Nagoya, Japan. *International Journal of Epidemiology*, 17: 814–820, 1988, 1994.

Ogden J. and Fox P.: Examination of the Use of Smoking for Weight Control in Restrained and Unrestrained Eaters. *International Journal of Eating Disorders*, 16(2): 177–185.

O'Neill, Glasgow R., and McCaul K.: Component Analysis in Smoking Prevention Research: Effects of Social Consequences Information. *Addictive Behaviour*, 8: 419, 1983.

Page RM, Allen O, Moore L, and Hewitt C: Weight Related Concerns and Practices of Male and Female Cigarette Smokers and Non-smokers. *Journal of Health Education*, 24(6): 336–346, 1993.

Peto R., Lopez A.D., Boreham J., Thun M., Heath C., Doll R.: Mortality From Smoking World-wide. *British Medical Bulletin*, 52:12–21, 1996.

Pianenza M. seller E., Tyndale R : Nicotine Metabolism Reduces Smoking, *Nature*,393: 750, 1998.

Pierce J. and Gilpin E.: How Long Today's Adolescent Smokers Be Addicted to Cigarettes? *American Journal of Public Health*, 86:253–256, 1996.

Pomerleau O.F.: Individual Differences in Sensitivity to Nicotine: Implications for Genetic Research on Nicotine Dependence, *Behaviour and Genetics*, 25:161–177, 1995.

Prokhorov AV, Alexanderov A.A.: Tobacco Smoking in Moscow School Students. *British Journal of Addiction*, 87: 1469–1476, 1992.

Sabol S.Z., Nelson M.L., Fisher C., Gunzerath L., Brody C.L., Hu S., Sirota L.A., Marcus S.E., Greenberg B.D., Luvas IV F.R., Benjamine J., Murphy D.L. and Hamer D.H.: *A Genetic Association for Cigarette Smoking Behaviour*. Health Psychology: *American Psychological Association*, 1999.

Sahakian B., Jones G., Levy R., Gray J. and Warburton D.: The Effects of Nicotine on Attention, Information Processing and Short-term Memory in the Patients of Dementia of the Alzheimer's Type. *British Journal of Psychiatry*, 154:797–800, 1989.

Seaton M. and Vesell E.: Variables Affecting Nicotine Metabolism, *Pharmacology and Therapeutics*, 60:461–500, 1993.

Severson H.H. and Lichtenstein E.: Smoking Prevention Programmes for Adolescents: Rationale and Review. In: Krasnegor N and Cataldo M (Eds.) *Child Health and Behaviour*, New York, Wiley, 1986.

Shields J.: Monozygotic Twins Brought Up Apart and Brought Up Together. *Oxford University Press:* London, 1962.

Silvis G., and Perry C.: Understanding and Deterring Tobacco Use Among Adolescents. *Paediatric Clinics of North America*, 34: 363–379, 1987.

Smith G.M.: Personality and Smoking: A Review of the Literature. In: WC Hunt (Ed) *Learning Mechanisms in Smoking*, Aldine, Chicago, 1974.

Spear S.F. and Akers R.L.: Social Learning Variables and the Risk of Habitual Smoking Among Adolescents: The Muscatine Study. *American Journal of Preventive Medicine*, 1988.

Stone S., and Kristeller J.: Attitudes of Adolescents Towards Smoking Cessation, *American Journal of Preventive Medicine*. 8: 221.1, 1992.

Townsend J.L., Roderick P. and Cooper J.: Cigarette Smoking By Socio-economic Group, Sex and Age: Effects of Price, Income and Health Publicity. *British Medical Journal*, 309 (6959): 923–926, 1994.

United States Department of Health and Human Services (USDHHS) Public Health Services. *Drug Abuse and Drug Abuse Research. The Triennial report to Congress from Secretary*, Department of Health and Human Services. Washington DC, *US Government Printing Office, DHHS Publication* No. (ADM) 87–1486, 1987.

United States Department of Health and Human Services (USDHHS): *The Health Benefits of Smoking Cessation*. Surgeon General's Report, *US Government Printing Office: Washington DC*, 1990.

Warburton D.M.: Nicotine: An addictive Substance or a Therapeutic Agent? *Progress in Drug Research*, 33:9–41.

Wiecha J.M.: Differences in Patterns of Tobacco Use in Vietnamese, African-Americans, Hispanic, and Caucasian Adolescents in Worcester, Massachusetts. *American Journal of Preventive Medicine*, 12: 29–37, 1996.

Weekey C.K., Klesges R.C. and Reylea G.: Smoking as a Weight Control Strategy and its Relationship to Smoking Status. *Addictive Behaviour*, 17:259–271, 1992.

World Bank: Development in Practice – Curbing the Epidemic – Governments and Economics of Tobacco Control. The World Bank: Washington DC, 1999.

World Health Organization: *Women and Tobacco*, WHO, Geneva, Switzerland, 1992.

Zhu S.H., Sun J., Billings S., Choi W. and Malarcger A.: Predictors of Smoking Cessation in US Adolescents. *American Journal of Preventive Medicine* 16: 202–207, 1996.

CHAPTER 7

# Women and Children: Victims of Passive Smoking

*The increasing awareness that Environmental Tobacco Smoke (ETS) is harmful to health places an onus on governments to safeguard public health by providing legislation to protect the general public from passive (involuntary) smoking.*

— World Health Organization, 2002.

Prevalence of tobacco smoking, in the past and to a great extent during the current times, has been a custom and addiction of men, leaving women and children to form the majority of world's passive or involuntary smokers (Samet and Yang, 2001). Approximately 1.3 billion people or a third of world's population, estimated to be smoking tobacco[1], make involuntary inhalation of tobacco smoke almost unavoidable throughout the world. Exposure to environmental tobacco smoke (ETS) is strongly associated with a number of adverse effects, particularly those involving the respiratory tract. Given that more than a thousand million adults smoke worldwide, WHO estimates that approximately 700 million, or almost half of the world's children are exposed to environmental tobacco smoke (ETS). This high exposure, along with the evidence that ETS causes illness in children, suggests that ETS constitute a substantial public health threat for children (WHO, 1999).

One's own home is the predominant location for smoking, and women and children are exposed to tobacco smoke as they carry out their daily lives – sitting together in the living room, eating and even while sleeping. This may be worsened by exposure at work place, at school and in transport. Consequently, in many countries, women and children cannot avoid inhaling tobacco smoke and this is particularly so in many of the Asian countries like India and the Pacific region, where majority of men are smokers (WHO, 1997).

1 World Resources Institute, United Nations Environment Programme. United Nations Development Programme, World Bank, World Resources, (1998), A Joint Publication by World Resources.

## Environmental Tobacco Smoke

The inhalation of tobacco smoke by nonsmokers has been variously referred to as "passive smoking", or "involuntary smoking" or "secondhand smoke". Cigarette smoke contains particles and gases generated by combustion of tobacco, paper and additives at a very high temperature. The smoke that is inhaled by the nonsmokers contaminates indoor space as well as outdoor environment and has often been referred to as "environmental tobacco smoke" (ETS). ETS is a mixture of side stream smoke released by the smoldering cigarette, contaminants emitted during the puff and the mainstream smoke that is exhaled by the smoker[2].

There are substantial similarities and differences between the mainstream smoke and side-stream smoke components of ETS (Guerin *et al.,* 1992). The main differences arise due to the differences between the temperature of combustion of the tobacco, pH, and the degree of dilution with air accompanied by a corresponding rapid decrease in temperature. Mainstream smoke is generated at a higher temperature than side-stream smoke (800–900° C as against 600° C). Mainstream smoke has a lower pH (6.0–6.7) than side-stream (6.7–7.5).

Side-stream being slightly alkaline contains more ammonias, is depleted of acids, contains greater quantities of organic bases and contains lesser hydrogen cyanide than mainstream smoke. Differences in mainstream smoke and side-stream smoke are also ascribable to the differences in oxygen content (16% in mainstream smoke as against 2% in side-stream smoke). Because side-stream smoke is generated at lower temperature and more reduced conditions than mainstream smoke, many carcinogens and other toxicants are produced in greater amounts in side-stream smoke than in mainstream smoke (Claxton and Morin, 1989).

After its production, side-stream smoke is rapidly diluted in air. Nicotine is predominantly in particle phase in mainstream smoke but is found mainly in gas phase in side-stream smoke and thus rapidly diluted in the air. The particle size range for side-stream smoke is typically 0.01–1.0 micro m., while the mainstream smoke particle size range is typically 0.1–1.0 micro m (Guerin *et al.,* 1992). These differences in size distributions in side-stream smoke and mainstream smoke particles, as well as the different breathing patterns of smokers and nonsmokers, have implications for deposition pattern of particles in various regions of human respiratory tract. It is estimated that about 47% to 90% of mainstream smoke particles are deposited in the respiratory tract while for side-stream smoke 10% deposition has been reported. The risks arising from the deposited ETS material in the respiratory tract are not simply proportionate to the amount of material deposited. The site of deposition, presence of sensitive cells, solubility, clearance mechanism and other physiological factors all have a major influence on potential for risk to health.

ETS is a complex mixture of several thousand compounds containing more than 4000 chemicals in the suspended particulate matter and gases. More than 50 chemicals found in tobacco smoke are carcinogenic,[3] such as 4-aminobiphenyl, 2-naphthylamine, benzene, nickel

[2] Health Effects of Exposure to Environmental Tobacco Smoke. National Cancer Institute. Smoking and Tobacco Control Monograph, No. 10, 2002.

and a variety of polycyclic aromatic hydrocarbons and N-nitrosamines. A number of irritants such as ammonias, oxides of nitrogen, sulphur-dioxide and aldehydes, and cardiovascular toxicants, such as carbon monoxide and nicotine are also present.

ETS is a known human carcinogen classified as "A" carcinogen[4]. exposing the non-smokers to increased risk of lung cancer and coronary heart disease[5].

In terms of human exposure to ETS in a given enclosed indoor space, there may be persons receiving individual exposure considerably greater than the average.

Staff members working in a bar may receive more side-stream and mainstream smoke due to their close proximity to smokers sitting at the bar than the staff members working on the floor of the bar. An infant in the lap of a smoking mother may receive more smoke than an infant lying in the cradle. The space, e.g. inside a room in a residence or an office area, which has a relatively uniform concentration of ETS during the time spent is referred to as its microenvironment. Environmental tobacco smoke (ETS) is an inherently dynamic mixture that changes in characteristics and concentration from the time it is formed and the distance the smoke has traveled. The smoke particles change in size and composition as gaseous components are volatilized and moisture content changes; gaseous element of ETS may be absorbed on to materials, and particle concentration drops with both dilution and impaction on surfaces. Exposure to ETS in a microenvironment is described as the weighed sum of the concentration of ETS in an environment where time is spent. A useful framework for considering exposure to ETS is offered by the micro-environmental model that describes personal exposure to ETS as the weighed sum of the concentrations of the ETS in the microenvironment where time is spent and the weight supplied by the time spent in each (Jaakkola and Jaakkola, 1997).

Those most affected by secondhand smoke are children. Because their bodies are still developing, exposure to the poisons in the form of ETS exposes children to various health-risks. Young children, whose lungs are not fully developed are particularly susceptible to ETS, leading to serious respiratory problems such as severe asthma, lower respiratory tract infections, middle ear infection and Sudden Infant Death Syndrome (SIDS). For children, microenvironments are constituted by home, transportation, public places and even the school, while for women, home and work place could be the microenvironments. Interplay of the family members within home may heighten exposure to ETS because of the frequency of physical proximity of parents and children and of spouses within the home[6].

---

3 National Toxicology Programme, US Department of Health and Human Services, Public Health Service. 10th Report on Carcinogens. Publication No. 99-4645, 2004.

4 Exposure to environmental tobacco smoke and cotinine levels—Fact sheet. Tobacco Information and Prevention Source, 2004. http://www.cdc.gov/tobacco/research–data/environmental/factsheet–ets.htm

5 Respiratory Health Effects of Passive Smoking: Lung Cancer and other disorders. US Environmental Protection Agency, Washington DC, EPA/600/6-90/006F, 2004.

6 Women and Smoking: A Report of the Surgeon General. US Department of Health and Human Services. Office of the Surgeon General, US, 2004.

## Indicators of ETS Exposures

In 1995 about 1.157 billion people performed the act of tobacco smoking and consumed approximately 6 trillion cigarettes world-wide. The smoke generated through the smouldering tobacco rods could not have gone without its effect on those who were exposed to it. It is reasonable to assume that ETS exposure is prevalent and is an important public health problem, particularly in developing countries where men smoke substantially more than women (49% vs 9%). Given the wide-spread use of tobacco, it is well known that ETS exposure is common throughout the world.

Assessment of exposure to ETS is essentially in epidemiological investigations of the health impact of ETS and also in evaluating the effectiveness of strategies to reduce exposure. Exposure can be assessed in a number of ways including direct and indirect methods. Within the framework set by the micro-environmental model, there are a number of useful indicators of exposure to ETS which include:

- Direct measurement of exposure
- Biomarkers (which are reflective of dose).
- Surrogate measures

***Table 1: Indicators of ETS exposure***

| *Measure* | *Indicator* |
|---|---|
| Indirect measures | Report of ETS exposures: Home and Workplace |
| | Smoking in the household |
| | —Number of smokers |
| | —Parent smoking |
| | —Number of cigarettes smoked |
| | Smoking in the workplace |
| | —Presence of ETS |
| | —Number of smokers |
| Direct measures | Concentration of ETS components |
| | —Nicotine |
| | —Respirable particles |
| | —Other markers |
| | Biomarker concentrations |
| | —Cotinine |
| | —Carboxyhemoglobin |
| Surrogate measuxz | Prevalence of smoking in men and women |

**Source:** *Women and Tobacco Epidemic: Challenges for the 21st Century, WHO, 2001.*

Indirect measures include self-reported exposure and descriptions of the source of ETS, such as smoking in relevant microenvironments, most often the home and the work place. The components of ETS include a number of irritating and odiferous gaseous components, such as aldehydes. Nonsmokers typically identify the odour of ETS as annoying, and the threshold for detecting ETS is at low concentration (Samet *et al.*, 1991). Self-reported exposure to ETS is a useful indicator although questionnaire reports of intensity of exposure are of uncertain validity. Questionnaires used to measure passive smoking generally use WHO definition which says: exposure for at least 5 minutes per day more than one day per week (WHO, 1999). Other determinants of ETS concentration, room volume, air exchange and removal are not readily determined by questionnaires and are usually assessed only for research purposes. Table 2 provides data from a number of recent population-based studies that have used questionnaires to characterize exposure. Some of these studies were national in scope like the national sample in China, Australia and United States and others were from states of specific localities. Several of these studies incorporated cotinine as a biomarker. In the studies in the developing countries, close to half of the children and adolescents are exposed to ETS, primarily at home. In a nationwide survey in China in 1996, 53.58% reported exposure to ETS. The prevalence rate of ETS exposure in women (57%) was higher than in men (45%). The highest prevalence of exposure to ETS was in women during reproductive age range (60%), indicating a higher exposure in the younger than in the older age groups. The majority of passive smokers were exposed to passive smoking every day, with 71.2% reporting exposure at home, 25.0% reporting in their work environment and 32.5% in public places.

The Behavioural Risk Factor Surveillance System in the USA estimated the prevalence of ETS exposure at 37 percent in men and women over 18 years of age in 1993 and at 31 percent in 1997.

Direct measurement of ETS is done by various traces: acrolein, aromatic hydrocarbons, carbon monoxide and nicotine, oxides of nitrogen, nitrosamines and inhalable particles (Marconi and Seifert, 1995). Usually, just one compound in ETS is monitored because it is neither practical nor possible to monitor the full range of compounds. The most widely used marker compounds for assessing the percentage and concentration of ETS in the indoor air are vapour-phase nicotine and respirable suspended particle mass. Respirable suspended particles are present in large quantities in ETS, and levels in indoor air are a useful marker for the particulate phase of ETS. Even under conditions of low smoking rate, easily measurable increase in respirable suspended particles have been recorded above background levels (Repace and Lowrey, 1980). Concentration of suspended particulate matter (particularly of <2.5 mic.m) can be 2-3 times higher in homes with smokers than in homes with no smokers (Spengler *et al.*, 1981). Cigarette smoking is the most important factor determining the level of suspended particulate matter and respirable sulfates and particles in indoor air (Dockery and Spengler, 1981).

Biomarkers are measured in biological materials such as blood, urine or saliva for tobacco smoke constituents or their metabolites. Biomarkers should be specific to nicotine and they include (a) nicotine and cotinine (b) thiocynate and carboxyhaemoglobin (c) metabolites of a tobacco-specific carcinogens, namely 4-(methylnitrosamino)-1-(3-pyridyl)-1-butanone (NNK) and (d) biomarkers of genotoxicity namely protein and DNA adducts.

Cotinine, a metabolite of nicotine, is a highly specific indicator of exposure to ETS in nonsmokers (Benowitz, 1999). Cotinine level also offers a highly specific and sensitive indicator of ETS exposure. In nonsmokers, half life of cotinine is about 20 hours, so that the level of cotinine offers a measure of exposure to ETS over several days. Cotinine can be readily measured in blood, urine and even in saliva with either radio-immunoassay or chromatography. Since nicotine is highly specific for tobacco smoke, serum cotinine levels track exposure to tobacco smoke and its toxic constituents. In 1991, data showed that nearly 90% of the US population had measurable levels of cotinine in their blood[7]. The Centres for Disease Control and Prevention's National Report on Human Exposure to Environmental Chemicals[7] found more than a 75% decrease in median cotinine levels for non-smokers in the United States since 1991.

Children and teenagers, 3–19 years old, had higher levels of cotinine than did adults[8]. Carboxyhemoglobin that is formed by combination of haemoglobin with carbondioxide is a far less sensitive and specific measure that is of little utility for involuntary smoking, but is a more valid indicator of active smoking. There could be many other conditions where exposure to carbon dioxide can take place.

Prevalence of smoking in men and women is the one and only useful indicator available for many countries. Among adults, smoking tends to aggregate within couples so that the proportion of nonsmoking women married to smokers is not necessarily estimable under the independent assumption of smoking among husbands and wives. It provides a measure of likelihood of exposure. For Asian countries where smoking rate among men is very high, majority of women are exposed to tobacco smoke at home.

Data from a 1988 nationwide survey in USA shows that one half of children there under 5 years of age are exposed to tobacco smoke (Overpeck and Moss, 1991) and more than a quarter of the children begin their exposure even before birth. 42% of these children lived in a household with a smoker. The prevalence of exposure is almost double in the lower socio-economic groups in comparison to higher socio-economic groups. As the children grow, non-household sources of exposure to ETS become important (Greenberg *et al.,* 1991). 58% of the newborn babies were exposed to ETS from smoking, primarily by the fathers and less frequently by the mothers (Zhang *et al.,* 1992). For older children,

---

7 Cenres for Disease Control and Prevention Cigarette Smoking among adults —United States, 1992, and changes in the definition of current cigarette smoking. MMWR, 1994;43:342–346.

8 Exposure to environmental tobacco smoke and cotinine levels – Fact sheet. Tobacco Information and Prevention Service, 2004. http://www.cdc.gov/tobacco/research data/environmental/factsheet ets.htm.

40-70% children were exposed to ETS (Somerville *et al.*, 1988; Ware *et al.*, 1984; Dijkstra et al., 1990 and Sherril *et al.*, 1992).

***Table 2: Prevalence of environmental tobacco smoke (ETS) exposure –population-based studies***

| *Reference* | *Study Design & Population* | *Results* |
|---|---|---|
| Coultas *et al.*, 1987 | Cross-sectional study,2029 Hispanic children in New Mexico | Prevalence=39% 18yrs+, 48%13-17 yrs, 46% 6-12 yrs,54%<5 yrs |
| Somerville *et al.*, 1988 | Cross-sectional study, 4337 children 5-11 yrs in England & 766 in Scotland | Prevalence =42% in England & 60% in Scotland |
| Chilmonczyk *et al.*, 1990 | Cross-sectional study, aged 6-8 weeks in greater Portland | 41% infants lived in a smoking household with urinary cotinine levels>10ug/L |
| Overpeck and Moss, 1991 | Cross-sectional study, 5,356 children<5 yrs | 50% of all US children <_5 yrs exposed to prenatal maternal smoking and/or domestic ETS |
| Borland *et al.*, 1992 | Cross-sectional, 7301 nonsmokers | 31.3% reported exposure at work |
| Jaakkola *et al.*, 1994 | Population-based cross-sectional, random sample of 1003 children, 1-6 yrs in Finland | 25.2% ETS exposure at home, |
| Burns and Pierce, 1992 | Cross-sectional, head of the house in 32135 homes in California. | 32.2%, 5-11 yrs children and 36.5% adolescents 12-17 yrs exposed to ETS at home. |
| Jenkins *et al.*, 1992 | Cross-sectional telephonic interview with 1579 English speaking adults and 183 adolescents (12-17 yrs) in California | 46% male nonsmoker adults exposed to ETS at work, 15-23% at other locations, 35% female nonsmoker adults at work and 20% at home and 13% at other locations, 13% adolescents at outdoor locations. |
| Pletsch PK, 1994 | Cross-sectional, 4256 Hispanic women 12-49 yrs | 31-62% for Mexican-Americans, 22-59% for PuertoRicans and 40-53% for Cuban-Americans. |
| Yang GH *et al.*, 1996 | Cross-sectional, 122700 records, 15 yrs and older from China | Prevalence for males=45.5%, for females=57%. |
| Pirkle JL *et al.*, 1996 | Cross-sectional, 9744 adults | Prevalence for males=43.5%, females=32.9%, 87.9% had detectable serum cotinine levels |
| Kauffmann F *et al.*, 1983 | Cross-sectional, 7818 adults, 25-49yrs, from 7 cities of France | Prevalence for males=4.2%, females=49.7% |
| Ware *et al.*, 1984 | Cohort study, nonsmoking children with respiratory illness in 6 US communities, 6-9 yrs | Prevalence=68%;maternal smoking associated with 20-35% increase in children respiratory illness rate |

*Contd...*

| *Reference* | *Study Design & Population* | *Results* |
|---|---|---|
| Greenberg *et al.*, 1989 | Questionnaire based cross-sectional study, mothers of 433 infants in North Carolina | 55% live in a household with at least one smoker, 42% infants exposed, cotinine detected in the urine sample of 60% |
| Dijkstra *et al.*, 1990 | Cohort study, nonsmoker children, 6-12 yrs, Netherlands | Prevalence=66%, ETS at home, disturbed lung function, wheeze |
| Thompson B *et al.*, 1995 | Cross-sectional, 20801, US employees from 114 worksites | 52.4% reported exposed to ETS at work |
| Brenner *et al.*, 1997 | Cross-sectional, 974 blue collar employees of South Germany | >60% exposed to ETS at work |
| Lam TH *et al.*, 1998 | Questionnaire based cross-sectional study, 6304 students 12-15 yrs, from 61 schools of Hong Kong | 51.3% living in a household with at least one smoker, 38% fathers and 3.55 mothers were smokers. |
| Steyn K *et al.*,1997 | 394 pregnant women from Johannesburg | 70% lived with a smoker |

***Source:*** *Women and Tobacco Epidemic: Challenges for the 21st Century, WHO, 2001.*

The cost of exposure of the children and adults to ETS has been estimated in the developed countries and the urban areas of the developing countries such as China and South Africa. These studies confirm the prediction of widespread exposure to ETS from the prevalent estimates of active smoking revealing that women and children represent the predominant exposure groups.

## Adverse Health Effects of Passive Smoking

ETS is likely to have the same health risk profile as that established for smoking. There is sufficient data to provide evidence that exposure to ETS causes adverse effects on human health. This evidence emphasizes the need of having policies and practices to reduce exposure to ETS in general and whereever possible, smoking should not be allowed where non-smokers are affected. It is evident from various epidemiological studies that passive smoking exposes an individual to several health risks involving various systems of the body. These studies have directly assessed the association of measures of ETS exposure with disease outcome.

The causality of associations between ETS exposure and health outcome are judged not only on the basis of epidemiological evidence but also on the basis of epidemiological and toxicological studies. US Surgeon General's (SG) Report (1984)[9] on involuntary smoking, US National Research Council[10] Report published in 1986, the Risk Assessment Report by

9 US Department of Health and Human Services(1984): The Health Consequences of Smoking—Chronic Obstructive Lung Disease – A Report of the Surgeon General. Washington, DC; US Government Printing Office.

10 National Research Council, Committee of Passive Smoking (1986) Environmental Tobacco Smoke: measuring exposure and assessing health effects. National Academy Press, Washington DC.

the Environmental Protection Agency[11] (EPA) in 1992, the comprehensive review of the California Environmental Protection Agency (CALEPA)[12] published in 1992 and many others (Table 3) involved systematic evaluation of the effect of ETS on nonsmokers to reach overall conclusion with regard to the evidence on ETS exposure and causation of disease. The causal conclusions were reached as early as 1986, the International Agency for Research on Cancer, the US Surgeon General and the US National Research Council[12] found involuntary smoking a cause of lung cancer in nonsmokers (Table 4).

***Table 3: Adverse effects from exposure to tobacco smoke***

| *Health Effect on the Body* | *SG (1984)* | *SG (1986)* | *EPA (1992)* | *CALEPA (1997)* | *UK (1998)* |
|---|---|---|---|---|---|
| Increased prevalence of respiratory illnesses | Yes/a | Yes/a | Yes/c | Yes/c | Yes/c |
| Decrement in pulmonary functions | Yes/a | Yes/a | Yes/a | Yes/a | |
| Increased frequency of bronchitis, pneumonia | Yes/a | Yes/a | Yes/a | Yes/c | |
| Increase in chronic cough, phlegm | | Yes/a | | | |
| Increased frequency of middle ear effusion | | Yes/a | Yes/c | Yes/c | Yes/c |
| Increased frequency of asthmatic episodes and symptoms | | Yes/c | Yes/c | | |
| Risk factor for new asthma | | | Yes/a | Yes/c | |
| Risk factor for SIDS | | | | Yes/c | Yes/a |
| Risk factor for lung cancer in adults | | Yes/c | Yes/c | Yes/c | Yes/c |
| Risk factor for heart disease in adults. | | | | Yes/c | Yes/c |

***Source:*** *WHO Report on ETS, 1999 Yes/a - association Yes/c – Cause*

## Adverse Effects of ETS Exposure on Children

Because many young children spend a large proportion of their time indoors, they may have significant exposure to environmental tobacco smoke. ETS causes a number of adverse effects in the exposed children. Exposure to ETS was found to be a cause of slightly reduced birth weight, lower respiratory tract illnesses, chronic respiratory symptoms, middle ear disease and reduced lung function. Maternal smoking is cited as a major cause of sudden infant death syndrome (SIDS).

***Fetal effects:*** Active smoking by mothers results in a variety of adverse health effects in children resulting from trans-placental exposure of the fetus to tobacco smoke components. Maternal

11 US Environmental Protection Agency (1992). Respiratory Health of passive smokers: lung cancer and other disorders. US Government Printing Office (EPA/600/006F), Washington DC.

12 California Environmental Protection Agency (1997). Office of the Environmental Health Hazard Assessment. Health effects of exposure to environmental tobacco smoke. California Environmental Protection Agency, California.

smoking reduces birth weight and increases the risk for SIDS. ETS exposure of non-smoking mothers is associated with reduced birth weight as well, although the extent of reduction is far less than that for active maternal smoking during pregnancy[13]. In a recent meta-analysis, the summary estimates of the reduction of birth weight associated with paternal smoking was only 28 grams (Windham *et al.,* 1999). A study carried out on urban pregnant women in South Africa found that 70 percent lived with at least one smoker and approximately 8–9% women actually thought that passive smoking and active smoking were either good for their health or had no effect on their health or that of their babies (Steyn *et al.,* 1997).

***Table 4: Studies investigating ETS exposure & lung cancer in pacific rim***

| | | |
|---|---|---|
| Koo *et al.*, 1985 | Case control study, 78 cases of 'never smoked' females from 1977 to 1980 and 137 'never smoked' female controls in Hong Kong. | No significant increase in relative risk(RR),RR<br>Squamous cells=1.75<br>Attributable risk(AR) (%)=34.7<br>RR large cells=1.44,AR=23.8<br>RR small cells=1.10,AR=6.6 |
| Lam *el al.*, 1987 | Case control study, 445 Chinese female lung cancer patients and 445 healthy controls from 1983 –1986 in Hong Kong | RR=1.65,95% CI=1.16, 2.35 significant trend with daily amount smoked by the husband. |
| Wu-Williams *et al.*, 1990 | Hospital-based case control study, 965 female cases and 959 controls from 1985 – 1987 in the Shenyang and Harbin districts, China | RR=0.7(95% CI=0.6, 0.9) for nonsmokers who live with a spouse who smoked in Harbin, no dose response relationship except for father's smoking in the presence of index case. |
| Liu Z *et al.*, 1991 | Hospital-based case-control study, 110 lung cancer patients and 426 controls from 1985 – 1986 in China | Nonsmoking females OR=0.77 (95% CI=0.30, 1.96) |
| Liu Q *et al.*, 1993 | Hospital-based case-control study, 224 male and 92 female lung cancer patients matched with hospital controls from 1983 – 1984 in Guangzhou, China. | OR=2.9 (95% CI=1.2, 7.3) for >_20 cigarettes/day smoked by husband, OR=0.7 (95% CI= 0.2, 2.2) for 1 – 19 cigarettes per day; C2=4.5, P=0.03 for trend test. |
| Du YX *et al.*, 1996 | 6,000 lung cancer deaths over past 9 years in Guangzhou, China; 2 studies: (1) 120 participants (28 males,92 females) (2) 72 'never smoked' females cases. | ETS exposure not statistically associated |
| Yuan *et al.*, 1996 | Review of Epidemiological investigations | No ETS exposure association |

*Contd...*

[13] Anonymous Cigarette Smoking among reproductive-age women — behavioural risk factor surveillance system (1987) MMWR Morbo Mortal Weekly Report.

| | | |
|---|---|---|
| Koo LC, Ho JH, 1996 | 4 Epidemiological studies over past 15 years in Hong Kong | ETS exposure moderately high in Hong Kong (36% currently smokers at home). |
| Ko Y-C *et al.*, 1997 | Hospital-based case-control study, 117 lung cancer females (106 nonsmokers) and 117 hospital controls from 1992 – 1993 in Kaohsiung, Taiwan | Odds Ratio (OR)=1.3,95% CI=0.7,2.5 for spouse smoking, OR=1.0,95% CI=0.4, 2.3 for cohabitant smokers. |
| Wang TJ, Zhou, 1996 | Meta-analysis of 6 case-control studies, 767 cases and 1193 controls from Shanghai, Guangzhou, Shenyang, Harbin, Xuanwei and Hong Kong | Overall OR= 0.91 (95% CI=0.75,1.10), c2=4.51 P>0.25, no significant dose response relationship. |
| Shen XB *et al.*, 1998 | Case-control study, 70 adenocarcinoma lung cancer cases and 70 controls in Nanjing, China | No statistical association with ETS exposure; risk factors include chronic lung disease (OR=3.90), and family tumour history (OR=4.36) |

***Source:*** *Women and Tobacco Epidemic: Challenges for the 21st Century, WHO, 2001.*

Health effects of ETS exposure on a newborn child include SIDS and further, it has adverse effects on the child's neuro-psychological development and physical growth. A number of components of ETS that may produce these effects include nicotine and carbon monoxide. Possible long-term health effects of fetal ETS exposure include increased risk for childhood cancers of the brain, leukemia and lymphomas, among others.

***Perinatal health effects:*** These health effects include reduced fetal growth, and congenital abnormalities. Low birth rate was first reported in 1957 to be associated with maternal smoking (Ernst and Zibrask, 1998), and subsequent studies have found that maternal cigarette smoking during pregnancy is causally associated with low birth weight. Low birth weight is also reported in the infants of nonsmoking women exposed to passive tobacco smoking during pregnancy (Martin and Bracken, 1986 and Rubin *et al.,* 1986). A strong association was demonstrated with growth retardation, with the risk ranging from 1.2 to 2.6 for those exposed compared with those non-exposed. The finding of ETS constituents in the urine of newborn infants of nonsmoking mothers (Jordanov, 1990), and the established causal association between active maternal smoking and reduced birth weight has led to the conclusion that ETS exposure in nonsmoking mothers during pregnancy causes a small reduction in birth weight.

***Postnatal health effects:*** ETS exposure due to parental smoking may lead to postnatal health effects, including increased risk of SIDS, reduced physical development, decrements in cognition and behaviour and increased risk for childhood cancers.

***Sudden Infant Death Syndrome (SIDS):*** SIDS refers to the unexpected death of a seemingly healthy infant while asleep. Maternal smoking during pregnancy is causally associated with SIDS but evidence on passive smoking (i.e. post-birth) and its association with SIDS is inconclusive although there are some indications of increased risk. Recently, a growing body of evidence links exposure to environmental tobacco smoke to sudden infant death syndrome[14]. This relationship seems to be independent of low birth weight and gestation age.

***Cancers:*** ETS exposure is a known risk factor for childhood cancers. However, the evidence is limited and does not support conclusions about the causal nature of observed associations. However, a recent study on 144 infants in the age group between 3 to 12 months who lived in homes where parents smoked found that 67 (46.5%) babies had a carcinogenic chemical NNAL in their urine. It was further noted that the babies having NNAL positive urine were exposed to at least 76 cigarettes per week (Hecht *et al.,* 2006).

***Lower respiratory tract illnesses in childhood:*** Lower respiratory tract illnesses are extremely common in childhood and there is increased risk of lower respiratory tract illness in infants with parents who smoked (Strachan *et al.,* 1997). There is significant increase in the incidence of bronchitis and pneumonia during the first year of life in children with parents who smoked. The first effect of passive smoking to be documented in children was increased rate of illnesses affecting the lower respiratory tract. A positive correlation between the presence of a smoker in the home and the incidence of perceived disease in children, is well established (Cameron, 1967). Harlap and Davis (1974) detected that pregnant smokers gave birth to babies who were more likely to be hospitalized for bronchitis and pneumonia during the first year of their life than were those whose mothers did not smoke.

Rantakallio (1978) showed that among children younger than one year, those with mothers who smoked cigarettes were almost four times as likely to be hospitalized as were the infants of the nonsmoking mothers. During the first five years of life, pneumonia and bronchitis were twice as likely and acute nasopharyngitis and sinusitis in the upper respiratory tract were about 1.5 times as likely to develop in children whose mothers smoked.

Colley *et al* (1974) found a consistent gradient in the incidence of pneumonia and bronchitis in the child's first year of life in relation to parents' smoking habits. Infants with both parents smoking were more than twice as likely to have pneumonia and bronchitis as were in infants with parents who did not smoke.

Pneumonia and bronchitis in an infant's first year of life increase with increasing maternal smoking in an approximately linear manner: increase of five cigarettes a day resulted in an increase of 2.5 to 3.5 incidents of lower respiratory illness per hundred children at risk.

***Respiratory symptoms and illness in children:*** There is a greater frequency of the most common respiratory symptoms such as cough, phlegm and wheeze in the children of

[14] Environmental tobacco smoke: A Hazard to Children. Pediatrics 99 (4), 1997.

smokers. These subjects are generally school going children. Cook and Strachan (1997) demonstrated an increased risk of respiratory symptoms in children whose parents smoked. They found increased frequency of wheeze, chronic cough, chronic phlegm and breathlessness. Having both parents smoke was associated with the highest level of risk.

***Childhood asthma:*** Environmental tobacco smoke may cause asthma as a long-term consequence of increased occurrence of lower respiratory tract infections in early childhood or through other patho-physiological mechanisms, including inflammation of the respiratory epithelium (Samet *et al.*, 1983 and Tager, 1988). Maternal smoking during pregnancy also reduces ventilatory function measured shortly after birth (Hanrahan *et al.*, 1992). These observations suggest that in utero exposures from maternal smoking may affect lung development and may increase risk not only for asthma but also for more severe lower respiratory illnesses.

Involuntary smoking worsens the status of those with asthma. Murray and Morrison (1986) and Murray and Morrison (1989) evaluated asthmatic children and found that the level of lung function, symptom frequency and responsiveness to inhaled histamines were adversely affected by maternal smoking. Asthmatic children with mothers who smoke tobacco are more likely to use asthma medications.

***Middle-ear disease in children:*** A positive association between ETS and otitis media has been consistently demonstrated in the studies with prospective cohort design but not as consistently in case control studies. The first two years of life are the peak age of risk for middle ear disease. Exposure to ETS has been consistently associated with recurrent otitis media and not with increased incidence of single episodes of otitis media. Kraemer and his associates (1983) in their case controlled study of risk factors for persistent middle ear effusions demonstrated that children who lived in households where more than three packs of cigarettes were smoked per day were more than four times as likely to be admitted to the hospital for tympanostomy tube placement than were children whose parents did not smoke.

Iversen and his colleagues (1985) studied children up to seven years of age and found that middle ear effusion was about 60% more likely to develop in children whose parents smoked. They estimated the overall fraction of middle ear effusion attributable to passive smoking to be 15%. There is an increased risk of middle ear effusion in children between 6–24 months of life who are exposed to environmental tobacco smoke (Etzel *et al.*, 1992).

## Health Effects of Involuntary Smoking on Adults

***Lung cancer:*** Association between involuntary smoking and risk of lung cancer has been documented. The principal epidemiological evidence that ETS increases the risk of lung cancer in nonsmokers comes from studies of nonsmoking women married to smokers where the number of cigarettes smoked per day by the husband is a common surrogate for ETS exposure. Lung cancer from passive smoking increases with the number of years of exposure and the strength of exposure (Hackshaw *et al.*, 1997). This has been established with meta-analysis after controlling for potential sources of bias and confounding. The excess risk is of the order of 20%, for women and 30% for men.[15] Reports from Japan (Hirayama, 1981) and Greece (Tricholoulos *et al.*, 1981) indicate increased lung cancer risk in nonsmoking women married to cigarette smokers.

The association of involuntary smoking with lung cancer derives biologic plausibility from the presence of carcinogens in side-stream smoke and the lack of documented threshold dose for respiratory carcinogenesis in active smokers. Moreover, genotoxic activity and the ability to damage DNA, has been demonstrated for many components of ETS (Lofroth, 1989). Experimental exposure of nonsmokers to ETS leads to their excreting 4-(methylnitrosamino)-1-(3-pyridyl)-1-butanol(NNAL), a tobacco specific carcinogen, in urine (Hecht *et al.*, 1993). Nonsmokers exposed to ETS also have increased concentrations of adducts of tobacco related carcinogens that are detectable binding of carcinogens of DNA of white blood cells (Crawford *et al.*, 1994). Significantly increased risk for nonsmoker men has also been demonstrated, married to wives who smoked 1–19 cigarettes and 20 or more cigarettes daily (Hirayama, 1984). Trichopoulos *et al.*, (1981) also demonstrated increased cancer risk in nonsmoking women married to cigarette smokers.

A meta-analysis of the 31 studies classifies ETS as class "A" carcinogen i.e. a known human carcinogen.[16] Overall, the analysis found a significantly increased risk for cancer in never smoking women married to smoking men. The most recent meta-analysis (Hackshaw *et al.*, 1997) included 37 published studies. The excess risk of lung cancer in smoker married to nonsmokers was estimated to be 24 percent.

***Passive Smoking and Lipid Profile:*** Passive smoking has also been reported to alter lipid profile in adolescents. Feldman and associates (1991) in their study of nonsmoking students found that those with elevated plasma cotinine concentrations had an 8.9% greater ratio of total cholesterol to high-density lipoprotein cholesterol and 6.8% lower high-density lipoprotein cholesterol than those with lower plasma cotinine concentrations. The nonsmoking students with increased cotinine levels had exposure to tobacco smoke in their environment. This may shed light on the mechanism of increased risk of coronary heart disease in passive smokers.

***ETS and Coronary Heart Disease (CHD):*** Causal association between active smoking and fatal and nonfatal CHD outcomes has long been demonstrated. Active cigarette smoking is known to:

---

15 International Agency for Research on Cancer (IARC) 2002.

16 International Agency for Research on Cancer (1986) IARC Monograph on the Evaluation of the Carcinogenic Risk of Chemicals to Humans: Tobacco Smoking. Vol. 38 Lyon France: World Health Organization International Agency for Research on Cancer.

- Increase the risk of cardiovascular disease by promoting atherosclerosis.
- Increase the tendency to thrombosis.
- Cause spasm of the coronary arteries
- Increase the likelihood of cardiac arrhythmias.
- Decrease the oxygen carrying capacity of blood.

It is biologically plausible that passive smoking could be associated with increased risk for CHD through the same mechanisms considered relevant for active smoking. Garland *et al* in 1985 demonstrated for the first time that smoking may increase risk for CHD and since then about 20 studies have shown an association between Environmental Tobacco Smoke and Cardiovascular disease. These studies assessed both fatal and nonfatal cardiovascular heart disease outcomes, and most used self-administered questionnaires to assess ETS exposure. Law *et al* (1997) estimated the excess risk from ETS exposure as 30 percent at age 60 years.

***Respiratory symptoms and illnesses in adults:*** Cross-sectional studies on an association between respiratory symptoms in nonsmokers and involuntary exposure to tobacco smoke have been found to cause acute respiratory morbidity. The acute responses of asthma to ETS have been assessed by exposing the persons with asthma to tobacco smoke in a chamber. In their study, Stankus *et al* (1998) reported 21 asthmatics having exacerbation of asthma with exposure to tobacco smoke.

Lung functions in adults: Exposure to passive smoking has been associated with several lung function measures. However, these findings are not consistent and further research is warranted because of widespread exposure at work place and home.

It is not only the smoke produced that causes harm to the environment, tobacco growing itself harms the environment. It leads to the degradation of the environment caused by the tobacco plant leaching nutrients from the soil, pollution from the pesticides and fertilizers and deforestation as a result of fire curing of some common varieties of tobacco. A recent study that assessed the amount of forest and woodland consumed annually for curing tobacco concluded that about 5% of total deforestation in various growing countries was due to tobacco cultivation.

No doubt, environmental tobacco smoke places an individual to the risk of a variety of morbidity which can be prevented. Children are more vulnerable to this risk where parents or other elders in the house smoke and unknowingly raise their children to be unhealthy citizens. Exposure of children to environmental tobacco smoke is associated with increased rates of lower respiratory illness and increased rates of middle ear effusion, asthma and sudden infant death syndrome. Exposure during childhood to environmental tobacco smoke may also be associated with development of cancer during adulthood.

## Interventions to Control ETS Exposure

Everyone has a right to breathe healthy air therefore it is the responsibility of every government to protect its citizens from the harmful and polluted air with tobacco smoke (WHO, 2000). Following the basic laws of physics, environmental tobacco smoke rapidly diffuses throughout the room. At a ventilation rate of one air change per hour it can take more than three hours for 95% of the smoke in a typical room to dissipate once smoking has ended. This indicates that using ventilation to eliminate environmental tobacco smoke in indoor spaces presents a considerable task to ventilation engineering professionals (Repace, 1994). Air quality may not be the same throughout the ventilated space. Secondhand smoke is not satisfactorily cleared out with the help of ventilation mechanism especially in the hospitality venues such as bars, restaurants etc. Interventions need to be targeted at behavioural intervention of those responsible for ETS and enactment of legislation.

***Models and strategies for intervention:*** It is unlikely that a home, where an individual spends his personal life, will ever become the subject of legislation to minimize environmental exposure to tobacco. Interventions to reduce the exposure of women and children in the home require changes in the smoking behaviour of men – fathers and husbands. In many cultures, it may not be acceptable for a wife to ask her husband to stop smoking. In the rural northern India, majority of men smoke either *hookah* or *beedis, and* enjoy social sanction for their smoking behaviour. However, some women organizations have started expressing their collective resentment against drinking and smoking of their husbands[17].

If it continues, it may lead to social awakening among people against the harmful effects of ETS and may lead to individual behaviour changes. Such approaches to behaviour changes have to be culture specific. The theories of behaviour changes can be classified into three broad groups, which are useful as a foundation for developing interventions to reduce exposure to ETS at home (Glanz, 1997).

The first group is based on interpersonal theories of health behaviour: the health belief model, the reasoned action and its companion, planned behaviour, the theories of health and coping. These theories explain the formation and change of individual health behaviour with perceived susceptibility, perceived benefits and barriers, cues to action and self-efficacy.

The second group focuses on models of interpersonal health behaviour which include social cognitive theory, social support and social network, and provider-patient communication. The social cognitive theory includes two key concepts: (i) Cognitive frame

[17] The Report on Tobacco Control in India (2004) Edited by Reddy KS and Gupta PC. Ministry of Health and Family Welfare, Government of India, Centres for Disease Control and Prevention USA and the World Health Organization.

of reference of the individual and (ii) the processes by which the individual's cognitive frame could be changed. The social cognitive theory is a dynamic, multi-component theory proposing that the individuals derive an enhanced sense of self-efficacy or confidence over their health behaviour. The social cognitive theory can guide the development of a finely targeted intervention.

The third group relates to the role of organizations, social institutions and communities in health enhancement. These theories can help professionals understand the health behaviour of large groups, communities, organizations and can guide health promotion and education interventions. Mass media can play a crucial role.

These health promotion theories are reflected in the Ottawa Charter[18] which puts forward five actions:

- Developing public health policies
- Creating a support environment
- Strengthening community action
- Developing individual skills
- Orienting health services.

A two level approach is needed in programmes intended to reduce ETS exposure in the homes. At the individual level, smokers need to learn that their smoking harms not only themselves but also their families (Table 5).

At the community level, programmes are needed to (i) make smoking at home unacceptable, particularly in the presence of children (ii) draw on governmental and nongovernmental resources including mass media (iii) tap governmental action for public places and work environment, housing and building quality improvement for increasing exchange of indoor air with outdoor air. Some of the principal strategies:

- National and state level governments can enact laws to ban smoking in public places such as hospitals, schools, offices etc. There should be effective implementation of the law after it is issued. Several states[19] in India have enacted such laws but their effective implementation is yet to come.·
- There should be plan to disseminate information through the mass media or by health lebel warnings.
- The programnme should provide support through community empowerment.

---

18 Ottowa Convention as quoted in Women and Tobacco Epidemic: Challenges for the 21st Century. (2001) World Health Organization, Geneva, Switzerland.

19 Report on Tobacco Control in India by Government of India, Centre for Disease Control and Prevention USA and the World Health Organization.

Special populations such as minorities and people at low socio-economic and educational level should be targeted. Small community projects can be developed such as smoking cessation intervention for pregnant women etc.

*Table 5: Strategies for prevention of ETS exposure*

| *Location* | *Community level* | *Individual level* |
|---|---|---|
| Public places And Work places | Legislate and implement smoking ban<br>Communicate information on ETS exposure<br>Set up smoking areas<br>Improve ventilation in all buildings | Monitor and advise smokers<br>Discourage children and adolescents from smoking<br>Help smokers quit |
| Home | Information on ETS exposure risk to parents & pregnant women through mass-media<br>Improve ventilation equipment<br>Campaign for tobacco-free families<br>Change smoking practice around children | Teach parents and pregnant women the risks of ETS<br>Teach parents to stop visitors to smoke in the presence of children |

**Source:** *Women and the Tobacco Epidemic—Challenges for 21st century, WHO publication, 2001.*

## Current interventions to reduce ETS exposure at global and regional levels:

*Legislation for reducing exposure to ETS at work-sites and public places:*

A growing body of legislation and regulations against smoking in public places and work place as well as decline in social acceptability of smoking in public are important developments. Currently many countries are developing and implementing comprehensive legislation that restricts smoking in many public settings (Tables 6 and 7).

Since the 1970s, accumulating evidence on the health risks of involuntary smoking has been accompanied by a wave of social action regulating tobacco smoking in public places in the United States. Laws at federal and state levels have been enacted. There is no federal law restricting smoking at public places, however, control measures have largely taken place at state and local levels. Several states have passed extremely stringent smoking regulations, while some cities have virtually banned all smoking in public places before 1995.

*Table 6: Current tobacco control strategies in the South-east Asia*

| *Countries* | *Strategies for protection of nonsmokers* |
|---|---|
| Bangladesh | Administrative measures to create smoke free areas have been implemented in hospitals, public transport, elevators, theatres, cinemas and government premises. Some other work places have taken voluntary measures to ensure smoke-free areas. |
| South Korea | Smoking is prohibited in restaurants, shops and railway waiting rooms. |

*Contd...*

| *Countries* | *Strategies for protection of nonsmokers* |
|---|---|
| India | In 1990, through an executive order, the government implemented a prohibition on smoking in all health care establishments, government offices, educational institutions, air-conditioned railway cars, buses and domestic air flights. |
| Indonesia | By regulation all health facilities educational institutions cinema halls are tobacco smoke-free, but no regulation; domestic flights of less than two hours are smoke free. No law for smoking in buses and trains. |
| Maldives | Smoking is banned in government office buildings. |
| Myanmar | Smoking is banned in hospitals and theatres & prohibited by administrative measures in public transport. |
| Nepal | Smoking was banned in public places in 1992. |
| Sri Lanka | Some control in place. |
| Thailand | Since 1976, smoking is banned in public places, since 1985, in cinema halls, since 1988, in cabinet meetings, in government house, ministries. Non-smokers' Health Protection Act in 1992. |

***Source:*** *Women and the Tobacco Epidemic—Challenges for the 21st century WHO, 2001*

There is no overall evaluation of legislation; it is believed that legislation can reduce ETS exposure to different extents and levels. Marcus *et al.* (1992) reported that employees in workplaces that allowed smoking in numerous locations were more than four times more likely to have detectable cotinine concentration than were those in workplaces with bans on smoking. Brownson *et al.* (1995) found a slight decline in ETS exposure of nonsmokers after enforcement of Clean Indoor Air Legislation, between 1990 and 1993.

***Table 7: Current tobacco control strategies in the Western Pacific Regions***

| *Country* | *Strategy to protect non-smokers* |
|---|---|
| Australia | 1988-ban in all work places of the Federal government, in all public and private sectors, successful legal action. |
| Brunei | No |
| Cambodia | Partial ban |
| China | 1949: ban smoking in public vehicles, 1986: in sub-ways; 1983: domestic flights 1995: all flights, health ministry offices; 1994: Shanghai declared all indoors tobacco free, 1995: Beijing declared all indoors tobacco free. |
| Cook Island | Partial ban |
| Fiji | Smoking is banned by regulation |
| Japan | Partial ban |
| Kiribati | Some regulation on smoking in public places |

*Contd...*

| | |
|---|---|
| Lao People's Democratic Republic | Some voluntary measures |
| Malaysia | Ban in government offices, flights |
| Marshall | No |
| Micronesia | Partial ban |
| Mongolia | Ban |
| Nauru | No |
| New Zealand | Ban |
| Niue | Partial ban |
| Palau | 1992 legislation passed banning smoking within government buildings |
| Papua New Guinea | 1987 Act prohibits smoking in many public places |
| Philippines | Smoking is banned voluntarily in many hospitals; 1995: law mandates that all public and private elementary and high schools and colleges become smoke free. |
| Republic of Korea | 1989: set up smoking areas, smoking partially banned in public places, 1994: banned sale of duty-free cigarettes in all flights |
| Samoa | Partial ban |
| Singapore | 1970: law restricting smoking in public places, 1989: banned smoking in domestic flights. |
| Solomon Island | Partial ban |
| Tonga | 1987: ministry of health banned smoking in all hospitals, partial ban in other public places. |
| Tuvalu | No |
| Vanuatu | Partial ban |
| Vietnam | Law on health protection adopted in 1989, no smoking in halls, cinemas, theatres, 1995: banned smoking in all health facilities, smoking banned in domestic flights, in other ministries. |

***Source:*** *Women and Tobacco Epidemic: Challenges for the 21st Century, WHO, 2001*

## Health Education and Information to Protect Children from ETS Exposure

Dissemination of the findings of scientific evaluation should be the foundation of any intervention strategy. In addition, the ability of the government to take action to prevent children from exposure to ETS at home and in family day care settings is a must, which is so far quite limited. The Environmental Protection Agency (EPA) had some success in its initiative to communicate health risks of ETS exposure.

## Projects to Prevent ETS Exposure in various Target Populations

Some countries have comprehensive projects to reduce ETS exposure. Family day care is generally a locally run initiative by the local council, family and community services. Area health service workers need to approach the supervising authority to assist in developing a policy of not smoking when caring for the children. Strategies that can be used in implementing nonsmoking policies (Graham-Clarke and Nathan, 1996) are:

- Holding workshops for caregivers focusing on positive role modeling, health effects of passive smoking, possibility of future liability, effects of nonsmoking policy.
- Circulating information on health effects of passive smoking in relation to children.
- Developing formal agreements with caregivers as part of duty to the children that home is free from tobacco smoke.
- Conduct unannounced home inspections.
- Issuing written caution and counseling.

Projects at the local level can be successful in reducing ETS exposure with good design and implementation with the focus on protecting children.

Greenberg *et al* (1994) conducted a randomized controlled trial to determine whether a home based intervention programme could reduce infant passive smoking and lower respiratory illness. Among 121 infants of the smoking mothers, there was a significant difference in the trends over the year between the intervention and the control group in amount of exposure to tobacco smoke. There are few reports of evaluations of intervention from developing countries , however, the experiences of these reports cannot be applied directly to other countries due to differences in culture and social norms.

***Comprehensive intervention action:*** It is important for the developing countries to combine interventions to reduce ETS exposure with more comprehensive tobacco control actions. Countries like India, which are facing the threat of rising active tobacco smoking and inevitable increase in passive smoking that will follow should have a comprehensive programme to save the passive smokers from preventable victimization. The intervention in Thailand has adopted comprehensive tobacco control programme to effectively control tobacco menace.

*Benefits of smoke-free home*:

- Smoke-free home is safe for women and children.
- Smoke-free home smells much better.
- In a smoke-free home food tastes better.
- Curtains, walls and widow mirrors etc. of the house remain clean.
- It will not offend the non-smoking visitor.

Environmental tobacco smoke contributes significantly in polluting the environment making it unfit for healthy living. Our children deserve clean air to breathe and it becomes our duty and commitment to provide them smoke-free atmosphere.

## REFERENCES

Annonymous Cigarette Smoking Among Reproductive-age Women- Behavioural Risk Factor Surveillance System: *MMWR Morbidity Mortalality Weekly Reporter*, 91:719–23, 1989.

Benowitz N.L.: Biomarkers of Environmental Tobacco Smoke. *Environmental Health Perspective.* 107(suppl.2): 329–340, 1991.

Benowitz N.L.: Cotinine as a Biomarker of Environmental Tobacco Smoke Exposure. *Epidemiological Review.* 18:188–204, 1999.

Borland R., Pierce J.P., and Burns D.M.: Protection from Environmental Tobacco Smoke in California. the Case for a Smoke-free Work Place *Journal of American Medical Association. (JAMA)* 268:749–752, 1992.

Brenner H., Born J and Novak P.: Smoking Behaviour and Attitude Towards Smoking Regulations and Passive Smoking in the Workplace. *Preventive Medicine.* 26:138–143, 1997.

Brownson R.C., Davis R.M. and Jackson-Thompson J.: Environmental Tobacco Smoke and Awareness: the impact of state-wide clean indoor air law and the report of US EPA. *Tobacco Control.* 4: 132–138, 1995.

Burns D., and Pierce J.P.: Tobacco Use in California 1990–1991 Sacramento, CA: California Department of Health Services, 1992.

California Environmental Protection Agency: Office of the Environmental Health Hazard Assessment. Health Effects of Exposure to Environmental Tobacco Smoke. California: *California Environmental Protection Agency*, 1997.

Cameron P.: The Presence of Pets and Smoking As Correlates of Perceived Disease*m. Journal of Allergy*, 40:12–15, 1967.

Chilmonczyk B.A., Knight G.J. and Palomaki, G.E.: Environmental Tobacco Smoke Exposure During Infancy. *American Journal of Public Health.* 80: 1205–1208, 1990.

Claxton L.D. and Morin R.S.: A Genotoxic Assessment of Environmental Tobacco Smoke (ETS) Using Bacterial Bioassay. *Mutation Research*, 222: 81–99, 1989.

Colley J.R., Holland W.W. and Corckhill R.T.: Influence of Passive Smoking and Parental Phlegm on Pneumonia and Bronchitis in Early Childhood. *Lancet*, 2:1031–1034, 1974.

Cook D.G. and Strachan D.P.: Parental Smoking and Prevalence of Respiratory Symptoms and Asthma in School Age Children. *Thorax.* 52: 1081–1094, 1997.

Coultas D.B., Howard C.A. and Peake G.T.,: Salivary Cotinine Levels and Involuntary Tobacco Smoke Exposure in Children and Adults in New Mexico. *American Review of Respiratory Disorders.* 136: 305–308, 1987.

Crawford F.G., Mayer J. and Santella R.M.: Biomarkers of Environmental Tobacco Smoke in Pre-school Children and Their Mothers. *Journal of National Cancer Institute.*86: 1398–1402, 1994.

Cummings M: Passive Smoking Study, Memorandum to D. Collia,OSHA, from M. Cummings, 1994.

Dijkstra l., Houthuijs D. and Brunekreef B.: Respiratory Health Effects of the Indoor Environment in A Population of Dutch Children. American *Review of Respiratory Disorders.* 142: 1172–1178, 1990.

Dockery D.W. and Spengler J.D.: Indoor–Outdoor Relationship of Respirable Sulfates and Particles. *Atmosphere and Environment,*15: 335–343, 1981.

Du, YX,Cha and Q. Chen, X.W.: An Epidemiological Study of Risk Factors for Lung Cancer in Guangzhou, China. *Lung Cancer* 14(suppliment 1) S9 – S37, 1996.

Ernst A., and Zibrask J.D.: Carbon Monoxide Poisoning, *New England Journal of Medicine.* 339:1603–1608, 1998.

Etzel R.A., Pattishall E.N., Haley N.J., Fletcher R.H. and Henderson F.W.: Passive Smoking and Middle Ear Effusion Among Children in Daycare. *Paediatrics,* 90:228–232, 1992.

Garland C., Barret-Connor E. and Suarez L.: Effect of Passive Smoking on Ischaemic Heart Disease Mortality of Nonsmokers: A Prospective Study. *American Journal of Epidemiology.* 121: 645–650, 1985.

Glanz K: Community and Group Intervention Models of Health Behaviour Change. In: Glanz K., Lewis F.M., Rimer B.K. Eds. Health Behaviour and Health Education, Theory, Research and Practice. . 2 Ed. San Francisco, C.A.: Jossey Bass Publishers. 237–238, 1997.

Graham-Clarke P. and Nathan S.: NSW Health Promotion Survey 1994. Best Practice for Reducing the Prevalence of Smoking in the Areas of NSW. *National Centre for Health Promotion,* 1996.

Greenberg R.A., Bauman K.E. and Glover L.H.: Ecology of Passive Smoking By Young Infants. *Journal of Paediatrics.* 114: 774–780, 1989.

Greenberg R.A., Bauman K.E. and Strecher V.J.: Passive Smoking During the First Year of Life. *American Journal of Public Health.* 81:850–853, 1991.

Greenberg R.A., Strecher V.J. and Bauman K.E.: Evaluation of Home-based Intervention Programme to Reduce Infant Passive Smoking and Lower Respiratory Illness. *Journal of Behavioural Medicine.* 17: 273–290, 1994.

Guerin, M.R., Jenkins, R.A. and Tomkin, B.A.: The Chemistry of Environmental Tobacco Smoke: Composition and Measurement. Centre for Indoor Air Research, eds. Chelsea, MI: Lewis Publishers, Inc., 1992.

Hackshaw, A.K. Law, M.R. and Wald, N.J.: The Accumulated Evidence on Lung Cancer and Environmental Tobacco Smoke. *British Medical Journal* 315:980 – 988, 1997.

Hanrahan J.P., Tager I.B. and Segral M.R.: The Effect of Maternal Smoking During Pregnancy on Early Infant Lung Function. *American Review of Respiratory Disorders.* 145: 1129–1135, 1992.

Harlap S. and Davies A.M.: Infant Admissions to the Hospital and Maternal Smoking. *Lancet,*1: 529–532, 1974.

Hecht,S.S., Carmella, S.G. and Murphy, S.E.: A Tobacco Specific Lung Carcinogen in the Urine of Men Exposed to Cigarette Smoke. *New England Journal of Medicine* 329:1543 – 1546, 1993.

Hecht S.S., Carmella S.G. and Murphy S.E.: Carcinogens in the Smokers' Babies. *Cancer Epidemiology, Biomarkers and Prevention,* 15:988–992, 2006.

Hirayama T.: Non-smoking Wives of Heavy Smokers Have a Higher Risk of Lung Cancer: A Study from Japan. *British Medical Journal* (clinical research edition). 282: 183–185, 1981.

Hirayama, T.: Cancer Mortality in Nonsmoker Women with Smoking Husbands Based on a Large Scale Cohort Study in Japan. *Preventive Medicine*. 13680 – 690, 1984.

International Agency for Research on Cancer: IARC Monographs on the Evaluation of the Carcinogenic Risk of Chemicals to Humans: Tobacco Smoking. Vol. 38 Lyon France: World Health Organization International Agency for Research on Cancer (IARC), 1986.

Iverson M., Birch L., Lundqvist G.R. and Elbround O.: Middle Ear Effusion in Children and the Indoor Environment: An Epidemiological Study. *Archives of Environmental Health*, 40:74–79, 1985.

Jaakkola N., Ruotsalainen, R. and Jaakkola J.J.K.: What are the Determinants of Children's Exposure to Environmental Tobacco Smoke at Home. *Scandinavian Journal of Social Medicine*. 22:107–112, 1994.

Jaakkola M.S. and Jaakkola J.J.K.: Assessment of Exposure to Environmental Tobacco Smoke. *European Respiratory Journal*. 10:2384–97, 1997.

Jenkins PL, Phillips TJ and Mulberg E.J.: Activity Patterns of Californians: Use of and Proximity to Indoor Pollutant Sources. *Atmosphere and Environment*. 26A: 214–218, 1992.

Jordonov J.S.: Cotinine Concentrations in Amniotic Fluid and Urine of Smoking, Passive Smoking and Nonsmoking Pregnant Women At Term and in the Urine of Their Neonates on First Day of Life. *European Journal of Paediatrics*, 149: 734–737, 1990.

Kaufmann F., Tessier J.F. and Oriol P.: Adult Passive Smoking in the Home Environment: A Risk Factor for Chronic Airflow Limitation. *American Journal of Epidemiology*. 117: 269 – 280, 1983.

Koo, L.C., Ho, J.H. and Lee, N.: An Analysis of Some Risk Factors for Lung Cancer in Hong Kong. *International Journal of Cancer*. 38:149 – 157, 1985.

Koo, L.C. and Ho, J.H.: Diet as a Confounder of Association Between Air Pollution and Female Lung Cancer: Hong Kong Study on Exposure to Environmental Tobacco Smoke, Incense and Cooking Fumes As Examples. *Lung Cancer*, 14 (supplement. 1) S47 – S51, 1996.

Ko Y.C., Lee, C.H. and Chen, M.J.: Risk Factors for Primary Lung Cancer Among Nonsmoking Women in Taiwan. *International Journal of Epidemiology*. 26:24 – 31, 1997.

Kraemer M.J., Richardson M.A. and Weiss N.S.: Risk Factors for Persistent Middle Ear Effusions: Otitis Media, Catarrh, Cigarette Smoke Exposure, and Atopy. *Journal of American Medical Association* (Jama), 249:1022–1025, 1983.

Lam, TH, Kung, ITM and Wang, LM: Smoking, Passive Smoking and Histological Types of Lung Cancer in Hong Kong Chinese Women. *British Journal of Cancer* 56:673 – 678, 1987.

Lam T.H., Chung S.F. and Betson C.L.,: Respiratory Symptoms Due to Active and Passive Smoking in Junior Secondary School Students in Hong Kong. *International Journal of Epidemiology*. 27:41–48, 1998.

Law, M.R., Morris, J.K. and Wald, N.J.: Environmental Tobacco Smoke Exposure and Ischaemic Heart Disease: An Evaluation of the Evidence. *British Medical Journal* , 315:973 – 980, 1997.

Lofroth G: Environmental Tobacco Smoke: Overview of Chemical Composition and Genotoxic Components. *Mutation. Research*. 222: 73–80, 1989.

Liu, Q. Sasco, A.J. and Riboli, E.: Indoor Air Pollution and Lung Cancer in Guangzhou People Republic of China. *American Journal of Epidemiology* 137:145 – 154, 1993.

Liu, Z.Y. he, X.Z. and Chapman, R.S.: Smoking and Other Risk Factors in Xuanwei China. *International Journal of Epidemiology* 20:26 – 31, 1991.

Marcus B.H., Emmons K.M. and Abrams D.B.: Restrictive Workplace Smoking Policies: Impact on Nonsmokers' Tobacco Exposure. *Journal of Public Health Policy*. 13: 42–51, 1992.

Maroni M. and Seifert B.: A Comprehensive Reference Book: *Indoor Air Quarterly*. Elsevier Publication, 1995.

Martin T.R. and Bracken M.B.: Association of Low Birth Weight with Passive Smoke Exposure in Pregnancy. *American Journal of Epidemiology*. 124: 633–642, 1986.

Murray, A.B. and Morrison, B.J.: the Effects of Cigarette smoking from the Mother on Bronchial Responsiveness and Severity of Symptoms in Children with Asthma. *Journal of Allergy and Clinical Immunology*. 77:575 – 581, 1986.

Murray, A.B. and Morris, B.J.: Passive Smoking By Asthmatics: Its Greater Effect on Boys Than on Girls and on Older Than on Younger Children. *Pediatrics*. 84451 – 459, 1989.

National Research Council, Committee on Passive smoking: Environmental Tobacco Smoke: Measuring Exposure and Assessing Health Effects. Washington, DC: National Academy Press, 1986.

Overpeck M.D. and Moss A.J.: Children's Exposure to Environmental Cigarette Smoking Before and After Birth. Hyattsville MD: UD Department of Health and Human Services, 1991.

Pierce J.P.E.N., Farkas A.J. and Cavin S.W.: Tobacco Use in California: An Evaluation of the Tobacco Control Programme. 1989–1993. LA Jolla CA: Cancer Prevention and Control, University of California San Diego, 1994.

Pirkle J.L. , Flegal K.M. and Bernert J.T.: Exposure of US Population to Environmental Tobacco Smoke. the Third National Health and Nutrition Examination Survey, 1988–1991. 275:1233–1240, 1996.

Pletsch P.K.: Environmental Tobacco Smoke Exposure Among Hipsanic Women of Reproductive Age. *Public Health Nursing*. 11:229–235, 1994.

Rantakallio P.: Relationship of Maternal Smoking to Morbidity and Mortality of the Child Up to the Age of Five. *Acta Paediatrica Scandinavia*, 67:621–631, 1978.

Repace J.L.: Risk Management and Passive Smoking At Work and At Home. *St Luis University Public Law Review*, 13(2): 763–785, 1994.

Repace J.L. and Lowrey A.H.: Indoor Air pollution, Tobacco Smoke and Public Health. *Public Science*, 208:464–472, 1980.

Rubin D.H., Krasinikoff P.A. and Leventhal J.M.: Effect of Passive Smoking on Birth-weight. *Lancet*. 2: 415–417.

Samet J.M., Cain W.S. and Leaderer B.P.: Environmental Tobacco Smoke. In: Samet JM, Spengler JD, eds. *Indoor Air Pollution: A Health Perspective*. 131–169, 1991.

Samet J.M., Tager I.B. and Speizer F.E.: The Relationship Between Respiratory Illnessin Childhood and Chronic Airflow Obstruction in Adulthood. *American Review of Respiratory Disorders*. 127:508–523, 1983.

Samet J.M. and Yang G.: Passive Smoking, Women and Children. Women and the Tobacco Epidemic: Challenges for the 21st Century. World Health Organization in Collaboration with Institute for Global Tobacco Control and Johns Hopkins School of Public Health, 2001.

Shen, X.B. Wang, G.X. and Zhou, B.S.: Relation of Exposure to Environmental Tobacco Smoke and Pulmonary Adenocarcinoma in Nonsmoking Women: A Case Control Study in Nanjing. *Oncology Report.* 5:1221 – 1223, 1998.

Sherrill D.L., Martinez F.D. and Lebowitz M.D.: Longitudenal Effects of Passive Smoking of Passive Smoking on Pulmonary Function in Newzealand Children. *American Review of Respiratory Disorders.* 145:1136–1141, 1992.

Somerville S.M., Rona R.J., and Chinn S.: Passive Smoking and Respiratory Conditions in Primary School Children. *Journal of Epidemiology and Community Health.* 42: 105–110, 1988.

Spengler J.D., Dockery D.W. and Turner W.A.: Long-term Measurement of Respirable Sulfates and Particles Inside and Outside Homes. *Atmosphere and Environment*, 15:23–30, 1981.

Stankus, R.P., Menan, P.K. and Rando, R.J: Cigarette Smoke-sensitive Asthma: Challenger studies. *Journal of Allergy and Clinical Immunology.* 82:331 – 338, 1998.

Steyn K., Yach D. and Stander I.: Smoking in Urban Pregnant Women in South Africa. *South African Medical Journal.* 87:460–463, 1997.

Strachen, D.P. and Cook, D.G.: Health Effects of Passive Smoking. Parental Smoking and Lower Respiratory Illness in Infancy and Early Childhood. *Thorax.* 52:905 – 914, 1997.

Tager I.B.: Passive Smoking-bronchial Responsiveness and Atopy. *American Review of Respiratory Disorders.*138: 507–509, 1988.

Thompson B., Emmons K. and Abrams D.: ETS Exposure in the Work Place. Perceptions and Eactions by Employees at 114 Work Sites. *Journal of Occupational and Environmental Medicine.* 37:1363, 1995.

Trichopoulos D. and Kalandidi A., Sparros L.: Lung Cancer and Passive Smoking. *International Journal of Cancer.* 27: 1–4, 1981.

US Department of Health and Human Services: The Health Consequences of Involuntary Smoking: A Report of the Surgeon General. Washington DC: US Government Printing Office (DHHS) Publication No.(CDC) 87–8398, 1986.

US Environmental Protection Agency: Respiratory Health Effects of Passive Smoking: Lung Cancer and Other Disorders. Washington, DC: US Government Printing office. (EPA/600/006F), 1992.

Wang, T.J., Zhou, B.S., Shi, J.: Lung Cancer in Nonsmoking Chinese Women: A Case Control Study. *Lung Cancer* 14 (Supplement 1) S93 – S98, 1996.

Ware J.H., Docker D.W. and Spiro A. III: Passive Smoking Gas Cooking and Respiratory Health of Children Living in Six Cities. *American Review of Respiratory Disorders.* 129: 366–374, 1984.

Windham G.C., Eaton A. and Hopkins B.: Evidence for an Association Between Environmental Tobacco Smoke Exposure and Birth Weight: A Meta-analysis and New Data. *Paediatric and Perinatal Epidemiology.* 13: 35–37, 1999.

World Health Organization: Tobacco or Health: A Global Status Report. WHO, Geneva, Switzerland, 1997.

World Health Organization: International Consultation on Environmental Tobacco Smoke and Child Health. Consultation Report, WHO, Geneva, Switzerland, 1999.

World Health Organization: Environmental Tobacco Smoke (Chapter 8.1). WHO Air Quality Guidelines for Europe. WHO, 2000.

World Health Organization, Women and the Tobacco epidemic: Challenges for the 21st Century. WHO, Geneva, Switzerland, 2001.

World Health Organization: International Agency for Research on Cancer, Tobacco Smoke and Involuntary Smoking. IARC Monograph Vol. 83, 2002.

World Resources Institute, United Nations Environment Programme, United Nations Development Programme, World Bank, World Resources: 1998) A joint Publication by World Resources Institute, The United Nations Environment Programme, the United Nations Development Programme and the World Bank, New York: Oxford University Press.

Wu-William, A.H., Dai, X.D. and Blot, W.: Lung Cancer Among Women in Northeast China. *British Journal of Cancer*. 62:982 – 987, 1990.

Yang G.H., Lixin F. and Zhengjing H.: Smoking and Health in China: National Prevalence Survey of Smoking Pattern. Eds. Beijing China Science and Technology Press, 1996.

Yuan, J.M., Ross, R.K. and Wang X.L.: Morbidity and Mortality in Relation to Cigarette Smoking in Shanghai, China. *Journal of American Medical Association (JAMA)*. 275:1646 – 1650, 1996.

Zhang J., Savitz D.A. and Schwingl P.J.: A Case-control Study of Parental Smoking and Birth Defects. *International Journal of Epidemiology*. 21: 273–278, 1992.

# CHAPTER 8

# Tobacco Use and Medical Morbidity

*"Smoking harms almost every organ of the body, causes several diseases and reduces the health of the smoker in general……."*

— US Surgeon General's Report, 2004

Historically, the strength of opposition to the tobacco use waxed and waned. The arguments against tobacco use traditionally involved appeals to a combination of religious, moral and aesthetic principles, with little or no emphasis on the health consequences. Till recently, anti-tobacconists were a feeble and ever-dwindling minority whose argument against tobacco use was entirely derived from the fact that tobacco was neither necessary for sustenance of life nor did it play any nutritional role in human body. A feature of the present situation, however, is that anti-tobacco sentiment is firmly anchored in widely accepted medical evidence. There is an authentic inference that tobacco consumption leads not only to a varied range of morbidity but also shortens life span and causes premature deaths in a significant number of consumers. According to a WHO estimate 59.1 million disability adjusted life years (DALYs) are attributable to tobacco every year (Goswami *et al.*, 2005). Tobacco consumption is responsible for the death of 1 in 12 adults causing about 5 million premature deaths every year, of which around 4 million occur in males. Tobacco causes 50% of these deaths during middle age robbing about 22 years of normal life expectancy. By 2020 about 10 million yearly deaths will take place due to tobacco related diseases of which 7 million will occur in developing countries alone[1]. However, despite clearly evident health-risks, today, a significant number of world populations consume tobacco. It is estimated that one-third of world's adult population, about 1.3 billion people consume tobacco in one form or the other and this number is likely to rise to 1.6 billions in 2020s if the current trend continues.

---

1 Tobacco Control: Country Profile (Second Edition, 2003 page 3).

The health effects of smoking in a population only become fully pronounced about half a century after the habit is adopted by a sizeable percentage of young adults. The risk increases as the amount and duration of smoking increases. To begin with, smoking was adopted first by the men of the developed countries followed by the women of the developed countries and the men of the developing countries and only recently have the women of the developing world taken to smoking (Ernst, 2001). Reports on the ill effects of tobacco began to pour in by the beginning of the 20$^{th}$ century and most of what is known about the health effects of tobacco relates to the smoking of manufactured cigarettes. Although in some areas, of the world, use of other forms of tobacco is also common and smoking is of relatively recent origin in these areas, information on the ill effects of such a use is scanty. Therefore, the most of the work on the ill effects of smoking comes from the developed countries where the prevalence of smoking is more than a century old. However, consumption of tobacco in any form exposes an individual to the risk of a wide range of morbidity and premature death (Gajalakshmi *et al.*, 2000). Increasing use of tobacco and its related health problems are a great concern in the world today. Now, it is well established that overall mortality rates for cigarette smokers are 60 to 80% higher than the non-smokers. Tobacco use in the form of smoking is the leading preventable cause of disability and death.

Raymond Pearl of John Hopkins University, in 1938, was the first to demonstrate statistically that the non-smokers lived longer than the smokers. Only 46% of the heavy smokers lived beyond 60 years of age as against 67% of non-smokers (Ashton and Stepney, 1982). Subsequently known carcinogens were identified in the tobacco smoke (Van Proosdij, 1960). In 1939, the first scientific study was published linking lung cancer with tobacco smoking, and during the 1950s and 1960s, conclusive evidence was finally made available that cigarette smoking was the most important cause of lung cancer as well as a major factor in coronary heart disease, chronic bronchitis, emphysema, and other diseases.

In view of the strong scientific evidence that tobacco consumption was hazardous the UK Royal College of Physicians' Report (1962) and US Surgeon General's Advisory Committee Report (1964) warned against the ill effects of tobacco. Health warnings started appearing on various tobacco products to inform the consumers of the harmful effects of the products they were using while the media took the lead in creating awareness among general public.

The tobacco sub-system, one of the most powerful economic and political forces in US on the other hand had succeeded in keeping the health question a low priority item on the government's agenda by playing off one government agency against the other. The tobacco industry kept on challenging the validity of the health reports refusing to accept the results that were long accepted by all health scientists. Amidst this tug of war between tobacco lobby and scientific evidence, in United States of America, there was a rise in cigarette consumption between 1963 and 1973 despite unprecedented governmental and health agency efforts to curb the menace. US Surgeon General's Advisory Committee Report (1964) and the anti-cigarette campaigns did have one major effect, however. Vast majority of smokers turned from plain to filter tip cigarettes and from high-tar-high-nicotine to low tar-low-nicotine brands. Between 1920 and 1950, cigarette nicotine levels remained 35–40 milligrams, whereas subsequently levels were lower and carcinogenic tars were reduced (Ashton and Stepney, 1982).

## Tobacco and Medical Morbidity

Nicotine is the main chemically active constituent in tobacco responsible for a number of patho-physiological changes in the body. Nicotine not only causes damaging effects it also leads to tolerance to its own action. Nearly 3000 chemicals have been identified in smokeless tobacco, while close to 4000 are present in tobacco smoke. The US Surgeon General's Report of 1985[2] documents that cigarette and other forms of tobacco are not only addicting because of nicotine, but they contain over 43 carcinogens (Ezzati and Lopez, 2003) causing cancer and cigarette smoking in particular causes cancer of lung, oropharynx, larynx, oesophagus, pancreas, kidney and uterine cervix (see appendix).

Cigarette smoking increases the risk of chronic obstructive pulmonary diseases and cardiovascular diseases. Recent epidemiological evidence suggests that cigarette smoking is also deleterious to the gastrointestinal tract. It increases the incidence and relapse rate of peptic ulcer and delays its healing process (Ma *et al.*, 1999). More recent evidence points to the relationship between smoking and cancers of the stomach, liver and colon (Michael, 2002). The US Surgeon General's Advisory Committee Report, 2004 reveals that smoking harms almost every organ of the body, causes several diseases and reduces the health of the smoker in general[3]. Tobacco-related health consequences are described below in Table 1:

*Table 1: Health consequences related to tobacco exposure*

| |
|---|
| ***Heart and blood vessel diseases*** |
| • Atherosclerosis, coronary heart disease.<br>• Cerebrovascular diseases.<br>• Abdominal aortic aneurysm. Peripheral vascular disease (may cause gangrene in legs).<br>• Erectile dysfunction or impotence (atherosclerosis and endothelial dysfunction of the internal pudendal and penile arteries). |
| ***Cancers*** |
| • Cancerous lesions with proven association: cancers of the bladder, cervix, oesophagus, kidney, larynx, lung, oral cavity, and pharynx, pancreas, stomach, and leukaemia.<br>• Cancerous lesions with suspected association: Cancer of colorectum, liver and breast.<br>• Precancerous lesions: Leucoplakia, erythroplakia of the oral cavity. |
| ***Respiratory diseases*** |
| • Chronic Obstructive Pulmonary Disease: chronic bronchitis.<br>• Acute respiratory illnesses: Pneumonia, bronchitis and other respiratory infections. |

*Contd...*

---

2 A Report of the Surgeon General, US Department of Health & Human Services Publication No. (CDC) 89–8411, 1989.

3 Reddy KS and Gupta PC (2004) Report on Tobacco Control in India. Supported by Government of India, Centre for Disease Control and Prevention, USA and World Health Organization, Geneva.

- Respiratory effects mediated in utero; reduced respiratory function in infants.· Respiratory effects in childhood and adolescence: decreased physical fitness, unfavourable lipid profile, potential retardation in the growth of lungs,
- Respiratory effects in adulthood: acceleration in age-related decline in lung function.·
- Other respiratory effects: Increased cough, phlegm, wheezing and dyspnoea.

*Reproductive effects*

- Foetal death and still birth: Sudden Infant Death Syndrome (SIDS).
- Fertility: delayed conception.
- Low birth weight: Foetal growth restriction.
- Pregnancy complications: premature rupture of membranes, placenta praevia, and preterm delivery.

*Other effects*

- Cataract.
- Diminished health status.
- Low bone density among post-menopausal women, peptic ulcer, peridontitis.
- Root-surface dental caries.

***Source:*** *Reddy KS and Gupta PC (2004) Report on Tobacco Control in India. Supported by Government of India, Centre for Disease Control and Prevention and World Health Organization.*

## Tobacco and Carcinogenesis

Nicotine and carcinogens found in tobacco are inalienable partners. The patho-physiological consequences of tobacco use exposure include tissue destruction contributing to lung disease, cellular changes contributing to cancer and cellular and molecular reinforcing effects leading to dependence. The addiction property of nicotine precipitates and perpetuates people to consume tobacco products and once the patho-physiological consequences of tobacco use have occurred, it may no more be a matter of personal choice to abstain from tobacco than to reverse metastatising lung cells. A nicotine-dependent individual voluntarily continues to consume cigarettes and its carcinogens. The toxic effects studied are based on various assays, cell culture studies, animal experiments and tests on humans. These effects are classified as follows[4]:

1. Mutagenicity
2. Carcinogenicity
3. Genetic Damage

[4] International Agency for Research on Cancer. IARC Monographs on Evaluation of the Carcinogenic Risks of Chemicals to Humans. Tobacco Smoke and Involuntary Smoking. Vol.83. Lyon; IARC Press 2004.

### 1. Mutagenicity

In earlier studies nicotine was generally considered as a weak carcinogen (William *et al.*, 2004). In this regard, *mutagenicity* of nicotine has been widely studied. Nicotine is a potential, genotoxic compound and depending on dose and time, it can induce sister-chromatid exchange and chromosome aberration in CHO cells at concentrations achievable in saliva of tobacco chewers (Trivedi *et al.*, 1990). An ethanolic extract of the *pandharpuri* brand of chewing tobacco and *masheri* (Bhide *et al.*, 1984 and Niphadkar *et al.*, 1996), extracts of *beedi* tobacco (Bagwe and Bhisey, 1995) and *beedi*/cigarette smoke condensates (Pakhale and Bhide, 1984 and Shirname, 1985) were found to be *mutagenic* in the Ames assay that used *Salmonella typhimurium* strains for detecting the *mutagenic* activity of chemicals. Urine samples from *masheri* users (Govekar and Bhisey, 1993), tobacco chewers and *beedi* industry workers, and gastric fluid from tobacco chewers (Niphadkar *et al.*, 1994) were also found to be *mutagenic*. Recently, more sensitive *mutagenicity* assay methods are employed to study the *mutagenic* properties of nicotine. Dose dependently nicotine could form adducts with liver DNA, lung DNA, histone $H^1/H^3$, Hb, and albumin in mice (Wu *et al.*, 1997). The levels of PAH-induced DNA adducts that can lead to *mutations* were higher in the skin of the mice administered total particulate matter from the smoke of *beedi* (Thapliyal *et al.*, 2004).

Studies show that *Beedi*/cigarette smoke condensates, and ethanol extract of *Pandharpuri* tobacco induced *mutation* in Chinese hamster $V_{79}$ cells and increased micronucleated cell frequency in mouse bone marrow cells (Pakhale and Bhide, 1984). In another study an extract of snuff inhibited the growth of mouse tongue epithelial cells in culture (Gijare *et al.*, 1990).

A single, 24-hour treatment of hamster tracheal epithelial cells in culture with an extract of *beedi* tobacco decreased the growth rate of cells, with respect to untreated control cells, increased the rate of DNA synthesis, ornithine decarboxylase activity and the number of cells in DNA synthesis phase. Repeated exposure to the extract, however, leads to a significant increase in cell number, suggesting that chronic inhalation of tobacco dust among *beedi* industry workers may stimulate proliferation of the tracheal cells and thereby increase the risk for the development of pulmonary disorders including cancer (Shah *et al.*, 2001). Cotinine, an important metabolite of nicotine is also *mutagenic*. Nicotine potentates the *mutagenic* effect of cotinine with or without S9 by exerting its xenotoxic effect through metabolic conversion to cotinine.

### 2. Carcinogenicity

Nicotine-derived tobacco specific nitrosamines (TSNAs) are the alkaloids that are structurally related to nicotine and give rise to carcinogens. Of these 43 such carcinogens identified in tobacco smoke, N-nitrosonornicotine (NNN) and 4-methyl-nitrosamino-1-butanone (NNK) are the prominent ones (Table 2). In the urine of an experimental animal treated with nicotine, NNN, N'-nitrosoanabasine (NNB), and N'-nitrosoanatabine (NAT), all of which are carcinogenic nicotine-derived nitrosoamines, was found (Carmella *et al.*, 1997). Tobacco-specific nitrosamines are formed during fermentation and curing of tobacco.

*Table 2: Nitrosamines in cigarette smoke*

| Tobacco-specific nitrosamines |
|---|
| N′-Nitrosonornicotine (NNN) |
| N′-Nitrosoanabasine (NAB) |
| N′-Nitrosoanatabine (NAT) |
| 4-(Methylnitrosamino)-1-(3-pyridyl)-butanone (NNK) |
| 4-(Methylnitrosamino)-1-(3-pyridyl)-1-butanol (NNAL) |
| 4-(Methylnitrosamino)-4-(3-pyridyl)-1-butanol (iso-NNAL) |
| 4-(Methylnitrosamino)-4-(3-pyridyl)-1-butyric acid (iso-NNAC) |

***Source:*** *William et al., (2004) The Pharmacological Action of Nicotine on the Gastrointestinal Tract. Pharmacological Sciences; 94:351*

Tobacco smoke is rich in naphthalene and polycyclic aromatic hydrocarbons (PAH), which are known carcinogens and produce serious adverse effects on the body. Studies from India show high levels of benzapyrene in *masheri*, snuff and chewing tobacco (Nair *et al.*, 1987 and Bhide *et al.*, 1984).

Cancer promoting effect of nicotine is found to be dependent upon EGF receptor (EGFR) and c-Src phosphorylation and upregulation of 5-lipooxygenase(5-LOX) expression. EGFR and c-Src are, respectively, membrane and intracellular tyrosine kinases mediating many important mitogenic signals, while 5-LOX is pertinent to the metabolism of arachidonic acid. Inhibitors of EGRF, c-Src, and 5-LOX all significantly abolish the nicotine induced tumour growth (Ye *et al.*, 2004).

The effect of nicotine on cell proliferation has also been studied in non-epithelial cells. Snuff application to hamster cheek pouch resulted in increased incidence of tumours in the forestomach and not in the cheek pouch (Gijare *et al.*, 1990). Application of an extract of *masheri* to the skin of the back induced skin tumours in 20% of mice (Bhide *et al.*, 1987), while application of an extract of *beedi* tobacco promoted the growth of skin papillomas induced by a tumour-initiating carcinogen (Bagwe *et al.*, 1994). Experimentally, tumours are induced in the liver, forestomach and oesophagus of mice treated with *beedi* smoke condensate (Pakhale *et al.*, 1988 and Doll *et al.*, 1994).

*Apoptosis* is crucial in carcinogenesis by which cells accumulate when the rate of cell death is lower than the cell division. Suppressed *apoptosis* also renders the cell more readily to accumulate genetic lesions and tolerate DNA mistakes. It is also proposed that *apoptosis* actively takes part in the process of immune surveillance, growth factor/hormone independence, *angiogenesis*, metastasis, chemoresistance and radioresistance (Reed, 2002). Evidences indicate that nicotine can suppress *apoptosis* induced by tumour necrosis factor (TNF), ultra violet light, chemotherapeutic drugs, and calcium ionophore in a variety of species and tissues, including tumour cell types related to tobacco use (Wright *et al.*, 1993). Mitogen-activated protein kinase, specifically extracellular signal- regulated kinase, and subsequent over expression of anti-apoptotic protein bcl-2 are proposed to be the major signaling pathway for nicotine-induced suppression of *apoptosis* (Heusch and Maneckjee, 1998).

*Angiogenesis* is the growth of new blood vessels from the preexisting vasculature by budding and sprouting of endothelial cells. Tumour growth is highly dependent on the balance between cell formation and cell death at the tumour site, and tumourigenesis highly relied on the new blood vessels supplying the required nutrients in supporting tumour growth in the tissue. The growth of a solid tumour is *angiogenesis* dependent (Folkman, 1992). Nicotine accelerates the growth of tumour supported by increased neovascularization. The crucial role of nicotine in *angiogenesis* is confirmed by molecular and cellular evidence. Nicotine increases endothelial cell growth and tube formation *in vitro* and accelerated fibrovascula growth *in vivo* (Heeschen *et al.,* 2001). Nicotine also upregulates vascular endothelial growth factor (VEGF), MMP-2, and MMP-9, and of which are important mediators in *angiogenesis,* in colon cancer xenograft in nude mice when the cancer cells were pretreated with nicotine before inoculation (Ye *et al.,* 2004). Cigarette smoke increases ulcerative colitis-associated colonic adenoma formation in mice, which was associated with increased *angiogensis* (William *et al.,* 2004). The increased blood vessel count is also accompanied by upregulation of VEGF expression (Liu *et al.,* 2003). Nicotine may, therefore, in part play a key role in this process.

***3. Genetic Damage in Humans***

The frequency of chromosomal damage denoted by chromatid breaks and gap type aberrations is found to be significantly higher among those who chew tobacco with other ingredients such as betel nut (Adhvaryu *et al.,* 1986 and Trivedi *et al.,* 1993) or tobacco with lime (Mahimkar *et al.,* 2001), *Masheri* users and those who chew tobacco with containing betel quid or *gudhaku,* a tobacco-containing chewing product (Bhisey *et al.,* 1999). Chromosomal damage is known to occur at a higher frequency in the lymphocytes of smokers, workers in cigarette factories (Umadevi *et al.,* 2003) and those engaged in processing of tobacco for manufacture of *beedis* (Mahimkar and Bhisey 1995). Micronucleated cells are more commonly seen in the buccal epithelial cells of tobacco users or those with occupational exposure to tobacco (Nair *et al.,* 1991; and Bagwe and Bhisey, 1993).

## Magnitude of Cancer

More than 10 million people are diagnosed to be suffering from cancer annually worldwide and it is estimated that by 2020, there will be 15 million new cancer cases every year. Cancer causes 6 million deaths every year, or 12% of all deaths globally. Tobacco-related cancers in the developed countries account for about 90% of all cancers among men and 70% among women. Oral cancer accounts for one-third of all cancer cases and 90% of oral cancer cases occur because of tobacco chewing. In 1995, an estimated one-third of all cancer deaths in developed countries (47% of male cancer deaths and 14% of female cancer deaths) were attributable to smoking. Population-based Cancer Registries in India reveal that 56.4% cancer cases in males and 44.9% in females are clearly associated with tobacco use[5]. Cancers at different sites in the body related to tobacco use are:

### Tobacco use and Lung Cancer

Lung cancer is the first major concern related to tobacco smoke. It is well established that lung cancer is generally rare in populations where smoking prevalence has been low and that it tends to increase following increase in smoking prevalence. Risk of cancer occurrence increases with duration and amount of smoke exposure and decreases with smoking cessation (England *et al.,* 1996). Longer smoking history and more often smoking increase the risk of developing cancer (Dikshit and Kanhere, 2000).

As cigarette smoking had become increasingly popular after the First World War, reports on lung cancer began to pour in. During the first two decades of twentieth century, lung cancer was not that common, however, its incidence increased significantly in Americas and Europe as the cigarette consumption became popular. By the 1950s, lung cancer had become a leading cause of deaths among men in many developed countries. The careful epidemiological studies by Doll and Hill in the UK (Doll and Hill, 1952) and Wynder and others in the USA (Wynder *et al.,* 1956) showed a clear statistical association between smoking and cancer. By the 1970s and 1980s, lung cancer mortality rates became higher among men in developing countries, as well as among women in many developed regions where female cigarette smoking was already well established.

Current smokers (more than 19 cigarettes per day) have 13.7 times greater risk of developing lung cancer than those who have never smoked. Atypical bronchial epithelium has been found in 98% of current smokers, 67% of ex-smokers, and 26% of people who have never smoked[6]. Quitting decreases the risk over time from the point of quitting. After 10 years of abstinence, the risk of lung cancer is about 30 to 50% of the risk of continuing smoking. A case control study from India reveals that ever-smoking men have a five fold higher risk and ever-smoking women have a two and a half fold higher risk of developing lung cancer compared to non-smokers (Gupta *et al.,* 2001). Chronic tobacco dust inhalation among *beedi* industry workers that stimulates the proliferation of tracheal cells, increase the risk for the cancer (DeAngelis, and Flanagin, 2004).

### Oral Cavity Cancer and Tobacco Use

Indian studies recognize tobacco use as a major cause of cancer in Indian population. Association of smokeless tobacco use with oral cancer was pointed out as early as 1908

---

5 National Cancer Registry Programme (NCRP) Two year report of the population-based cancer Registries, 1997-1998, Bangalore, Indian Council of Medical Research, Coordination Unit, 2004.

6 US Department of Health and Human Services. The Health Benefits of Smoking Cessation, Centre For Disease Control, Centre for Chronic Disease Prevention and Health Promotion, Office on Smoking and Health. DHHS Publication No (CDC) 90-8416, 1990, pp75-92.

(Pindborg *et al.*, 1968 and Niblock, 1902). Subsequent Indian studies on tobacco use have also showed ample evidence of its association with cancer both in smoking and smokeless form. Smoking of tobacco in India is mainly in the form of *beedis,* followed by cigarettes, *hookah, chillum, chutta* etc. Use of smokeless tobacco in Indian population is in the form of *khaini, mainpuri* tobacco, *mawa, paan masala* etc. More recently through a variety of epidemiological and clinical studies (Gupta, Murali and Bhonsle, 1996), chewing of *paan* with tobacco has been reported to be associated with oral cancer (Gupta, Murti and Bhosle, 1996). The case-control studies reveal that the risk of oral cancer increases with the use of tobacco in various forms in comparison to nonuse. Smoking increases the risk of oral cancer relative to nonsmokers, and chewing of tobacco causes higher risk of oral cancer than smoking. In a study, *paan*-tobacco user males had 6-fold greater risk of oral cancer than nonusers (Balaram *et al.*, 2002). In another study, women chewing *paan*-tobacco had a 46 times higher risk than the women who did not chew tobacco.

### Tobacco Use and Cancer of Oesophagus

Both tobacco chewing and smoking increase the risk of developing oesophageal cancer several fold (Nayar *et al.*, 2000). Tobacco chewing increases 3-fold risk than non-chewing and *beedi* smoking a 4-fold risk. The risk of cancer in the lower third of the oesophagus for *paan*-tobacco chewers was 6.6-fold greater than for non-chewers. *Beedi* smoking in males is a significant risk factor for the cancer of all the three segments of the oesophagus, but confers a 7-fold greater risk for the upper third compared to that of non-smokers (Nandakumar *et al.*, 1996). Case controlled studies show that both tobacco chewing and smoking increase the risk of developing oesophageal cancer several-fold.

### Larynx Cancer and Tobacco Use

*Beedi* smoking is a significant risk factor for laryngeal cancer, with around 230% greater risk as compared to non-smokers (Rao *et al.*, 1999). *Beedi* smoking has emerged as a significant risk factor for laryngeal cancer (Sankaranarayanan, 1990) and the risk increases seven folds in individuals who have been smoking for 20 years or more in comparison with the nonsmokers.

### Cancer of the Cervix and Tobacco Use

A direct association between *paan*-tobacco chewing and cervical cancer has been reported. A dose-dependent direct association of *paan*-tobacco chewing with invasive cervical cancer is observed in women (Rajkumar *et al.*, 2003). In a study, 54% of the women with the habit of *paan*-tobacco chewing had cervical dysplasia (Chakrabarti *et al.*, 1990).

Cancers of gall bladder (Dutta *et al.*, 2000), urinary bladder (Notani *et al.*, 1996) and penis (Harish and Ravi, 1995) have been reported to be associated with tobacco use.

## Smoking and Ulcerogenesis

Cigarette smoking increases both the incidence and relapse of peptic ulcer diseases and also delays ulcer healing in humans (Ma *et al.*, 1999). Integrity of gastric and duodenal mucosa is maintained by interplay and balance between defensive and aggressive factors. Nicotine may tilt the balance favouring aggressive factors but attenuating defensive factors.

***Gastric acid secretion*** is regarded as one of the major aggressive factors in ulcer formation. Chronic nicotine administration, at least 25mg/kg body weight for ten days, increased gastric secretion volume and acid output stimulated by pentagastrin or bethanechol in pylorus-ligated animals. Chronic nicotine administration can lead to increased muscarine receptor sensitivity, and consequently, basal acid secretion (Wong and Ogle, 1995). It was also noted that pH during lunch hour after nicotine was significantly lower than that after placebo, suggesting that nicotine might impair postprandial gastric neutralization (Lindell *et al.*, 1992). Similarly, acute nicotine treatment has the ability to dose-dependently abolish the depressing effects of ethanol on acid secretion and gastric secretory volume (Cho *et al.*, 1990). Intravenous administration of nicotine stimulates basal gastric output by direct effect on parietal cells and potentates the histamine-mediated response in the isolated cell model (Albinus *et al.*, 1988). However, all these findings are not conclusive, contradictory findings have been reported (Leung, 1994).

***Helicobacter pylori-induced ulcer*** **:** *Helicobacter pylori (H. pylori)* and cigarette smoking are two major risk factors for gastroduodenal ulcers but the interaction between them on ulcerogenesis are complex. It was found that the *H. pylori* infection was positively associated with cigarette smoking (Hamajima *et al.*, 2002) and the success rate of *H. pylori* was significantly lowered if the patient continues to smoke during medication (Matsuo *et al.*, 2003). Cigarette smoking might exacerbate disease progression in *H. pylori*-positive subjects. Cigarette smoking might lead to progression of atrophic gastritis and intestinal metaplasia in patients infected with *H. pylori* (Nakamura *et al.*, 2002). Nicotine has the ability to potentate the vacuolating toxin activity of *H. pylori* in gastric cells (Endoh and Leung, 1994).

***Pepsinogen and vasopressin secretions*** have completely different actions on gastric mucosa. Pepsin bears powerful mucolytic properties and is recognized as crucial aggressive agent in the pathogenesis of peptic ulcer disease (Pearson *et al.*, 1986). Pepsin secretion correlates with serum pepsingen-1, the endocrine component of pepsinogen secreted by the chief cells and it is proposed that nicotine directly stimulates pepsinogen secretion probably via nicotine receptors on the gastric chief cells.

***Vasopressin*** can cause vasoconstriction and provoke platelet aggregation, leading to an impaired tissue blood supply. Endogenous vasopressin plays an aggressive role in the development of gastroduodenal ulceration. Incidence of peptic ulcer is lower in vasopressin-deficient patients and different ulcerogenic substances can increase intramucosal vasopressin levels. Nicotine chewing gum induces non-osmotic vasopressin release in humans suggesting that by stimulating noradrenalin release in the supraoptic nucleus, nicotine facilitates vasopressin release from the neurohypophysis. The action is mediated at least in part by increased cytosolic $Ca^{2+}$ and activation of cAMP-dependent proteinkinase A (Shioda *et al.*, 1997).

***Gastric mucosa blood flow*** plays an important role in the protection of mucosal barrier in the stomach. Disturbances in blood perfusion in the gastric mucosa result in the formation of erosions and ulcers. Therefore, ulcerogenicity of nicotine is mediated through the reduction of mucosal blood flow. Chronic administration of nicotine markedly reduces gastric mucosal blood flow in experimental animals (Eastwood, 1997). Centrally administered nicotine has an inhibitory effect on mucosal blood flow and high dose of nicotine (25 mg/ml) in drinking water potentates the decrease of gastric mucosal blood flow induced by ethanol (Cho *et al.,* 1990).

***Mucosal restitution:*** Gastric mucal surface is prone to an easy damage by wear and tear and capable of repairing rapidly after injury and restores through restitution and regeneration. During restitution, epithelial cells spread and migrate to reseal superficial wounds after injury, a process independent of cell proliferation. Nicotine suppresses the process of mucosal restitution through inhibition of rnithine decarboxylase, a key enzyme responsible for production of endogenous polyamines, and down-regulation of expression of voltage-gated potassium ion channel (Shin *et al.,* 2002).

***Mucus secretion:*** Evidences favour the proposition that nicotine is ulcerogenic, it can not be protective against gastric damage by enhanced mucus production. Ethanol consumption is associated with depletion of mucosal mucus followed by chronic gastritis. Acute intragastric nicotine administration was found to offer acute protection against ethanol-induced gastric injury.

***EGF and Prostaglandins:*** Salivary gland is one of the major sources of EGF. Salivary EGF level is usually 5-10 times more than found in the blood or gastric juice (Konturek *et al.,* 1989). EGF is important in maintaining gastrointestinal mucosal integrity and ulcer healing. EGF decreases not only the gastric secretion and increases bicarbonate/mucus secretion it also enhances mucosal blood flow. It is demonstrated that nicotine reduces the salivary EGF level associated with the pathogenesis of smoking-related peptic ulcer disease. Prostaglandin inhibits gastric acid secretion and exerts protective action including those on mucosal blood flow and mucus secretion in gastric mucosa. Prostaglandin $E^2$ synthesis in the gastric mucosa of smokers, was found to be decreased. Acute and chronic nicotine administration inhibits prostaglandin $E^2$ production and increase susceptibility to ulceration in stomach (Lindell *et al.,* 1997).

***Glutathione (GSH)*** is another protective mediator that provides different protective action against mucosal injury in gastrointestinal tract. A free radical scavenger, GSH is able to prevent cellular injury induced by oxidative stress. Nicotine is found to deplete intracellular GSH by augmenting stress-induced reduction in gastric GSH level and haemorrhagic ulceration in rodents (Wong *et al.,* 2002).

***Tobacco use and ulcerative colitis:*** There is reduced risk of ulcerative colitis in cigarette smokers in comparison with nonsmokers (Thomas *et al.,* 1995). Intermittent smokers find their symptoms improved with smoking (Rudra *et al.,* 1989); and a dose-response relationship exists, with a decreased risk of ulcerative colitis with the increasing amounts of cigarettes smoked (Lindberg, 1988). Cessation of smoking by individuals having smoked a greater number of cigarettes also confers a greater risk of developing ulcerative colitis (Boyko *et al.,* 1997). Nicotine has been examined as a possible pharmacological agent accounting for such an association and nicotine patches have been clinically tried in the treatment of ulcerative colitis (William *et al.,* 2004). After 6 weeks of treatment in a randomized, placebo controlled trials, rate of remission of ulcerative colitis doubled (Pullan *et al.,* 1994). Nicotine liquid enema was found to be beneficial in the treatment of distal colitis (Sandborn, 1997). Ex-smokers with ulcerative colitis also showed symptomatic improvement with nicotine gum (Lashner *et al.,* 1990). The addition of transdermal nicotine to treatment with mesalamine enema is beneficial to patients with distal ulcerative colitis refractory to rectal mesalamine alone.(Gulslandi *et al.,* 2002), however, relapse rate was comparable with placebo (Thomas *et al.,* 1995). It is suggested that nicotine is not effective as monotherapy. In a 6 weeks trial comparing transdermal nicotine (15 to 20 mg/day) with prednisolone (15 mg/day), only 30% patients had clinical and endoscopic improvement with nicotine versus 60% with prednisolone (Thomas *et al.,* 1998).

*Mechanism of the beneficial effect of nicotine on ulcerative colitis* is explained on the bases of several mechanisms, which include: effects on the epithelial mucus, gut motility, eicosanoid metabolism, and production of pro-inflammatory cytokines. Nicotine boosts up the mucin synthesis and thus provides a protective mucus layer in the colon (Finnie *et al.,* 1996). Nicotine also reduces circular muscle activity, predominantly through the release of nitric oxide (Green *et al.,* 2000). Nicotine also modifies eicosanoid-mediated inflammation in patients with ulcerative colitis. It is also found that nicotine reduced prostaglandin $F^{1\alpha}$, prostaglandin $F^{2\alpha}$, and 15-hydroxyeicosatetranoic acid levels in the rectal mucosa of rabbits (Zijlstra *et al.,* 1994). In addition, both *in vivo* and *in vitro* studies showed that nicotine inhibited proinflammatory cytokines including IL-1beta, IL-2, IL-8, IL-10, and TNF alfa production (Hodgson and Bhatti 1996). The amelioration of colonic inflammation was accompanied by upregulation of somatostatin and intestinal trefoil factor mRNA expression. Recent evidence also demonstrates the expression of nAChRs in colon epithelium (Richardson *et al.,* 2003). Therefore, it needs to be investigated whether the beneficial action of nicotine is mediated through the cholinergic receptors in the colon.

## Tobacco and Vascular Diseases

Cardiovascular diseases (CVD) as a group are the leading cause of death world over and more so in the developed countries. CVD is also the largest contributor to tobacco-related deaths, in terms of absolute numbers. In many countries, deaths due to CVD considerably outnumber cancer-related deaths.

Tobacco use, especially smoking, is associated with vascular diseases such as chronic heart disease (CHD), angina, sudden cardiac death (SCD), arrhythmias, stroke, peripheral artery disease (gangrene of the legs), abdominal aortic aneurysms, renal artery stenosis, cor pulmonale and erectile sexual dysfunction. Thus smoking affects the entire vascular system.

Smoking has a direct toxic effect on vascular endothelium, with induced degenerative changes. Smoking also increases the adherence of platelets to arterial endothelium, playing a direct role in acute coronary occlusions. Smoking reduces the high level of high-density lipoprotein HDL-C, which diminishes the protective effects of HDL-C on the development of arteriosclerosis, with an inverse relationship between level of smoking and level of HDL-C.

There is increased myocardial oxygen demand in smokers, which is critical at times of acute coronary occlusion. Smoking also is related to increased cerebrovascular disease, probably similar to mechanisms that increase atherosclerosis in smokers. The excess risk of vascular disease caused by smoking can be reduced by 50% in the first year of abstinence on smoking-cessation and after 15 years almost returns to the risk of people at the same age who never smoked.

Nicotine and carbon monoxide present in the tobacco smoke are responsible for the cardiovascular effects. Other chemicals present in tobacco smoke causing vascular injury include nitrogen oxide, hydrogen cyanide and tar, with cadmium, zinc and carbon disulphide being minor contributors (Gupta, 1987). Smoking causes endothelial dysfunction (blood vessels can not dilate normally), lipid alterations and platelet activation leading to a prothrombotic state (Tsiara, Elisa and Mikhailidis, 2003). Tobacco use also increases the risk and severity of vascular disease by increasing the risk of diabetes, which itself damages the blood vessels by accelerating atherosclerosis.

Smokers have 2.87 times increased risk of coronary heart disease (CHD) compared to non-smokers. In a study, individuals smoking more than 40 cigarettes per day had a 9 times increased risk of CHD compared to those who never smoked. There is a dose-response relationship between the quantity of cigarettes smoked and cardiovascular morbidity (Rogot and Murray, 1980). The risk increases with the number of cigarettes smoked and the duration of smoking. About 48% of all myocardial infarction (MIs) cases in young and middle-aged Italian women were attributed to cigarette smoking (Gramenzi *et al.*, 1989).

Women who use contraceptives have a particularly elevated risk of coronary heart disease if they smoke (Pais *et al.,* 1996). Women who smoke also have elevated risk of ischaemic stroke and subarachnoid haemorrage, carotid atherosclerosis and death from ruptured abdominal aortic aneurysm.

Passive smokers (whose spouses smoke), are exposed to an increased risk (30%) of ischaemic heart disease (IHD). Nonsmokers exposed to second-hand smoke have a 25% excess risk of chronic heart disease compared with nonsmokers not exposed to smoke. A significant dose-response relationship is found (He *et al.,* 1999). A ban on public smoking was found to be associated with a reduced incidence of hospital admissions for acute myocardial infarction and within 6 months of ban enforcement number of admissions fell significantly compared to the same period before the law enforcement (Sargent, Shepard, and Glantz, 2004). These studies point towards a clear association between tobacco use and cardiovascular diseases. However, there are no Indian studies that have looked into the effects of second hand smoke.

According to a WHO Report, 16.7 million people died due to cardiovascular diseases constituting 29.2% of the total global deaths in 2002 and 80% of these deaths occurred in developing countries. By 2010, cardiovascular diseases will be the leading cause of death in the developing countries. In 1990, 17% of the total mortality due to cardiovascular deaths occurred in India alone (Reddy and Yusuf, 1998). CVD-related deaths in India are expected to rise from 3 million in 2000 to 4.8 million in 2020 (Leeder *et al.*, 2004). By 2020, about 42% of the total deaths in India are expected to be due to cardiovascular causes. During the period 2000-2030, about 35% of all deaths due to CVD in India are projected to occur in the age group of 35–64 years, an age group that shows maximum morbidity and mortality due to adverse effects of tobacco smoking. Lower-middle class and urban poor are becoming the worst victims in India.

## Tobacco and Lung Disease

There is a strong association between tobacco smoking and lung diseases. Smoking is associated with increased airway responsiveness (Woolcock *et al.*, 1987). It is hypothesized that smoking leads to chronic obstructive lung disease by causing airway and alveolar inflammation due to chronic chemical irritation, then bronchial narrowing with airway hyper-responsiveness, and finally breakdown of lung parenchyma, resulting in emphysema (Sparrow *et al.*, 1987). Decreased pulmonary functions occur with smoking, with increased association with asthma and chronic bronchitis. Passive smoke exposure increases risk of respiratory infections, and asthma.

***Chronic obstructive pulmonary disease (COPD)*** is a leading cause of morbidity and mortality worldwide (Hurd, 2000) and tobacco smoking is the most important cause of the development of COPD. Tobacco smoking accounts for 80–90% of the cases of COPD. Based on epidemiological, clinical and laboratory data from various studies (Serthi and Rochester, 2002), there has been a definite causal relationship between COPD and tobacco. This relationship was first established in the 1960s through several population-based epidemiological studies[7]. COPD occurs due to inflammation of the lung tissue and exposure to toxins in the tobacco smoke. Smoke particulates and gases present in tobacco smoke cause inflammation and swelling of respiratory tract resulting in narrowing of respiratory tubes and obstruction to airflow and trapping of air into lungs. Tobacco chemicals also initiate several enzymatic reactions causing damage to the lung tissue. Both the airway narrowing and lung damage progress, especially in the presence of continued smoking. In chronic smokers irreversible lung damage occurs resulting in respiratory disability, failure and premature death.

Several hospital-based studies from North India in 1960s reveal the prevalence of chronic bronchitis to be 2.5% of total indoor patients (Viswanathan, 1964). COPD accounted for 31% of the outpatient attendance in 1952–1954 in Punjab (Wig, Guleria and Bhasin, 1964). Epidemiological studies of 1990s reported prevalence data from cross-sectional community surveys. The overall prevalence of COPD was found to be 5% in males and 2.8% in females in a cross-sectional study from Haryana (Jindal, 1993).

---

[7] United States Public Health Service. Smoking and Health: Report of the Advisory Committee to the Surgeon General of Public Health Service, Washington DC: United States Public Health Services, Washington DC, Publication No. 1103.

*Table 3: Prevalence of chronic obstructive pulmonary disease (COPD)*

| Authors | Population studied | Total Number | Prevalence of COPD (%) M | F | Ratio of Smokers: nonsmokers (Males) |
|---|---|---|---|---|---|
| Viswanathan 1964 | Patna | 15,900 | 2.1 | 1.3 | 7.4 |
| Wig *et al.*, 1964 | Delhi (Urban) | 2366 | 3.1 | 1.9 | 8.8 |
| | Delhi (Rural) | 1406 | 8.4 | 2.4 | 4.7 |
| Jindal, 1993 | Chandigarh | 1473 | 5.0 | 2.7 | 9.6 |
| Sikand *et al.*, 1966 | Delhi | 14,460 | 3.3 | 2.6 | 5.9 |
| Bhattacharya *et al.*, 1975 | Lucknow | 1140 | 6.7 | 4.5 | 1.7 |
| Joshi *et al.*, 1975 | Punjab (Industrial Workers) | 473 | 12.5* | | 5.3 |
| Viswanathan and Singh, 1977 | Delhi (Urban) | 993 | 8.0 | 4.3 | 4.1 |
| | Delhi (Rural) | | 4.7 | 3.5 | 9.6 |
| Thiruvengadam *et al.*, 1977 | Madras | 817 | 1.9 | 1.2 | 10.2 |
| Radha *et al.*, 1977 | Delhi | 2098 | 4.2 | 2.1 | 1.8 |
| Malik *et al.*, 1977 | Chandigarh | 1154 | 8.3 | 5.3 | 4.8 |
| Nigam *et al.*, 1982 | Jhansi (Rural) | 1424 | 8.1 | 4.5 | 1.4 |
| Malik, 1986 | Chandigarh(U) | 1450 | 10.8 | 1.65 | 11.0 |
| | Chandigarh(R) | 671 | 20.5 | 4.9 | 4.0 |
| Malik and Kashyap, 1988 | Himachal (R) | 446 | 21.7 | 19.0 | 5.5 |
| Behera and Malik, 1987 | Chandigarh (School teachers) | 681 | 3.3 | 2.1 | 1.6 |
| Ray *et al.*, 1995 | Tamil Nadu | 9946 | 4.1 | 2.6 | |

*Data for both combined

***Source:*** *Reddy KS and Gupta PC (2004) Report on Tobacco control in India. Supported by Government of India, Centre for Disease Control and Prevention, USA and World Health Organization.*

COPD accounted for 5.8 % of total deaths and it is expected that by 2020 death toll will rise to 9.3%. COPD is also a major cause of economic burden in both developed and developing countries (Sullivan *et al.*, 2000). Smoking cessation results in reduction in common respiratory symptoms, improved pulmonary functions even in people with COPD, and decreased by chronic respiratory disease.

## Tobacco and Reproductive Health Outcome

Smoking by mothers during pregnancy has been identified as the greatest single preventable cause of infant morbidity and mortality in the West. Smoking may have long-term effects on surviving children. In addition, several complications in the mother have been associated with maternal cigarette smoking (DiFranza and Lew, 1995) which may include abruptions, placenta praevia, abortions, retarded foetal growth, low birth weight and others.

Compared with nonsmoking women, smokers are more likely to experience primary and secondary infertility (Daling *et al.,* 1987 and Joesoef *et al.,* 1993) and delays in conceiving (Baird and Wilcox, 1985). The effects of maternal smoking during pregnancy encompass a wide spectrum — decreased foetal growth, spontaneous abortions, foetal deaths, pregnancy complications including those that predispose to pre-term delivery, and long-term effects on the surviving children. Studies show that with respect to pregnancy outcomes, women who smoke are at increased risk of premature rupture of membranes, abruptio placentae, placenta privia, (Hadley, Main and Gabbe, 1990) and lower average birth weight babies. Women who smoke are more likely to experience dysmenorrhoea (Wood; Larsen and Williams, 1997 and Sundell; Milsom and Andersch, 1990) and premature menopause. On average, women who are currently smokers go through menopause about 1-2 years earlier than nonsmoking women (Willett *et al.*, 1983).

There has been increasing evidence both from India and abroad indicating that the smoking men have a lower sperm count than non-smokers; the sperm quality of their semen is reduced and contains a higher proportion of malformed sperms, which also have reduced motility (Banerjee *et al.*, 1993 and Merino *et al.,* 1998). Smoking also increases the risk of impotence by around 50% for men in their thirties and forties. Thus, smoking causes impairment of reproductive health in male smokers as well.

## Effects of Smoking Mothers on Infants and Children

Nicotine, carbon monoxide (CO), heavy metals and polycyclic aromatic hydrocarbons (PAHs) present in tobacco smoke, cause reduced oxygen delivery to the foetal cells, decreased blood supply to the uterus and placenta, impaired organ development, retarded foetal growth and foetal toxaemia and disrupted endocrine system (Rowell and Clark, 1982).

Cigarette smoking by the women during pregnancy has long been considered an important independent risk factor for decreased birth-weight. Such babies are more likely to be small for gestational age (Cnattingius, 1997) and are at increased risk of stillbirth and perinatal mortality than are the infants of nonsmoking women. The infants of mothers who smoke during pregnancy have birth weights approximately 200–250 grams lower, on average, than infants born to nonsmoking women (Murphy, Butler and Petersen, 1996). Risks of stillbirths (Cnattingius, Haglund and Meirik, 1988), neonatal death, and Sudden Infant Death Syndrome (Dwyer, Ponsonby and Couper, 1999) are also greater among the offspring of women who smoke. Foetal death rates are 35% higher among women who smoked during pregnancy than those who were non-smokers[8]. Breastfeeding is less common or of shorter duration among women who smoke than among

[8] US Surgeon General's Advisory Committee Report, 2001 Washington DC, USA.

female nonsmokers and that smokers who breastfeed may produce less breast milk than nonsmokers (Horta, Victora and Menezes, 1997).

In a study, mothers of hyperkinetic children were found to be smoking more than 14 cigarettes a day during their pregnancy[9]. and these children were lesser in their mathematical and general ability as compared to the children whose mothers did not smoke during pregnancy[10]. Children born to women who smoked during pregnancy had more behavioural problems compared to the children whose mothers did not smoke during pregnancy and they performed poorer on intelligence tests. Learning and memory deficits in the offspring of the mothers exposed to nicotine during pregnancy were observed in animal studies as well as in humans (Roy 1994). Nicotine damages the brain cell quality of the foetus causing increased risk of conduct disorder in the child (Lauren *et al.*, 1997). Children of the mothers who smoked during their pregnancy still showed the harmful effects at age 14.

Exposure to second-hand smoking produces numerous effects on the health of children, particularly with respect to ear infections, lung function and asthma (these effects have been discussed elsewhere). Older children and adolescents who are active smokers have increased risk of respiratory illness, cough and phlegm production, slower rates of lung growth, reduced lung function and poorer lipid profiles than the nonsmoking counterparts.

## Tobacco and Oral Mucosal Lesions and Dental Diseases

Oral and Pharyngeal tissues come in contact with carcinogens present in smokeless tobacco products and tobacco smoke. In addition, tobacco-specific nitrosamines may be formed in the mouth through the process of nitrosation.

Tobacco use in any form has marked effects upon the soft tissues of the oral cavity, leading to precancerous lesions such as erythroplakia, and other oral mucosal lesions. Leucoplakia is the most common precancerous lesion associated with smoking and chewing tobacco. **Oral submucous fibrosis** (OSMF) is emerging as a new epidemic, especially among the youth.

OSMF is a premalignant condition characterized by slowly progressive chronic fibrotic disease of the oral cavity and oropharynx, in which the oral mucosa loses its elasticity and develops fibrous bands, which ultimately lead to difficulty in opening the mouth (Gupta *et al.*, 1998). OSMF is a high-risk precancerous condition and 4.5 to 7.6% of its lesions progress to become oral cancers (Pindborg *et al.*, 1984 and Murti *et al.*, 1984). The relative risk of malignant transformation of these lesions is because of continued tobacco use as compared to those who don't have any precancerous tobacco lesions. The increased malignant potential is due to generalized epithelial atrophy. In India, a higher occurrence of leucoplakia and carcinoma is reported in patients with OSMF. It is believed to be an important factor responsible for

[9] Canadian Psychiatric Association Journal, Vol. 20:183–187, 1975.

[10] British Medical Journal, Vol. 4:573–575, 1973.

increasing incidence of oral cancer in lower age groups (below 35 years of age) (Gupta *et al.*, 1998 and Gupta and Ray, 2002). The dramatic increase in OSMF among young people in India has been attributed to chewing *gutka* and *paan masala*.

### Smoking and Pulmonary Tuberculosis

Currently, one-third of the world's population is infected with tubercular bacillus and approximately 2 million individuals die each year of tuberculosis (TB), with more than 90% infections and deaths occurring in low- and middle-income countries. 80% of all new TB cases are seen in 23 countries; more than half are concentrated in 5 countries of Bangladesh, China, India, Indonesia and Nigeria (DeAngelis and Flanagin 2004). In India, pulmonary TB is highly prevalent and a major cause of death. Thus, ascertaining the role of smoking in the development and progression of TB is of great importance. Survey reports indicate that the overall prevalence of tuberculosis in India is 0.6% in rural areas and 0.4% in urban areas; 0.62% in males and 0.46% in females and increases with age. It is established that 2 million people in India develop TB each year (Dye *et al.*, 1999).

Studies reveal that there is an association between tobacco smoking and tuberculosis (Gajalakshmi *et al.*, 2003). The prevalence of TB is about three times as great among ever-smokers as among never-smokers and heavier the smoking, the greater the prevalence of tuberculosis among smokers. In smoker tuberculosis patients mortality is three times higher than nonsmoker TB patients (Gupta *et al.*, 2000 and Gupta *et al.*, 2001).

### Green Tobacco Sickness Among Tobacco Growers

Tobacco cultivation involves different practices such as sowing, transplanting of seedlings, topping of flowering buds, disbudding of axillary buds, harvesting of plants and leaves, separating of leaves, stringing and tying of leaves before they are kept in barns for curing, grading etc. These activities lead to smearing of thick, gummy plant sap on the hands of workers and other parts of their bodies that come in contact with tobacco leaves. This leads to absorption of nicotine through the dermal route. Workers engaged in various processes get cuts and abrasions on their palms and the skin around their nails gets peeled off, facilitating nicotine absorption (Lewin and Elvin, 1977). Tobacco growing in the fields or in an uncured state is called 'green tobacco.' This is toxic when in prolonged direct contact with the skin. Workers engaged in tobacco cultivation activities suffer from an occupational illness is known as **'green tobacco sickness' (GTS)**. The illness was first reported among tobacco workers in Florida, in 1970, as cropper sickness (Weizenecker and Deal, 1970). Later, absorption of nicotine from wet tobacco plants is found to be responsible for GTS. Since the sickness is self-limiting, treatment is not always necessary.

Green tobacco sickness is an acute form of nicotine toxicity and usually occurs several hours after continuous exposure to green tobacco leaves. The illness is characterized by headache, nausea, vomiting, giddiness, loss of appetite, fatigue, weakness and sometimes fluctuations in the blood pressure or heart rate lasting for 12–24 hours (Morgan, 1989). Although GTS is not reported to be associated with mortality or long-term morbidity, it causes considerable amount of discomfort to the sufferer.

India is the third country to have reported GTS among tobacco harvesters (Ghosh *et al.*, 1979). Headache, giddiness, nausea and vomiting were the four most common symptoms observed in all tobacco workers and GTS was found to be higher in *beedi* tobacco workers than the cigarette tobacco workers.

### Tobacco Related Deaths

Of all the diseases causally associated with smoking, lung cancer is the most well known, largely because in most populations, almost all lung cancer deaths are due to smoking. In 1930, lung cancer death rate for men in the USA was 4.9 per 100,000, in 1990; the rate increased to 75.6 per 100,000[11]. Smoking is responsible for 90% of all lung cancers. However smoking causes more deaths from other diseases than lung cancer. In 1995, there were 514,000 smoking caused lung cancer deaths in developed countries, compared to 625,000 smoking attributed deaths from heart and other vascular diseases in the same year. Cigarette kills 50% of all lifetime cigarette users and tobacco kills more than AIDS, drugs, road accidents, murder and suicide combined (Mackay and Eriksen, 2002).

Tobacco is estimated to have caused 3 million deaths a year in early 1990s and death toll is steadily increasing and it is currently responsible for the deaths of one in 12 adults worldwide (about five million deaths each year). If current smoking patterns continue, it will cause some ten million deaths each year by 2025[12]. 70% of these deaths will be in the developing countries alone.

In 1990s, about 25% of all male deaths in developing countries were due to smoking. In women of developing countries, percentage of all deaths caused by smoking increased more than six folds, from 2% in 1955 to 13% in 1995.

The South Asia (SA) region which includes 8 countries: Afghanistan, Bangladesh, Bhutan, India, Maldives, Nepal, Pakistan and Sri Lanka comprises world's 23% population, mortality rate due to cancer of trachea, lungs and bronchi is quite common in these countries and significantly higher among men and more so in the male smokers from Bangladesh (Figure 1). Smokeless tobacco poses serious health risks. The annual mortality from tobacco chewing in South Asia alone is 50,000 deaths. Mortality from cancer of lip, oral cavity and pharynx is higher among men and more so in the men of Sri Lanka. (Figure 2).

---

[11] Barry M (1991) New England Journal of Medicine; 324: 917–920.

[12] Tobacco Free Initiative (TFI), World Health Organization, 2004.

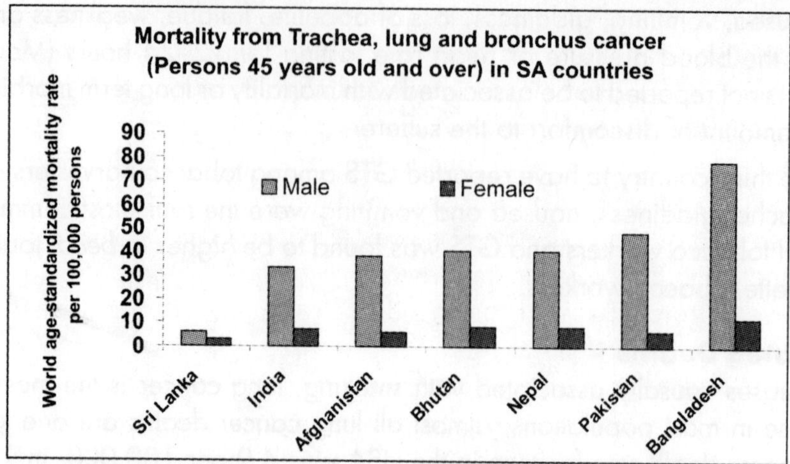


*Figure: 1: Standard death rate from trachea, lungs and bronchus cancer per 100,000 persons for SA countries in 1990.*

***Source:*** *Ferlay J; Parkin DM; and Pisani P (1998) GLOBOCAN I: Cancer incidence and Mortality worldwide. [CD-ROM]. International Agency for research on cancer.*

Recent epidemiological studies[13] reveal that India has 184 million tobacco users of which 20% smoke cigarettes, 40% smoke *beedi* and 40% use smokeless tobacco. Chewing habit being common, has exposed users to the risk of oral cancer. Smoking is responsible for 75% of all cases of chronic bronchitis and emphysema (Bhattacharya *et al.*, 1975).

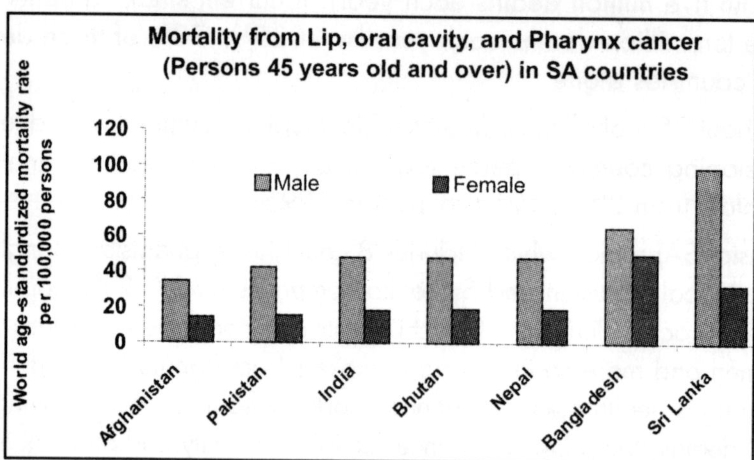


*Figure: 2: Standard death rate from lip, oral cavity and pharynx cancer per 100,000 persons for SA countries in 1999.*

***Source:*** *Ferlay J; Parkin DM; and Pisani P (1998) GLOBOCAN I: Cancer incidence and Mortality World-wide. [CD-ROM]. International Agency for Research on Cancer.*

[13] Indian Council of Medical Research Bulletin, November, 2000.

An average Indian smoker is middle-aged male unaware of health consequences of smoking contribute significantly to the national mortality and morbidity rates. In 1996, it was estimated that 800,000 people died from tobacco related diseases in India (NSSO, 1998) and that 150,000 cases of cancer, 4.2 million cardiovascular cases, and 3.7 million chronic respiratory disease cases were due to tobacco (CMR, 1996). Tobacco use is fast being recognized as a public health disaster in India (WHO, 2003). Further, the ubiquity of smokeless tobacco use has allowed some of the best estimates to be derived for the relationship between consumption and oral cancers. Prevalence of oral cancer in India is very high; around 33% of world's oral cancer occurs in India. Oral cancer caused by chewing tobacco accounts for about 50–70% of all cancers. In 1990, approximately 1.5% of total deaths in India were tobacco-related and tobacco consumption continues to grow at the rate of 2–3% per annum. If current trend continues, tobacco alone would lead to 13.3% of all deaths in India in 2020.

No doubt, tobacco trade offers bountiful revenue, provides employment to many and helps society with several economic 'benefits', but its devastating effects are enormous. Tobacco consumption is not only a major cause of morbidity and mortality, it imposes considerable costs, including both the direct costs of the health care and indirect costs of lost productivity.

It may cause property loss through fire, raise the cost of fire-protection measures, and lead to deforestation because of extensive use of wood in flue-curing process of tobacco preparation. Equally important are the real costs entailed in looking after the smokers during their illness, the loss of production and lower productivity on account of avoidable tobacco-related diseases and mortality, higher overall health and welfare spending, opportunity cost foregone consumption (Kabra, 1998).

Most effects of tobacco consumption manifest later and appear in future when tobacco-related disease victimizes the smoker, quality of life deteriorates, financial resources are diverted to the care of disease affliction and the longevity of life gets shortened. In fact, valuation of human life transcends any estimate of financial gains or costs and is a major factor for treating tobacco as a demerit good better termed as 'bad'. As Warner (1998) sums up, no 'economic' valuation' of life and longevity is possible as it is simply invaluable and beyond numerical figures. Globally and nationally, there is enough evidence regarding society's recognition of tobacco use as a menace and the need to go in for tobacco control.

## REFERENCES

Adhvaryu S.G., Bhat R.G., Dayal P.K., Trivedi A.H., Dave B.J. and Vyas R.C.: SCE Frequency in Lymphocytes of Tobacco/Betel Nut Chewing and Patients with Oral Sub Mucous Fibrosis. *British Journal of Cancer*, 53: 142–143, 1986.

Albinus M., Frisch G. and Klein S.: The Effects of Nicotine on Basal and Stimulated Gastric Secretion in Conscious Cat and in Isolated Guinea Pig Gastric Mucosal Cells.. Agents Actions, 23:289–292, 1988.

Ashton H. and Stepney A.: *Smoking: Psychology and Pharmacology*.tavistock Publications, London, 1982.

Bagwe A.N. and Bhisey R.A.: Occupational Exposure to Tobacco and Resultant Genotoxicity in *Beedi* Industry Workers. *Mutation Research*, 299: 103–109, 1993.

Bagwe A.N., and Bhisey R.A.: Occupational Exposure to Unburnt Beedi Tobacco Elevates Mutagenic Burden Among Tobacco Processors. *Carcinogenesis*, 15: 1095–1099, 1995.

Bagwe A.N., Ramchandani A.G., and Bhisey R.a.: Skin Tumour Promoting Activity of Processed *Beedi* Tobacco in Hairless S/Rv Cri-ba Mice. *Journal of Cancer Research and Clinical Oncology*, 120: 485–489, 1994.

Baird D.D. and Wilcox A.J.: Cigarette Smoking Associated With Delayed Conception. *Journal of American Medical Association*, 253:2979–2983, 1985.

Balaram P., Sridhar H., Rajkumar T., Vacarella S., Herrero R. and Nandkumar A. Oral Cancer in South India, the Influence of Smoking, Drinking, *Paan* Chewing and Oral Hygiene. *International Journal of Cancer*,98: 440–445, 2002.

Banerjee A., Pakrashi A., Chatterjee S., Ghosh S. and Dutta S.K.: Semen Characteristics of Tobacco Users in Indian. *Archives of Andrology*, 1: 35–40, 1993.

Behera D. and Malik S.K.: Chronic Respiratory Disease in Chandigarh Teachers. *Indian Journal of Chest Diseases and Allied Sciencs*,29:25–28, 1987.

Bhattacharya S.N., Bhatnagar J.K., Kumar S. and Jain P.C.: Chronic Bronchitis in Rural Population. *India Journal of Chest Diseases*, 17:1 7, 1975.

Bhide S.V., Kulkarni J., Nair U.j., Spiegelhalder B. and Preussmann R.: (1987) Mutagenecity and Carcinogenecity of *Masheri*, A Pyrolysed Tobacco Product, and its Content of Tobacco-specific Nitrosamines *Iarc Science Publication*, 84: 460–462, 1975.

Bhide S.S., Murdia U.S. and Nair J.: Polycyclic Aromatic Hydrocarbon Profiles of Pyrolysed Tobacco Products Commonly Used in India. *Cancer Letters*, 24: 89–94. 1984.

Bhisey RA, Bagwe AN, Mahimkar MB and Buch SC: Biochemical Monitoring of Beedi Industry Workers Exposed Occupationally to Tobacco. *Toxicology Letters*, 108: 259–265. 1999.

Boyko E.J., Koepsell T.D., Perera D.R. and Inui T.S.: Risk of Ulcerative Colitis Among Former and Current Cigarette Smokers. *New England Journal of Medicine*, 316:707–710. 1997.

Carmella S.G., Borukhova A., Desai D. and Hecht S.S.: Evidence For Endogenous Formation of Tobacco-specific Nitrosamines in Rats Treated Ith Tobacco Alkaloids and Sodium Nitrite. *Carcinogernesis*, 18:587–592, 1997.

Chakrabarti R.N., Dutta K., Ghosh K., and Sikdar S.: Uterine Cervical Dysplasia With Reference to the Betel Quid Chewing Habit. *European Journal of Gynaecology and Oncology*, 11:57–59, 1990.

Cho C.H., Chen B.W., Hui W.m. and Lam S.K.: The Influence of Acute or Chronic Nicotine Treatment on Ethanol-induced Gastric Mucosal Damage in Rats. *Digestive Diseases and Sciences*, 35:106–112, 1990.

CMR 1996.

Cnattingius S.: Maternal Age Modifies the Effect of Maternal Smoking on Intrauterine Growth Retardation But Not on Late Foetal Death and Placental Abruption. *American Journal of Epidemiology*, 145:319–323, 1997.

Cnattingius S., Haglund B. and Meirik O.: Cigarette Smoking as a Risk Factor For Late Foetal and Early Neonatal Death. *British Medical Journal*, 297:258–261, 1988.

Daling J., Weiss N., Spadoni L: Cigarette Smoking and Primary Tubal Infertility. In: Rosenberg M.j., Ed. Smoking and Reproductive Health. *Littleton Ma, Psg Publishing Company*. 40–46, 1987.

Deangelis C.D. and Flanagin A. Tuberculosis: A Call For Papers. Journal of American Medical Association, 292:1889. Available From Url:Http://Jama.ama-assn.org/Cgi/Content/Full/292/15/1889, 2004.

Difranza J.R. and Law R.A.: Effect of Maternal Cigarette Smoking on Pregnancy Complications and Sudden Infant Death Syndrome (Sids). *Journal of Family Practice*, 40:385–394, 1995.

Dikshit R.P. and Kanhere S.: Tobacco Habits and Risk of Lung Oesophageal and Oral Cavity Cancer: A Population-based Case-control Study in Bhopal (India). *International Journal of Epidemiology*, 29:609–611, 2000.

Dolls R. and Hill A.B.: A Study of the Aetiology of Carcinoma of Thelung. *British Medical Journal*, 2: 1271–1286, 1952.

Doll R., Peto R., Wheatley K., Gray R. and Sutherland I.: Mortality in Relation to Smoking: 40 Years Observations on Male British Doctors.british Medical Journal, 309: 901–911, 1994.

Dutta U., Garg P.K., Kumar R., Tandon R.K.: Typhoid Carriers Among Patients With Gallstones and at Increased Risk for Carcinoma of Gallbladder. *The American Journal of Gastroenterology*, 95:784–787, 2000.

Dwyer T., Poison A.L. and Couper D.: Tobacco Smoke Exposure at One Month of Age and Subsequent Risk of Sids, A Prospective Study. *American Journal of Epidemiology*, 149:593–602, 1999.

Dye C., Scheele S., Dollin P., Pathania V. and Raviglione M.: Global Burden of Tuberculosis: Estimated Incidence, Prevalence and Mortality By Country. *Journal of the American Medical Association*, 282:677–686, 1999.

Eastwood G.L.: Is Smoking Still Important in the Pathogenesis of Peptic Ulcer Disease? *Journal of Clinical Gastroenterology*, 25 Suppl. 1: S1–S7, 1997.

Endoh K. and Leung F.W.: Effects of Smoking and Nicotine on the Gastric Mucosa: A Review of Clinical and Experimental Evidence. *Gastroenterology*, 107:864–878, 1994.

Engeland A., Haldorsen T., Andersen A.: The Impact of Smoking Habits on Lung Cancer Risk: 28 Years Observation of 26,000 Norwegian Men and Women. *Cancer Causes Control*, 7:366–376, 1996.

Ernster M., Heishman S.J., Spurgeon L. and London E.D.: Smoking History and Nicotine Effects on Cognitive Performance. Neuropsychopharmacology, 25:313–319, 2001.

Ezzati M. and Lopez A.D.: Estimates of Global Mortality Attributable to Smoking in 2000. *The Lancet*, 362: 847–852, 2003.

Finnie I.A., Campbell B.J., and Taylor B.J.: Stimulation of Colonic Mucin Synthesis by Corticosteroids and Nicotine. Clinical Sciences, London, 91:359–364, 1996.

Folkman J.: What is the Evidence That Tumours Are Angiogenesis Dependent? *Journal of National Cancer Institute*, 82:4–6, 1992.

Gajalakshmi C.K., Jha P., Nguyen S. and Yurekali A.: Patterns of Tobacco Use, and Health Consequences. In: Jha P and Chaloupka F (Eds) *Tobacco Control Policies in Developing Countries.* Oxford University Press, New York, 2000.

Gajalakshmi V., Peto R., Kanak T.S. and Jha P.: Smoking and Mortality From Tuberculosis and Other Diseases in India: Retrospective Study of 43000 Adult Male Deaths and 35000 Controls. *the Lancet*, 362, 507–515, 2003.

Ghosh S.K., Parikh J.R., Gokani V.N., Kashyap S.K. and Chatterjee S.K.: Studies on Occupational Health Problems During Agricultural Operation of Indian Tobacco Workers: A Preliminary Survey Report. *Journal of Occupational Medicine*, 21:45–47, 1979.

Gijare P.S., Rao K.V.K., and Bhide S.V.: Modulatory Effects of Snuff, Retinoic Acid and Beta-carotene on Dmba Induced Hamster Cheek Pouch Carcinogenesis in Relation to Keratin Expression. *Nutrition and Cancer*, 14: 253–259, 1990.

Goswami Anil, Reddiah V.P., Kapoor S.K., Bir Singh, Dwivedi S.N. and Guresh Kumar: Tobacco and Alcohol Use in Rural Eldely Indian Population. Indian Journal of Psychiatry, 47:192–197, 2005.

Govekar R.B., and Bhisey R.A.: Mutagenic Activity in Urine Samples From Female Tobacco Habitués. Cancer Letters, 69: 75–80, 1993.

Gramenzi A., Gentile A., Fasoli M., D'avanzo B., Negri E., and Parazzini F.: Smoking and Myocardial Infarction in Women: A Case –Control Study From Northern Italy. *Journal of Epidemiology and Community Health*, 43: 214–217, 1989.

Green J.T., Richardson C. and Marshall R.W.: Nitric Oxide Mediates A Therapeutic Effect of Nicotine in Ulcerative Colitis. Alimentary Pharmacology and Therapeutics, 14:1429–1434, 2000.

Gupta D., Boffetta P., Goborieau V., Jindal S.K.: Risk Factors in Lung Cancer in Chandigarh, India. *The Indian Journal of Medical Research*, 113:142–150, 2001.

Gupta P.C., Aggarwal AN, Kumar S. and Jindal S.K.: Smoking Increases Risk of Pulmonary Tuberculosis. *Journal of Environmental Medicine*, 3:65–69, 2001.

Gupta P.C., Murti P.R. and Bhosle R.B.: Epidemiology of Cancer by Tobacco Products and the Significance of TSNA. *Critical Reviews in Toxicology*, 26:183–198, 1996.

Gupta P.C., Peto R., Parkin D.M., Sankarnarayanan R., Lopez A. and Jha P. Cohort Study for Tobacco-attributable Mortality in Mumbai, India. In: Dhillon I, Gupta P and Asma S (Eds) Evidence for A Causal Link Between Smoking and Tuberculosis. Proceedings of the International Scientific Expert Meeting on the Possible Causality Between Smoking and Tuberculosis. Thiruvanthapuram, Kerala India 2002, 2000.

Gupta P.C. and Ray C.S. Tobacco and Youth in South East Asia Region. *(Indian) Journal of Cancer*, 39:5–34, 2002.

Gupta P.C., Sinor P.N., Bhonsle R.B., Pawar V.S., and Mehta H.C.: Oral Submucous Fibrosis in India: A New Epidemic? *National Medical Journal of India,* 11:113–116, 1998.

Gupta S.P.: Smoking and Cardiovascular Disease. In: Sanghvi L.D. and Natani (Eds) Tobacco and Health, The Indian Scene.proceedings of Workshop, *Tobacco and Health,* Bombay, 1987.

Gusland M., Frego R., Viale E. and Testoni P.A.: Distal Ulcerative Colitis Refractory to Rectal Mesalamine: Role of Transdermal Nicotine Versus Oral Mesalamine. Canadian Journal of Gastroenterology, 16:293–296, 2002.

Hadley C.B., Main D.M. and Gabbe S.G.: Risk Factors For Preterm Premature Rupture of the Foetal Membranes. *American Journal Perinatal,* 379– 379, 1990.

Hamajima N., L. H., Matsuo K., Tajima K. and Tomonago S.: Helicobacter Pylori Seropositivity, the Interleukin B Polymorphism and Smoking Among First-visit Outpatients. Asian Pacific Journal of Cancer Prevention, 3:23–28, 2002.

Harish K, Ravi R.: The Role of Tobacco in Penile Carcinoma. *British Journal of Urology,* 75:375–377, 1995.

HE J., Vupputuri S., Allen K., Prerost M.R., Hughes J. and Whelton P.K.: Passive Smoking and Risk of Coronary Heart Disease – A Meta–Analysis of Epidemiologic Studies. *New England Journal of Medicine,* 340: 920–926, 1999.

Heeschen C., Jang J.J. and Weis M.: Nicotine Stimulates Angiogenesis and Promotes Tumour Growth and Atherosclerosis. Nature Medicine, 7:833–839, 2001.

Heusch W.l. and Maneckjee: Signaling Pathways in Nicotine Regulation of Apoptosis of Human Lung Cancer Cells. Carcinogenesis, 19:551–556. 1998.

Hodgson H.J. and Bhatti M.A.: Smoking and Quality of Life in Crohn's Disease – as Many Questions Answered as Unanswered. European Journal of Astroenterology and Hepatology, 8:1067–1069, 1996.

Horta B.L., Victora C.G. and Menezes A.M.: Environmental Tobacco Smoking and Breastfeeding Duration. *American Journal of Epidemiology,* 146:128–133, 1997.

Hurd S.: The Impact of Copd in Lung Health Worldwide, Epidemiology and Incidence, Chest, 117:1s–4s.59, 2000.

Jindal S.K.: A Field Study on Follow-up At 10 Years of Prevalence of Chronic Obstructive Pulmonary Disease and Peak Expiratory Flow Rate. *Indian Journal of Medical Research,* 89:20–26, 1993.

Joesoef M.R., Beral V. and Aral S.O.: Fertility and Use of Cigarette,Alcohol, Marijuana, and Cocaine. *Annals of Epidemiology,* 3:592–594, 1993.

Joshi R.C., Madan R.N. and Brash A.A.: Prevalence of Chronic Bronchitis in Industrial Population of North India. *Thorax,* 30:61–67, 1975.

Kabra K.: Some Neglected Aspects of Economics of Tobacco. In: Abedien I, *Et Al* (Eds) *Proceedings of the Conference on Economics of Tobacco Control: Towards an Optimal Policy Mix,* Applied Fiscal Research Centre Cape Town, University of Cape Town, 1998.

Konturek S.J., Bielanski W., Konturek J.W., Oleksy J. and Yamazaki J.: Release and Action of Epidermal Growth Factor on Gastric Secretion in Humans. Scandinavian Journal of *Gastroenterology,* 24:485–492, 1989.

Lashner B.A., Hanauer S.B. and Silverstein M.D.: Testing Gum for Ulcerative Colitis Patients. Experience with Single-patient Trials. *Digestive Diseases and Sciences*, 35:827–832, 1990.

Lauren S.W., Benjamin B.L., Rolf L., Stephanie M.G., Rachel A.G. and Benette L.L.: Smoking During Pregnancy Increases Conduct Disorder. *Archives of General Psychiatry*, 54: 670–676, 1997.

Leeder S., Raymond S., Grrenberg H., Liu H. and Esson K.: *A Race Against Time: The Challenge of Cardiovascular Disease in Developing Economies*, Columbia University, New York, 2004.

Leung F.W.: Dissociated Effect of Nicotine Pentagastrin-stimulated Acid Secretion and Blood Flow in the Rat Stomach. *Scandinavian Journal of Gastroenterology*, 29:782–785, 1994.

Lewin W.H. and Elvin-lewin M.P.F.: Medical Botany – Plants Affecting Man's Health. Willey Interscience: New York, 392–393, 1977.

Lindberg E., Tysk C., Andersson K. and Jarnerot G.: Smoking and Inflammatory Bowel Disease. A Case-control Study. *Gut*, 29:352–357, 1988.

Lindell G., Brudin L., Ohlin P. and Graffner H.: Does Nicotine Administration Influence Intragastric Acidity? *Scandinavian Journal of Gastroenterology*, 27:143–146, 1992.

Lindell G., Bukhave K., Lilja I., Madsen J.R. and Graffner H.: Acute Effects of High Dose Intragastric Nicotine on Mucosal Defense Mechanisms: an Analysis of Nicotine Prostaglandin E2, Phospholipase A2 and Phospholipids. *Digestive Diseases and Sciences'* 24:640–644, 1997.

Liu E.S., Ye Y.N. and Shin V.Y.: Cigarette Smoking Exposure Increases Ulcerative Associated Colonic Adenoma Formation in Mice. *Carcinogenesis*, 24:1407–1413, 2003.

Ma L., Chow J.Y.C., and Cho C.H.: Cigarette Smoking Delays Ulcr Healing: Role of Constitutive Nitric Oxide Synthase in Rat Stomach. *American Journal of Physiology*, 276:G238–G248. 1999.

Mackay J. and Eriksen M.: The Tobacco Atlas. World Health Organization, Geneva Switzerland, 2002.

Mahimkar M.B., Bhisey R.A.: Occupational Exposure to Beedi Tobacco Increases Chromosomal Aberrations in Tobacco Processors. *Mutation Research*, 334: 134–144, 1995.

Mahimkar M.B., Buch S.C., Samant T.a., Kapoor M.d. and Bhisey R.a.: Influence of Smokeless Tobacco Exposure on Detoxification Status and Chromosomal Damage in Male and Female Habitués. *Mutation Research*, 491: 111–117, 2001.

Malik S.K.: Profile of Chronic Bronchitis in North India: 1972–1981. *Lung*, 45:81–100, 1986.

Malik S.K., Jindal S.K. and Bansal S.: Chronic Bronchitis in Northern India. In: Vidhwanathan Or and Jaggi Op (Eds) *Advances in Chronic Obstructive Lung Disease*, New Delhi. Asthma and Bronchitis Foundation of India, 87–91, 1977.

Malik S.K. and Kashyap S.K.: Chronic Bronchitis in Rural Hills of Himachal Pradesh, *Indian Journal of Chest Diseases*, 2870–75, 1986.

Matsuo K., Hamajima N. and Ikehara Y.: Smoking and Polymorphism of Fucosyltransferase Gene Le Affect Success of H. Pylori Eradication With Lansoprazole, Amoxicillin, and Clarithromycin. *Epidemiology of Infections*, 130:227–233, 2003.

Merino G., Lira S.C. and Martinez-chequer J.C.: Effects of Cigarette Smoking on Semen Characteristics of A Population in Mexico. *Archives of Andrology*, 41:11–15, 1998.

Michael J.T., Henley S.J. and Eugenia E.C. Tobacco Use and Cancer: an Epidemiological Perspective for Genetici. *Oncogene*, 21:7307–7325.sts: 2002.

Morgan D.P.: Recognition and Management of Pesticide Poisonings, Environmental Protection Agency: Washington Dc (4th Edition), 1989.

Murphy N.J., Butler S.W. and Petersen K.M.: Tobacco Erases Thirty Years of Progress: Preliminary Analysis of the Effect of Tobacco Smoking on Alaska Native Birth Weight. *Alaska Medicine*, 38:31–33, 1996.

Murti P.R., Bhonsle R.B., Pindborg J.J., Daftry D.K., Gupta P.C. and Mehta F.S.: Malignant Transformation in Submucous Fibrosis Over A 17-year Period. *Community Dentistry and Oral Epidemiology*, 13:340–341, 1984.

Nair U.J., Pakhale S.S., Speigelhalder B., Preussmann R., and Bhide S.V.: Carcinogenic and Cocarcinogenic Constituents of *Masheri*, A Pyrolysed Tobacco Product. *Indian Journal of Biochemistry and Biophysics*,24: 257–259, 1987.

Nair U., Ube G., Nair J., Maru G.B., Bhide S.V. and Pieper R.: Evaluation of Frequency of Micronucleated Oral Mucosa Cells as A Marker For Genotoxic Damage in Chewers of Betel Quid With Or Without Tobacco. *Mutation Research*, 261: 163–168, 1991.

Nakamura M., Haruma K. and Kamada T.: Cigarette Smoking Promotes Atrophic Gastritis in Helicobacter Pylori Positive Subjects. *Digestive Diseases and Sciences*, 47:675–681, 2002.

Nandakumar A., Anantha N., Pattabhiram V., Prabhakaran P.s., Dhar M. and Puttaswamy K.: Importance of Anatomical Subsite in Correlating Risk Factors in the Cxancer of the Oesophagus—Report of A Case-control Study. *British Journal of Cancer*, 73:1306–1311, 1996

Nayar D. Kapil U. Joshi Y.K., Sundaram K.R., Srivastava S.P. and Shukla N.K.: Nutritional Risk Factors in Oesophageal Cancer. *The Journal of Association of Physicians of India*, 48:781–787, 2000.

Niblock W.J.: Cancer in India, *Indian Medical Gazette*, 27: 161, 1902.

Nigam P., Verma B.L. and Srivastav R.N.: Chronic Bronchitis in an Indian Rural Community. *Journal of the Association of Physicians of India*, 30:277, 1982.

Niphadkar M.P., Contractor Q. and Bhisey R.A.: Mutagenic Activity of Gastric Fluid From Chewers of Tobacco With Lime. Carcinogenesis, 15:927–931, 1994.

Niphadkar P.M., Bagwe A.N., and Bhisey R.A.: Mutagenic Potential of Indian Tobacco Products. *Carcinogenesis*, 11: 151–154, 1996.

Notani P.N., Shah P., Jayant K. and Balakrishnan V.: Occupation and Camcers of Lung and Bladder: A Case-controlled Study in Bombay. *International Journal of Epidemiology*, 22:185–191, 1996.

National Sample Survey Organization (NSSO), A Note on Consumption of Tobacco in India: Nss 50th Round, 1993–1994. *Sarvekshana* 1998 January- March, New Delhi: Department of Statistics, Ministry of Planning, Government of India, 1998,76–89.

Pais P., Pogue J., Gerstein H., Zachariah E., Savitha D., and Jayaprakash S.: Risk Factors For Acute Myocardial Infarction in Indians: A Case- Controlled Study. *The Lancet*, 348:358–36, 1996.

Pakhale S.S., and Bhide S.V.: Mutagenecity of Smoke Condensate of Beedi- an Indigenous Cigarette of India. *Mutagenesis*, 5: 1179–1181, 1984.

Pakhale S.S., Sarkar S., Jayant K. and Bhide S.V.: Carcinogenecity of Indian Beedi and Cigarette Smoke Condensate in Swiss Albino Mice, *Journal of Cancer Research and Clinical Oncology*, 114: 647–649, 1988.

Pearson J.P., Ward R., Allen A., Roberts N.B. and Tylor W.H.: Mucus Degradation By Pepsin: Comparison of Mucolytic Activity of Human Pepsin 1and Pepsin 3: Implications in Peptic Ulceration. Gut, 27:243–248, 1986.

Pindborg J.J., Mehta F.S., Gupta P.C. and Daftary D.K.: Prevalence of Oral Submucous Fibrosis Among 50,915 Indian Villagers, *British Journal Cancer*, 22: 646–654, 1968.

Pindborg J.J., Murti P.R., Bhonsle R.B., Gupta P.C., Daftry D.k. and Mehta F.S.: Oral Submucous Fibrosis as Precancerous Condition. *Scandinavian Journal of Dental Research*, 92:224–229, 1984.

Pullan R.D., Rhodes J. and Ganesh S.: Transdermal Nicotine For Active Ulcerative Colitis. New England Journal of Medicine, 330:811–815, 1994.

Radhatg, Gupta GK, Singh A and Mathur N: Chronic Bronchitis in an Urban Locality of New Delhi, an Epidemiological Survey, Indian Journal of Medical Research,66:273–285, 1977.

Rajkumar T., Franceschi S, Vaccarella S, Gajalakshmi, V, Sharmila, A, Snijders P.j.f.: Role of *Paan* Chewing and Dietary Habits in Cervical Carcinoma in Chennai, India. *British Journal of Cancer*, 88:1388–1391, 2003.

Rao D.N., Desai P.B. and Ganesh B.: Alcohol as an Additional Risk Factor in Laryngopharyngeal Cancer in Mumbai: A Case-control Study. *Cancer Detection and Prevention*,23: 37–44, 1999.

Ray D., Abel R. and Selvaraj K.G.: A 5-year Prospective Epidemiological Study of Chronic Obstructive Pulmonary Disease in Rural South India. *Indian Journal of Medical Research*,101:238–244, 1995.

Reddy K.S. and Gupta P.C. Report on Tobacco Control in India. Supported By Ministry of Health and Family Elfare, Government of India, Centre For Disease Control and Prevention, USA and World Health Organization, 2004.

Reddy K.S., Yusuf S.: Emerging Epidemic of Cardiovascular Disease in Developing Countries. *Circulation*, 97: 596–601, 1998.

Reed J.C. Apoptosis. In: Alison M. The Cancer Handbook. Ature Publishing Group: London, 119–134, 2002.

Richardson C.E., Morgan J.M. and Jasani B.: Effect of Smoking and Transdermal Nicotine on Colonic Acetylcholine Receptors in Ulcerative Colitis. Quarterly Journal of Medicine, 96:57–65, 2003.

Rogot E. and Murray J.L.: Smoking and Causes of Death Among US Veterans: 16 Years of Observation. *Public Health Reports*, 95:213–222, 1980.

Rowell P.P., Clark M.J.: The Effect of Oral Nicotine Administration on Foetal Weight and Placental Amino Acid Accumulation in Mice. *Toxicology and Applied Pharmacology*, 19: 30–38, 1982.

Roy T.S.: Effects of Prenatal Nicotine Exposure on the Morphogenesis of Somatosensory Cortex. Neurotoxicology and Teratology, 16(4), 1994.

Royal College of Physicians of London, *Smoking and Health*: Summary and a Report of the Royal College of Physicians London on Smoking in Relation to Cancer of the Lung and other Diseases. Pitman: London, 1962

Rudra T., Motley R., and Rhodes J.: Does Smoking Improve Colitis? *Scandinavian Journal of Gastroenterology* (Suppl.), 170:61–63, 1989.

Sandborn W.J., Trimaine W.J. and Leighton J.A.: Nicotine Tartrate Liquid Enemas For Mildly to Moderately Active Left-sided Ulcerative Colitis Unresponsive to First-line Therapy: A Pilot Study. Alimentary Pharmacology and Therapeutics, 11:663–671, 1997.

Sankaranarayanan R., Duffy S.W., Nair M.K., Padmakumary G., Day N.E.: Tobacco and Alcohol as Risk Factors in Cancer of the Larynx in Kerala, India. *International Journal of Cancer*, 45:879–882, 1990.

Sargent R.P., Shepard R.M. and Glantz S.A. Reduced Incidence of Admissions For Myocardial Infarction Associated With Public Smoking Ban, Before and After Study, *British Medical Journal*, 328: 977–983, 2004.

Serthi J.M. and Rochester C.L. Smoking and Obstructive Pulmonarydisease. *Clinics in Chest Medicine*,21:67–86, 2002.

Shah M.D., Ramchandani A.G., Mahimkar M.B., Potdar P.D., Bhisey A.N. and Bhisey R.A.: Effect of an Aqueous Extract of Beedi Tobacco on the Growth of Hamster Tracheal Epithelial Cells. *Toxicology Letters*,119: 1–9, 2001.

Shin V.Y., Liu E.S., Koo M.W., Luo J.C., So W.H. and Cho C.H.: Nicotinesuppresses Gastric Wound Repair Via the Inhibition of Polyamine and $K^+$ Channel Expression. European Journal of Pharmacology, 444:115–121, 2002.

Shioda S., Yada T., Muroya S., Takiga M. and Nakai Y.: Nicotine Increases Cytosolic $Ca^{2+}$ in Vasopressin Neurons. Neurosciences Research, 29:311–318, 1997.

Shirname L.P., Menon M.M. and Bhide S.V.: Comparison of Mutagenecity of Indian Cigarette and Beedi Smoke Condensates. *Indian Journal of Experimental Biology*, 23:145–148, 1985.

Sikand B.K., Pamra S.P. and Mathur G.P.: Chronic Bronchitis in Delhi as Revealed By Mass Survey. *Indian Journal of Tuberculosis*, 13: 94–101, 1966.

Sparrow D., O'connor G., Colton T., Barry C.l. and Weiss S.t.: The Relationship of Nonspecific Bronchial Responsiveness to the Occurrence of Respiratory Symptoms and Decreased Levels of Pulmonary Function. *American Review of Respiratory Disorders*,135:1255–1260, 1987.

Sullivan S.D., Ramsay S.D., Lee T.A.: the Economic Burden of Copd. *Chest*, 117:5s–9s, 2000.

Sundell G., Milsom L. and Andersch B.: Factors Influencing the Prevalence and Severity of Dysmenorrhoe in Young Women. *British Journal of Obstetrics and Gynaecology*, 97:588–594, 1990.

Thapliyal R. Dolas S.S., Pakhale S.S. and Maru G.B.: Evaluation of DNA Damage in Mice Topically Exposed to Total Particulate Matter From Mainstream and Sidestream Smoke From Cigarettes and Beedis. Mutagenesis, 19: 413–421, 2004.

Thiruvedgadam K.V., Ragav T.P. and Bhardwaj K.V.: Survey of Prevalence of Chronic Bronchitis in Madras City. In: Vishwanathan O.R. and Jaggi O.P. (Eds) *Advances in Chronic Obstructive Lung Diseases*, New Delhi, 1977.

Thomas G.A., Rhodes J. and Green J.T.: Inflammatory Bowel Disease and Smoking – A Review. *America Journal of Gastroenterology*, 94:144–149, 1998.

Thomas G.A., Rhodes J. and Mani V.: Transdermal Nicotine as Maintenance Therpy for Ulcerative Colitis. New England Journal of Medicine, 332:988–992, 1995.

Trivedi A.H., Dave B.J. and Adhvaryu S.G.: Monitoring of Smokeless Tobacco Consumers Using Cytogenetic End Points. Anticancer Research, 13: 245–250, 1993.

Trivedi A.H., Dave B.J. and Adhvaryu S.G.: Assessment of Genotoxicity of Nicotine Employing in Vitro Mammalian Test System. Cancer Letter, 54:89–94, 1990.

Tsiara S., Elisa M. and Mikhailidis D.P. Influence of Smoking on Predictors of Vascular Disease. *Angiology*, 54: 507–530. 2003.

Umadevi B., Swarna M., Padmavathi P., Jyothi A. and Reddy P.P.: Cytogenetic Effects in Workers Occupationally Exposed to Tobacco Dust. *Mutation Research*, 535:147–154, 2003.

Van Prosdij C.: Smoking: Its Influence on the Individual and Its Role in Social Medicine, Elsevier, Amsterdam, 1960.

Viswanathan R.: Chronic Bronchitis Emphysema Syndrome: Incidence Aetiology and Natural History. *Indian Journal of Chest Disease*, 6:171–182, 1964.

Vishwanathan R. and Singh K.: Chronic Bronchitis in Urban and Urban Delhi. In: Vishwanathan OR and Jaggi OP (Eds) *Advances in Hronic Obstructive Lung Diseases*, New Delhi. Asthma and Bronchitis Foundation of India,44–58, 1975.

Warner K.E.: Economics of Tobacco and Health: An Overview. In: Abedien I,*Et Al* (Eds). *Proceedings of the Conference on Economics of Tobacco Control, Towards an Optimal Policy Mix*. Applied Fiscal Research Centre, Cape Town, University of Cape Town, 1998.

Weizenecker R. and Deal W.B.: Tobacco Cropper's Sickness. *Journal of Florida Medical Association*, 57:13–14, 1970.

Wig K.L., Guleria J.S., Bhasin R.C., Holmes E. Jr, Vasudeva Y.L. and Singh M.: Certain Clinical and Epidemiological Patterns of Chronic Obstructive Lung Disease as Seen in Northern India. *Indian Journal of Chest Disease*, 6:183–194, 1964.

Willett W. Stampher M.J. and Bain C.: Cigarette Smoking, Relative Weight, and Menpause. *American Journal of Epidemiology*, 117:651–658, 1983.

Wong D., Koo M.W., Shin V.Y., Liu E.S. and Cho C.H.: Pathogenesis of Nicotine Treatment and Its Withdrawal on Stress-induced Gastric Ulceration in Rats. European Journal of Pharmacology, 434:81–86, 2002.

Wong D and Ogle CW: Chronic Parentrally Administered Nicotine and Stress OR Ethanol Induced Gastric Muciosal Damage in Rats. European Journal of Pharmacology, 292:157–162, 1995.

Wood C., Larsen C. and Williams R.: Social and Psychological Factors in Relation to Premenstrual Tension and Menstrual Pain. *Australian and New Zealand Journal of Obstetrics and Gynaecology*, 19:111–115, 1979.

Woolcock A.J., Peat J.K., Salome C.M., Yan K. and Anderson S.D.: Prevalence of Bronchial Hjyper-responsiveness and Asthma in Rural Adult Population. *Thorax,42:* 361–368, 1987.

World Health Organization, 2003 Who Frmework Convention on Tobacco Control (FCTC) Article 13. Available From url: http://www.who.int/framework/final_text/en/ (Accessed on 15th October 2004).

Wright S.C., Zhong J., Zheng H. and Larrick J.W.: Nicotine Inhibition of Apoptosis Suggests A Role in Tumour Promotion. *Fab Journal*, 7:1045–1051, 1993.

Wu X.H., Wang F.H., Liu Y.F., Lu X.Y., Wang J.J. and Lee K.: Histone Adduction With Nicotine: A Bio-ams Study. *Radiocabon*, 39:293–297, 1997.

Wynder E.L., Bross L.J., Cornfield J. and O'donnell W.E.: Lung Cancer in Women. *New England Journal of Medicine*, 255(24(: 1111–1121, 1956.

Wynder E.L. and Hoffman D.: Tobacco and Tobacco Smoke. Academic Press: New York, 1967.

Ye Y.N., Liu E.S., Shin V.Y., Wu W.K., Luo J.C. and Cho C.H. Nicotine Promoted Colon Cancer Growth Via Epidermal Growth Factor Receptor, C-sre, and 5–Lipoxygenase-mediated Signal Pathway. *Journal of Pharmacology and Experimental Therapeutics*, 308:66–72, 2004.

Zijlstra F.J., Srivastava E.D. and Rhodes M.: Effect of Nicotine on Rectal Mucus and Mucosal Eicosanoids. *Gut*, 35:247–251, 1994.

## APPENDIX I

## CHEMICAL CONSTITUENTS OF TOBACCO SMOKE CLASSIFIED OR IDENTIFIED FOR THEIR CARCINOGENICITY

Modified from California EPA Report (California Environmental Protection Agency, 1997) with the classifications of the chemicals in the European Union also included (column 2)

| *Organic Compounds* | *EU Classification* | *IARC Classification* |
|---|---|---|
| Acetaldehyde | Carc. Cat 3; R40, Xi, R36/37 | **2B** |
| Acetamide | Carc. Cat. 3; R40, Xn; R68 | **2B** |
| Acrolein | T+; R26, T; R24/25, C; R34 | **3** |
| Acrylonitrile | Carc. Cat. 2; R45, T, R23/24/25, Xi; R37/38-41, R43 | **2A** |
| 4-Aminobiphenyl | Carc. Cat. 1; R45, Xn; R22 | **1** |
| Aniline | Carc. Cat 3; R40, T; R48/23/24/25, Xn; R20/21/21 | **3** |
| o-Anisidine | Carc. Cat. 2; R45, Muta Cat. 3; R68, T;R23/24/25 | **2B** |
| Benz[a]anthracene 1,3 | Carc. Cat. 2; R45 | **2A** |
| Benzene | Carc. Cat. 1; R45, T; R48/23/24/25 | **1A** |
| Benzo[b]fluoranthene | - | **2B** |
| Benzo[j]fluoranthene | Carc. Cat. 2; R45 | **2B** |
| Benzo[k]fluoranthene | Carc. Cat. 2; R45 | **2B** |
| Benzo[a]pyrene | Carc. Cat. 2; R45 | **2A** |
| Butadiene | [Carc. Cat. 1]* | **B2** |
| Captan | Carc. Cat. 3; R40, T; R23, Xi; R41, R43 | **3** |
| Carbon disulfide | Repr. Cat. 3; R62-63T; R48/23, Xi; R36/38 | **3** |
| Carbon monoxide | Repr. Cat. 1; R61, T; R23-48/23 | **2B** |
| Chrysene | Carc. Cat. 2; R45, Muta. Cat. 3; R68 | **3** |
| DDT | Carc. Cat. 3; R40, T; R25-48/25 | **2B** |
| Dibenz[a,h]acridine | | **2A** |
| Dibenz[a,j]acridine | | **2B** |
| Dibenz[a,h]anthracene | Carc. Cat. 2; R45 | **2B** |
| 7H-Dibenzo[c,g]carbazole | | **2B** |

| Organic Compounds | EU Classification | IARC Classification |
|---|---|---|
| Dibenzo[a,e]pyrene | | 2B |
| Dibenzo[a,h]pyrene | | 2B |
| Dibenzo[a,i]pyrene | | 2B |
| Dibenzo[a,l]pyrene | | 2B |
| 1,1-Dimethylhydrazine | [Carc.Cat.2: R45] | 2B |
| 1-Naphthylamine | Xn; R22 | 3 |
| Formaldehyde | Carc. Cat. 3; R40, | 2A |
| Hydrazine | Carc. Cat. 2; R45 | 2B |
| Indeno(1,2,3,-cd)pyrene | - | - |
| 2-Naphthylamine | Carc. Cat. 1; R45Xn; R22 | 1 |
| Nicotine | T+; R27, T; R25 | |
| 2-Nitropropane | Carc. Cat. 2; R45Xn; R20/22- | 2B |
| N-(Methylnitrosamino) -1-(3-pyridyl)-1-butanone (NNK) | - | NC |
| N-Nitrosodi-n-butylamine | - | 2B |
| N-Nitrosodiethanolamine | - | 2B |
| N-Nitrosodiethylamine | - | 2A |
| N-Nitroso-n-methylethylamine | - | 2B |
| N'-Nitrosonornicotine | - | 2B |
| N-Nitrosopiperidine | - | 2B |
| N-nitrosdi-n-propylamine | - | 2B |
| N-Nitrosopyrrolidine | - | 2B |
| Styrene | Xn; R20, Xi; R36/38 | 2B |
| Toluene | Xn; R20, [Repro. Cat. 3; R63 | 2B |
| 2-Toluidine | - | 2B |
| Urethane | | |
| Carc. Cat. 2; R45 | | |
| Vinyl chloride | Carc. Cat. 1; R45 | 2B |
| ***Inorganic Compounds*** | | |
| Chromium V1 | Carc. Cat. 2; R49, R43 | 1 |
| Arsenic | T; R23/25 | 1 |
| Cadmium | Cadmium chloride & fluoride Carc.Cat.2,R45, Repro. Cat. 2, | 2A |

(Contd...)

| *Organic Compounds* | *EU Classification* | *IARC Classification* |
|---|---|---|
| | R60-61, Muta. Cat. 3, R68, T+R26, T; R25,T;48/23/25, Cadmium oxideCarc. Cat. 2, R49 | |
| Lead | Repro. Cat. 3, R63, Muta. Cat. 3, R68, T; R23/25, Repro. Cat. 1; R61T;48/23/25, Repro. Cat. 3; R62Xn; R20/22, R33 | **2B** |
| Nickel | Carc. Cat. 1; R45 | **1** |

# CHAPTER 9 Tobacco Use in Psychiatric Patients

*Psychiatric co-morbidity in tobacco users reveals various forms of psychopathology.*

— Le Crubie, 2000

Epidemiological and clinical studies have shown a positive correlation between smoking and psychiatric disorders (Lopes *et al.*, 2002). Psychiatric co-morbidity in tobacco users reveals various forms of psychopathology (LeCrubie 2000). The early work in this field tended to focus on character pathology, and various aspects of negative affect, such as neuroticism, hopelessness, and general emotional distress, all of which were found to be associated with smoking. It was speculated that the initiation of smoking was environmentally based but its maintenance was more related to psychopathology (Krammer, 2000).

Over time, studies have confirmed that tobacco dependence is extremely common among co-morbid psychiatric populations (Lang, 2004). Smoking rates are substantially higher among individuals with a lifetime history of mental illness than among individuals without such a history (Lasser *et al.*, 2000) and as such mental health problems are associated with significantly higher prevalence of tobacco use than the general population. Smoking rates are also seen to be higher (up to 70%) in alcohol and other substance abuse populations (Fiore *et al.*, 2000) and tobacco is considered to be a gateway drug for alcohol and other drug users. In a recent population survey in England, the Office of Population Censuses and Surveys (OPCS) found 16% of the population sample suffering from psychiatric morbidity, vast majority of which suffered from neurotic disorders such as mixed anxiety and depression (Meltzer *et al.*, 1995). About 0.5% of the sample had psychotic illness. Table 1 shows a breakdown of smoking prevalence among six categories of neurotic disorders and one category of psychotic disorder from this study sample. Smoking prevalence in the study sample was higher than the general population. Overall smoking prevalence for the study sample was 32% in the general population (National smoking prevalence in general population in 1993 and 1998 was 30% and 26% respectively). All categories of mental health problems had higher levels of smoking. 44% of those diagnosed as having any neurotic disorder were smokers. The highest smoking rates were among those with a diagnosis of psychosis.

For the neurotic disorders, a clear relationship is observed between smoking and the number of neurotic symptoms as measured by the revised version of the Clinical Interview Schedule (CIS-R). Score range of this schedule is from 0 to 57 and minimum score for any significant psychiatric morbidity is 12. Current smoking increased in a step-wise fashion from 28% for a CIS-R score of 0–5, to 34% for a score of 6-11, 42% for a score of 12–17 and 48% for a score of 18 plus. Higher scores are also associated with heavier smoking. Smoking prevalence also varies with the number of neurotic disorders. For those with one neurotic disorder, current smokers are found to be 43% and those with two or more 54% (Meltzer *et al.,* 1995).

Dose response relationship has also been observed between the number of psychiatric diagnoses and smoking in a recent US study (Lasser *et al.*, 2000).

***Table 1: Smoking prevalence by mental health problem***

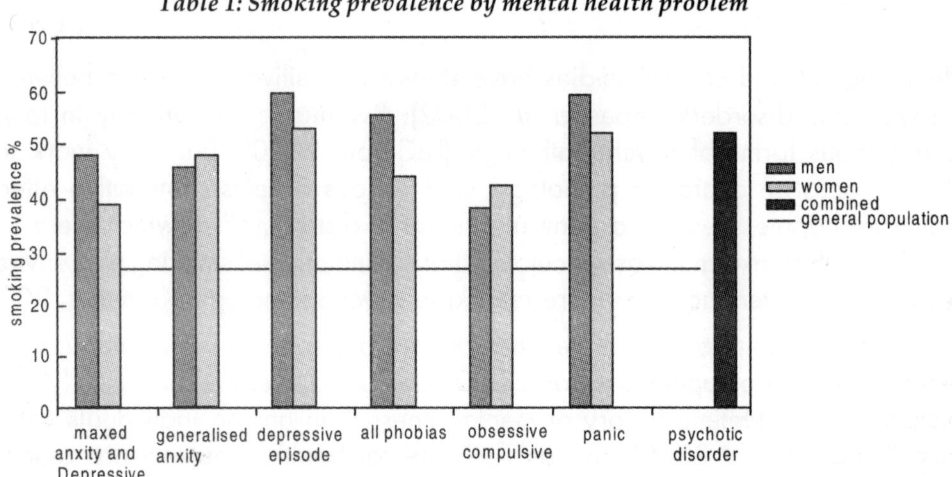


***Source :*** *Meltzer, H et al. OPCS Surveys of Psychiatric Morbidity in Great Britain Report 1 : The prevalence psychiatric morbidity among adults living in private households. London: HMSO 1995.*

## Smoking in the Inmates of Institutions

In 1996, the OPCS published a national survey of 1200 subjects residing in the psychiatric hospitals (Meltzer *et al.*, 1996) and a national survey of 1000 homeless subjects (Gill *et al.*, 1996). 70% of psychiatric hospital inmates had the diagnostic label of schizophrenia, schizo-affective psychosis or delusional disorder, 8% of the inmates had bipolar illness and 8% suffered from various types of neurotic disorders. Homeless subjects were given no psychiatric diagnosis.

The institutionalized inmates were found to have a high smoking rate: 74% in Schizophrenia, Schizo-affective and Delusional disorder group; 70% in Affective psychosis group and 74% in Neurotic disorder group. Among the homeless group of the study sample 70% of the subjects smoked tobacco (Table 2).

In an US survey nearly 45% of all cigarettes consumed, were smoked by the individuals suffering from some kind of psychiatric disorder or substance abuse disorder (Lasser *et al.*, 2000).

***Table 2: Cigarette smoking and psychiatric diagnosis in patients in institutions***

| | Schizophrenia delusional | Affective psychosis | Neurotic disorder | Homeless people |
|---|---|---|---|---|
| Cigarette smoking prevalence % | 74 | 70 | 74 | 70 |

OPCS Psychiatric Morbidity Study: Meltzer *et al*, 1996

## Relationship Between Smoking and Psychiatric Disorders

### *Schizophrenia*

Clinicians have observed for a long-time that schizophrenia patients are markedly prone to smoking tobacco (Lohr and Flynn, 1992). Of all psychiatric patients, schizophrenia patients smoke maximum. High prevalence of nicotine addiction in schizophrenics has the implications for the underlying neurobiology of schizophrenia (Kelly and McCreadie, 2000).

### *Prevalence of Smoking in Schizophrenia*

Number of schizophrenics who smoke is very high. The rate of smoking in these patients is at least two to three times higher than the general population. One study reports prevalence to be 88%, nearly three times the rate in the general population and higher than the elevated rates of smoking in patients with other psychiatric illnesses (Hughes *et al.*, 1986). Recent cross-sectional studies from different countries have reported high rates of smoking in patients with schizophrenia (Goff *et al.*, 1992; Chong and Choo, 1996). One large study of 360 state hospital in-patients, of whom 237 were diagnosed to be schizophrenics or schizo-affective disorder, found that the overall prevalence of smoking was 85%, and 93% in young male schizophrenics and schizo-affective disorder patients (de Leon *et al.,* 1995). Results of this study are slightly higher than those of the study of institutionalized patients carried out by the Office of Population Censuses and Surveys (OPCS) England wherein 74% schizophrenics (and patients with schizo-affective psychosis and delusional disorder) were found to be the current smokers (McNeill, 2001). Smoking rates may vary depending on the type of schizophrenia the individual is suffering from. A Greek study found that smoking rates differed between different subtypes of schizophrenia (Beratis *et al.,* 2001). Smoking occurs at much higher rates than other types of substance misuse or dependence, which have been shown also to be elevated among patients with schizophrenia. A recent meta-analysis of 42 worldwide studies across 20 countries (de Leon and Diaz, 2005) demonstrates an association between schizophrenia and current smoking with increased risk of starting smoking than the general population.

However, majority of smokers begin to smoke before the onset of schizophrenic illness. Kelly and McCreadie (1999) found that the average age when patients with schizophrenia started smoking was the same as in the general population, namely mid-teens; 90% of the patients who smoked had started smoking before their illness began.

There are also gender differences in the smoking pattern of schizophrenic smokers. In the OPCS study sample 62% of women with schizophrenia were current smokers compared to 78% of men schizophrenics (McNeill, 2001). One US hospital study found that male schizophrenic patients had the highest frequency of smoking followed by male non-schizophrenic patients, female schizophrenics and female non-schizophrenic smokers respectively (de Leon *et al.*, 1995).

Patients with schizophrenia are heavier smokers than people in general population and those with other psychiatric disorders. In their study, Kelly and McCreadie (1999) found that 68% of all schizophrenic smokers were heavy smokers (smoking 25 or more cigarettes daily) in comparison to 11% such smokers in the general population. In another study, Olincy *et al.*, (1997) found schizophrenic smokers to have much higher levels of nicotine metabolite cotinine in their blood in comparison to other smokers. Excessive smoking tends to be a life-long behaviour among schizophrenics and the proportion of those who quit is lower than in the general population. In a survey, only 8% ex-smokers were found to be schizophrenics in comparison to 31% ex-smokers in the general population (Kelly and McCreadie, 1999).

A recent study substantiates the above findings of greater frequency of heavy smoking and lower rate of smoking cessation in schizophrenics as compared to the smokers in the general population (de Leon and Diaz, 2005) however, worldwide smokers with schizophrenia and smokers with other severe mental disorders have relatively similar frequencies of heavy smoking and high nicotine dependence.

### *Why high prevalence of smoking in schizophrenia?*

Excessive rate of smoking among schizophrenia can be explained on the basis of three possible reasons: illness leads the patients to smoke, smoking is another risk factor for schizophrenia; or a third factor leads to both smoking and schizophrenia. The first possibility has received most attention. It has been suggested that smoking may be a marker of a more severe illness process (de Leon, 1996). Smokers are more often young and males; they have an earlier onset of illness, increased number of hospitalizations and receive higher doses of neuroleptic medication (Goff *et al.*, 1992; Ziedonis *et al.*, 1994). In addition, smokers have more severe symptoms with higher scores on the Brief Psychiatric Rating Scale (Overall and Gorham, 1962) for positive and negative symptoms (Goff *et al.*, 1992).

Some workers believe that smoking is used as a form of self-medication because nicotine can have a powerful impact on mood. Self-medication in psychiatric patients in general and in schizophrenia in particular is certainly an interesting and controversial topic (Hughes, 2000). Nicotine helps to regulate a dysfunctional mesolimbic dopamine system. It may increase dopamine release in the pre-frontal cortex and alleviate positive and negative symptoms (Dalack and Meador-Woodruff 1996). It has also been shown that nicotine administration enhances cognitive performance on a number of tasks. However, in general, patients with schizophrenia who smoke, report similar reasons to other smokers ("addicted", "for relaxation", "to calm down"), with only 17% reporting that smoking improved their psychotic symptoms (Kelly and McCreadie, 2000).

Schizophrenic patients smoke heavily as a result of snit-psychotic medication, which produces marked dopamine receptor blockade. Possibly, a very high level of smoking is necessary to overcome this blockade and to produce the reward effects. It has been shown that, compared with baseline, patients with schizophrenia smoke more after starting haloperidol (McEvoy *et al.*, 1995). A placebo-controlled study shows that after a single dose of haloperidol normal subjects smoked significantly more during the following hour as measured by blood nicotine levels (Dawe *et al.*, 1995).

Most patients who smoke begin to do so before the psychotic aspects of the illness appear, pre-morbid characteristics are perhaps important. It is important to note the patients who smoke were poorly adjusted socially as children than those who were not smokers.

A second explanation for the association between schizophrenia and smoking is that smoking is an aetiological risk factor for schizophrenia. It may be a possibility that repeated activation by nicotine of the mesolimbic system over a long time precipitates the onset of schizophrenia in vulnerable individuals. It is observed that the earlier the age of starting smoking, the earlier is the onset of psychotic illness in women (Kelly and McCreadie, 1999). Interestingly, nicotine acts like other drugs of addiction such as cocaine and amphetamines, activating the mesolimbic dopamine system (Pontieri *et al.*, 1996); this effect appears to be of critical importance for the reinforcing and the reward properties of the drug. Also, nicotine has been shown to increase burst activity in the dopamine neurons of the Ventral Tegmental Area (VTA), a form of firing pattern of these cells that is physiologically associated with basic motivational processes underlying learning and cognition (Iversen, 1996).

Third, genetic and/or environmental factors might predispose individuals to develop both schizophrenia and nicotine addiction. Much work in the genetics of both schizophrenia (Maier and Schwab 1998) and nicotine addiction (Clarke, 1998) has focused on the dopamine receptor system. A large number of world-wide studies describing current smoking in schizophrenia consistently suggest that schizophrenia patients from all countries share a biological factor that makes them more prone to smoke (de Leon and Diaz, 2005). Studies suggest that there may be genetic factors increasing the risk of both becoming a smoker and developing schizophrenia (Freedman *et al.*, 1997 and de Leon *et al.*, 2002). This model is supported by recent genetic studies (Leonard *et al.*, 2002 and Gurpregui *et al.*, 2005). Environmental factors are supposed to play an important role in smoking initiation.

### Morbidity and Mortality

Smoking remains the single greatest preventable cause of death globally. It appears to engender both general and specific health risks for patients with schizophrenia. Schizophrenic population has particularly high risk for smoking-related death and disease because of their typical low motivation to quit smoking and their high levels of dependence (George *et al.*, 2000). There is no doubt that cigarette smoking causes considerable morbidity and mortality, however, at present, there is no epidemiological data addressing smoking-related morbidity and mortality in schizophrenia. In schizophrenia life expectancy is estimated to be 20% lesser than in the general population. There is an increase in the deaths from natural causes and the most common causes are cardiovascular and respiratory diseases, both smoking related (Mortensen and Juel, 1993). The markedly elevated prevalence of smoking is clearly an important potential factor in explaining the elevated mortality in schizophrenia.

In view of these findings it can be concluded that smoking related fatal diseases are commoner among schizophrenics than among the general population (Brown *et al.*, 2000). These conclusions are further supported by a follow-up study of 1981 in which 370 schizophrenic smokers were followed for 12 years. During this period, 79 died, 73% from natural causes (which included smoking-induced diseases) and 24% from unnatural causes such as suicides or accidents. Standardized Mortality Rates (SMRs) were significantly raised for smokers (but not for non-smokers), and for smoking-related diseases. The SMR for lung cancer was twice the expected value.

### Medication and Side Effects

Smoking has been shown to decrease plasma levels of neuroleptics by inducing hepatic microsomal enzymes (Salokangas *et al.*, 1997). Therefore, the patients who smoke require larger doses of drugs than non-smokers to achieve the same therapeutic effect (Lohr and Flynn, 1992). It has also been reported that smokers have been prescribed neuroleptics at twice the daily dose of non-smokers while exhibiting significantly less neuroleptic-induced Parkinsonian symptoms. Spontaneous abnormal involuntary movements indistinguishable from tardive dyskinesia have also been reported in general population sample of older males who smoke (Nilsson *et al.*, 1997). It would seem likely, therefore, that there is an association between tardive dyskinesia and smoking in schizophrenia. However, some studies show that tardive dyskinesia is more common in smokers (Yassan *et al* 1987); and some studies show no relationship (Menzza *et al.*, 1991, Chiles *et al.*, 1993).

### Cognitive Functions

Research in normal smokers and in patients with schizophrenia has indicated that cigarette smoking or nicotine administration may improve cognitive functions, including memory, attention and spatial perception (Apud *et al.*, 2000). Schizophrenic patients exhibit an auditory sensory deficit characterized by diminished P50 (Levin *et al.*, 2001). Clozapine improves gating of P50-evoked response (West 2001) and it has been suggested that modulation of smoking by clozapine treatment may in part, be caused by similar mechanisms. The fact that these attention abnormalities also occur in non-psychotic relatives of schizophrenic patients suggests a genetic basis for this deficit. The P50 inhibition deficit in schizophrenia is linked to chromosome 15q13-14 in the region of the alfa-7 subunit gene (Ernst *et al.*, 2001). Postmortem studies have shown a reduction in the number of alfa-bungarotoxin-sensitive (alfa-7 containing) nAChRs in the hippocampal region of schizophrenic patients (Crocker, 2000), which appear to be secondary to polymorphisms in the alfa-7 promoter (McEvoy *et al.*, 1995). Another form of cognitive deficit associated with schizophrenia is latent inhibition, in which pre-exposure to a stimulus inhibits conditioning to that stimulus (McEvoy *et al.*, 1999). It has been suggested that smokers have enhanced latent inhibition, which is dependent upon the pre-exposure parameters (Procyshyn *et al.*, 2001).

Schizophrenic patients have impairments in other cognitive domains, including deficits in visuospatial working memory (VSWM), which is partly mediated by dopamine in the prefrontal cortex. Smoking abstinence differentially alters VSWM in schizophrenic versus control smokers, and cigarette smoking has beneficial effects on VSWM in schizophrenia but not controlled smokers (Combs and Advokat, 2000). Higher dose of nicotine patch improves reaction time, but not accuracy in a spatial rotation task, and also improves performance on a visual-match to a sample task in schizophrenic patients treated with haloperidol (Levin *et al.*, 1996).

## Bipolar Affective Disorder

According to the OPCS Survey, 70% of the institutionalized bipolar affective disorder patients smoked and within this group of smokers there is a high degree of dependence, 50% being heavy smokers with history of psychotic symptoms. Elevated rates of smoking in bipolar patients have also been observed in other studies (Hughes *et al.*, 1986) as well. In an Ireland study of 92 bipolar patients, smoking was found to be higher among those bipolar patients who had associated psychotic symptoms (Corvin *et al.*, 2001). Authors of this study believe that severity of psychosis is related to smoking behaviour.

## Depression

Patients suffering from major depression are more likely to smoke (George and Vessicchio 2001; Anda *et al.*, 1990). 56% of the patients currently suffering from depressive episode are found to be smokers (Meltzer *et al.*, 1995). Depression is more common among smokers than non-smokers (60% versus 15%) (Borreli *et al.*, 1996). Association between regular smoking in teenage girls and high levels of depression and anxiety has also been reported (Patton *et al* 1996). In addition as many as 30% of patients seeking smoking-cessation treatment may have a history of depression (Fiore *et al.*, 2000). Studies have also shown that people with major depression have difficulty when they try to stop smoking (Covey *et al.*, 1998). History of depression has a significant negative effect on success at quitting. Glassman *et al* (1988) found that subjects without a history of depression are more than twice as likely to quit smoking as those with history of depression. Symptoms of depression assessed at baseline predicted time to first cigarette smoked after attempting at quitting which illustrates symptoms of depression predicting failure to quit (Niaura *et al.*, 2001). More severe withdrawal symptoms are witnessed in the smokers who have history of depression. Smokers with the history of depression are more likely to experience more persistent withdrawal discomfort over a longer period of time (Covey *et al.*, 1997).

Nicotine may be effective in the treatment of depression. One of the better-accepted models of depression in the laboratory animals is "learned helplessness" in which the animal will not try to escape an unpleasant or painful event. This behaviour is thought to be the equivalent to a depressed human thinking that it is not worth protecting him/herself. High-dose nicotine reverses this behaviour in laboratory animals. There is also data showing that nicotine-patches given to non-smoker depressed patients for four days decreased their Hamilton Depression scores from 18 to 3, then, when patches were discontinued, the Hamilton score went back up to the baseline in four more days. There is also some evidence that cigarette smoke may have Mono-amine Oxidase Inhibition properties. Mono-amine Oxidase is significantly lower in smokers, but its activity returns to the level in non-smokers after smokers quit. Since nicotine does not have mono-amine oxidase inhibitory properties, it is felt that there is some other chemical in the cigarette smoke that functions as a mono-amine oxidase inhibitor (MAOI).

## Psychological Distress

The OPCS survey (Meltzer *et al.*, 1995) illustrates a smoking prevalence of 55% among people with **panic disorder** (52% among women and 59% among men). Higher rates of smoking are also witnessed in other countries as well (Amering *et al.*, 1999) though this finding is not consistent in men (Pohl *et al.*, 1992).

Smoking rates of 53 – 60%, and higher cigarette consumption, have been found among people with **post-traumatic stress disorder** (PTSD) (Beckham *et al.*, 1995 and Beckham *et al.*, 1997). Withdrawal symptoms due to nicotine abstinence are found to be more severe and intense in the individuals suffering from anxiety disorders, who had unsuccessfully tried to reduce their smoking frequency, than among those without such disorders (Breslau *et al.*, 1998).

OPCS survey of house-hold population (Meltzer, 1995) found 47% smoking rate among the Generalized Anxiety Disorder patients, 42% among those suffering from Mixed Anxiety and Depressive Disorder, 48% among those with Phobia and 40% among those with Obsessive Compulsive Disorder in the general population. Among those with any neurotic disorder 44% were current smokers, 43% of women and 47% of men in comparison to the general population with 29% smokers, 28% women and 30% men.

## Psychiatric Disorders of Childhood and Adolescence

### Attention Deficit Hyper-activity Disorder (ADHD)

Smoking is associated with adult and adolescent Attention Deficit Disorder (ADHD). Adults with ADHD show a greater smoking rate (40%) than the general population (26%) (Pomerleau *et al.*, 1995). Consistent with these adult rates, children with ADHD are twice as likely as children without ADHD to develop early drug use (including tobacco) (odd ratio=2.1) (Chilcoat and Breslau, 1997). The highest level of externalizing problems (rated on the Child Behaviour check-list) also increases the risk of early drug use. There is an emerging body of literature examining the therapeutic effects of nicotine on the symptoms of ADHD. Levin *et al* (1996) studied the acute effects of trans-dermal nicotine and placebo in adults with ADHD (both smokers and nonsmokers). They reported significant improvement in self-rated vigour and concentration and observer-rated illness severity for both subject groups. In addition, they found improvement in the speed of responding for both the smokers and nonsmokers, and a reduction in variability of reaction time for the smokers. Milberger *et al* (1998) reported that ADHD, particularly when co-morbid with other disorders (conduct disorder, major depression or anxiety disorder), predicted early initiation of cigarette smoking in a 4-year prospective study. In addition, smoking at 4-year follow-up was twice as high in adolescents with conduct disorder as in those without conduct disorder. In a study of delinquents with substance use disorders, the presence of ADHD and major depression predicted the severity of nicotine dependence (Riggs *et al.*, 1999).

Cigarette smoking is also associated with eating disorders (Pomerleau *et al.*, 1993) and substance use disorders (George and Vessicchio, 2001) and alcohol dependence. In fact, tobacco smoking is considered to be a gateway drug to other substances of abuse.

Nicotine appears to be effective in ADHD. It improves distractibility, impulsivity and other symptoms of ADHD. In animal models of ADHD, in which animals must discern between similar stimuli, high-dose nicotine causes the animals to be more accurate, and it is believed that this is the function of their becoming less impulsive. In the placebo-controlled studies of nicotine in ADHD patients, nicotine is found to be effective in both smokers and non-smokers (Coger *et al.*, 1996).

## Neuro-psychiatric Disorders

Nicotine receptors (nAChRs) are found throughout the central nervous system (CNS). These receptors are composed of two types of subunits, *alfa* and *beta*, of which nine *alfa* (*alfa*$^2$ to *alfa*$^{10}$) and three *beta* (*beta*$^2$ to *beta*$^4$) have been found in vertebrates (Gotti *et al.*, 1997; Lukas 1998 and Colquhoun and Patrick 1997). Nicotine innervation of the hippocampus, amygdale and frontal cortex has been demonstrated to be vital to memory function (Levin, 2002).

### Nicotine Receptor Stimulation and Cognitive-enhancement

Studies in humans have spanned several decades and consist mostly of experiments utilizing cigarettes to administer nicotine, usually to smokers deprived of cigarettes for some period of time. Though nicotine might improve performance in deprived smokers, it appears that this improvement is usually limited to restoring pre-deprivation performance, which clearly declines during cigarette withdrawal (Heishman *et al.*, 2002). Enhancement of normal non-deprived smokers and nonsmokers with nicotine has been more difficult to demonstrate. In studies with humans, nicotine has been shown to improve performance in smokers on attentionally and cognitively demanding vigilance tasks (Provost and Woodward, 1991). Smoking deprivation impairs cognitive performance and that re-administering cigarettes briskly relieves this performance decrement (Bell *et al.*, 1999). Utilizing electrophysiological assessment, nicotine administration to tobacco-dependent smokers improves power indices of electroencephalogram arousal, with shortened reaction times increasing P300 (evoked potential occurring 300 msec after stimulus representation) amplitudes (Knott *et al.*, 1999). Under conditions of superoptimal alertness, smokers who were administered nicotine showed improved and constant performance during a sustained choice reaction time task, suggesting that nicotine has an enabling effect on sustained cognitive effort, at least in this population (Davranche and Audiffren, 2002). Utilizing the strategy of administering a trans-dermal nicotine patch to smokers participating in a smoking withdrawal study showed no mitigation of cognitive effects of smoking cessation.

An intense relationship has been observed between some neuro-psychiatric illnesses with cognitive impairment and smoking such as:

### Mild Cognitive Impairment (MCI)

MCI is defined as a subjective and objective decline in cognitive function and function that does not need criteria for diagnosis of dementia (Petersen, 1995) and that represents a transitional state between the cognition of normal aging and mild dementia. Recent evidence indicates that people with mild cognitive impairment are at high risk for subsequently developing dementia (Petersen *et al.*, 1999). Amnestic mild cognitive impairment appears to represent the condition most likely to progress to Alzheimer's disease, whereas individuals who have multiple dementias or non-memory dementias impairment might progress to Alzheimer's disease and/or other types of dementias. By utilizing criteria for amnestic mild cognitive impairment, long-term follow-up studies have suggested that these individuals progress to dementia at a rate of approximately 12% per year. Stimulation of CNS nAChRs could be a promising strategy to ameliorate symptoms of mild cognitive impairment and/or slow or prevent progression to frank dementia. In a recent study of cognitive performance in patients with mild cognitive impairment, White and Levin, (2005) studied 10 subjects with MCI in a double-blind, placebo-controlled, crossover study.

### *Alzheimer's Disease*

In clinical studies, Newhouse *et al., (*1988) first showed evidence of improved cognitive functioning (decreased error) following intravenous injection of nicotine in Alzheimer's disease subjects. Two weeks of nicotine dermal patch treatment was found to significantly improve cognitive function in Alzheimer disease patients (Wilson *et al.,* 1995). These investigators found that the major effect of nicotine was to reduce error performance on the new learning phase of the repeated acquisition test – the same parameter on the same task (although performed differently) that Newhouse *et al.,* (1992) found to be specifically impaired after the nicotine antagonist mecamylamine. A four-week trial of trans-dermal nicotine in Alzheimer's disease showed significant improvement in attentional performance, as measured by continuous performance task, with consistent improvement in omission errors and improved consistency of reaction time (White and Levin, 1999). In a unique and not previously reported combination, the subjects that were treated with the cholinesterase inhibitor tacrine were administered nicotine; they showed decreased auditory-evoked potential latencies and increased visual evoked potential amplitude, suggesting improved sensory detection, attention and/or processing (Knott *et al.,* 2002).

In addition to direct stimulation of nAChRs, nicotine might provide cascading effects through stimulation of the release of a variety of transmitters involved in cognitive function, including acetylcholine, dopamine, norepinephrine, serotonin and glutamate (McGehee and Role 1995). Augmentation of activities of the remaining nAChRs might provide therapeutic benefit. However, loss of nAChRs in Alzheimer's disease could also limit the potential for nicotinic therapy. This might underlie the lack of nicotine effect in Alzheimer's disease and the limitations in the extent of improvement in studies of nicotine in Alzheimer's disease. Nicotine treatment might be more effective in older adults with less severe cognitive impairment and more nAChRs (LeHousezec, 1998).

### *Parkinson's Disease*

Changes in cholinergic systems in the Central Nervous System have been shown to occur in the brains of the patients suffering from Parkinson's disease. A loss of cholinergic cells in the basal forebrain nuclei has been described in Parkinsonism (Whitehouse, 1983). There is a marked reduction in cortical nAChR binding that parallels degree of dementia in Parkinson's disease and increasing age (Aubert *et al.,* 1992 and Morens *et al.,* 1995) and **Tourette's syndrome** (LeHousezec, 1998). It seems that nicotine has neuroprotective effect by alleviating the neurological impairment involved with these diseases (George and Vessicchio, 2001).

Preliminary findings of a study show that cognitive functioning of people with dementia improve after short-term (up to four weeks) nicotine administration and that an improvement has also been demonstrated in the symptoms of Tourette's syndrome following nicotine administration (White and Levin, 1999). Similarly, one initial case study has illustrated that long-term nicotine administration in the form of nicotine patch improved Parkinson's disease (Villafane *et al.*, 2001).

Nicotine holds great promise as a psycho-active drug. Smoking is associated with many psychiatric disorders, traits and symptoms. Generally, it increases concentration, decreases hunger, decreases anxiety and depression, and decreases anger. In the form of a cigarette, it also has an extremely effective delivery system. However, it is important to note that it has very small therapeutic index; the difference in dose between efficacy and toxicity is very small. As a result, nicotine's promise is not in the form of nicotine, but in the form of nicotine analogue yet to be developed. Psychiatric patients have very few behaviour re-enforcers and often have poor skills to get them. Moreover, psychiatric patients are often 'hypohedonic' in that they are less responsive to re-enforcers. Smoking must be one of the few and the best re-enforcers available.

## Substance Abuse

Among substance abusers, smoking rates are well above the population average (Budney *et al.*, 1993). Rates of alcoholics who smoke exceed 70%; they are more likely to be highly nicotine dependent than patients without such a co-morbid condition (Bobo *et al.*, 1998). Clinicians have been reluctant to encourage recovering alcoholics to try to quit smoking because of fears that smoking cessation may keep patients from completing their treatment for alcoholism, or that the stress of nicotine withdrawal will cause patients to relapse to drinking. However, treatment can be provided without necessarily leading to relapse with other substances (Campbell *et al.*, 1995).

## Why Do Psychiatric Patients Smoke More?

There may be more than one explanation for different types of mental health problems. Some of the hypotheses can be discussed under following headings:

1. Association of smoking and mental illness with deprivation.
2. The relationship of smoking and the environment.
3. Does smoking cause mental illness?
4. Does the illness cause smoking? Nicotine use as self-medication.
   (a) Relationship between nicotine and neuro-transmitters
   (b) Nicotine and depression
   (c) Nicotine and schizophrenia

(d) Links with negative symptoms-P-50 schizophrenia and other mental health problems.

(e) Nicotine and adult attention deficit hyperactivity disorder.

(f) Nicotine and cognition

(g) Interaction between nicotine and medication for schizophrenia.

  (i) Anti-psychotic medication for schizophrenia.

  (ii) Smoking and neuroleptics

  (iii) Smoking may reduce the side-effects

5. Difficulties with cessation and withdrawal effects

### 1. Association of Smoking and Mental Illness with Deprivation

Tobacco smoking has been observed to be concentrated in the most deprived groups of the society. A clear inverse relationship exists between smoking prevalence and social class[1].

*Table 3 : Cigarette smoking by deprivation in Great Britain GHS 1973 & 1998*

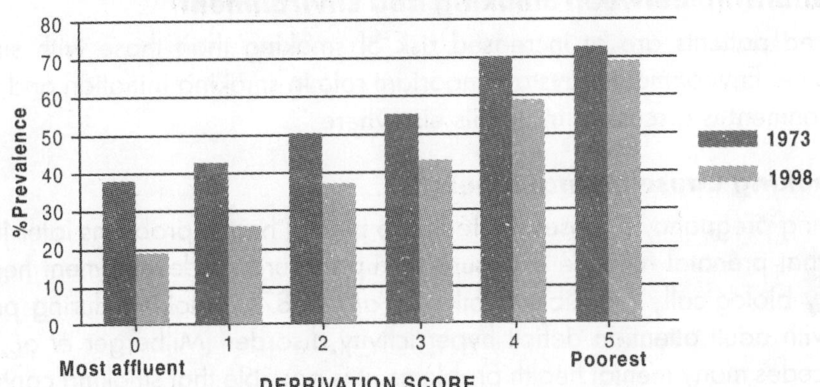


Table 3 shows smoking prevalence in relation to deprivation score (taking into account occupation, educational level, housing tenure, car ownership, unemployment, and living in crowded accommodation developed by Jarvis and Wardle in 1999). Smoking in more highly deprived groups has also been shown to have higher nicotine dependence levels as shown in Table 4.

A study has demonstrated that both social class and area level deprivation have independent association with mental health problems (Rasul *et al.*, 2001) and it is suggested that both personal disadvantage and the deprivation of the surrounding area are having an effect. Psychiatric patients smoke in a similar way to other deprived groups as a coping mechanism to deal with the stresses of their every day lives.

---

1 Office for National Statistics. Living in Britain: results from the 1998 General House-hold Survey. Stationery Office: London.

*Table 4 : Socio-economic status and dependance in smokers: saliva cotine levels in HALLS*

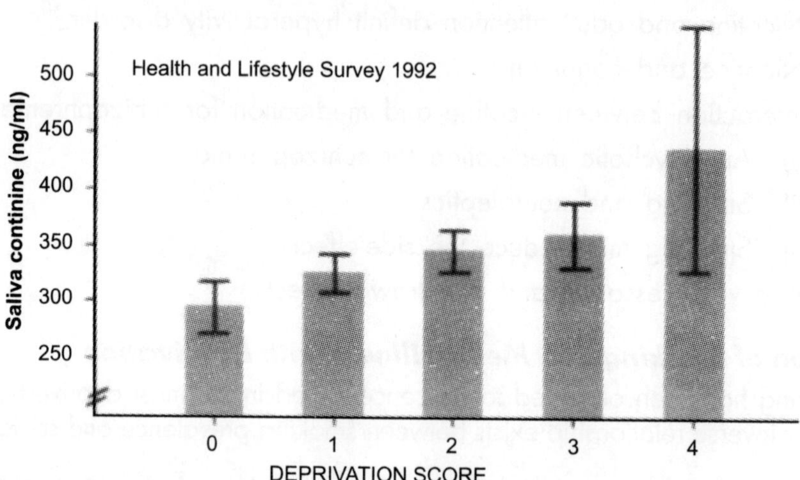


## 2. The Relationship Between Smoking and Environment

Institutionalized patients are at increased risk of smoking than those with similar illness staying at home. Environment plays an important role in smoking initiation and prevalence. Role of environment is discussed in details elsewhere.

## 3. Does Smoking Cause Mental Illness?

Smoking during pregnancy exposes the foetus to mental health problems later in life. There is evidence that prenatal nicotine exposure disrupts neuronal development hence making such a theory biologically plausible (Slotkin *et al.*, 1987). Smoking during pregnancy is associated with adult attention deficit hyperactivity disorder (Milberger *et al.*, 1998). As smoking precedes many mental health problems, it is possible that smoking contributes to or causes illness. This is also possible that there are common aetiologies (such as social, familial and individual risk factors) causing both smoking and mental illness, or that smoking is used to ameliorate symptoms of the illness before it becomes overt.

Smoking is found to predate the illness in many different diseases such as bipolar illness (Gonzalez-Pinto *et al.*, 1998) and schizophrenia (Hughes, 1999). Prospective data suggests that association between nicotine dependence and major depression probably have common factors that predispose to both disorders (Breslau *et al.*, 1992). In a five-year longitudinal study, a significantly increased risk for progression to daily smoking was found in the individuals who had history of major depression at the baseline (Breslau *et al.*, 1998).

In a follow-up study of 2000 US youth, tobacco smoking predicted a slight increase in the risk of subsequent onset of depressed mood, however, not associated with later initiation of cigarette smoking (Wu and Anthony, 1999).

## 4. Does the Illness Cause Smoking? Nicotine Use as Self-medication

Smoking is generally maintained when it has positive effect on the symptoms of the illness. A self-medication view is consistent with several hypotheses about the effects of nicotine: that it helps to alleviate some of the positive and negative symptoms of mental health problems; that it improves cognition; that it may also help to alleviate side-effects associated with anti-psychotic medications. In the first hypothesis where nicotine alleviates some of the symptoms, then abstinence from smoking and nicotine would result in increased symptoms on quitting (Breslau and Klein, 1999).

### *(a) Relationship between nicotine and neuro-transmitters*

Nicotine interacts with nicotine receptors on nerves throughout the body and brain. In the brain, nicotine acts on the acetylcholine receptors (nAchR) causing transmitter release and metabolism. Chronic nicotine use causes inactivation of the receptors which might cause increase in their numbers (Hughes; Hatsukami and Mitchell, 1986). The brains of smokers have increased number of high affinity nicotine receptors (Leonard and Bertrand, 2000).

Schizophrenics have lower number of nicotine receptors. Leonard hypothesized that this might be due to an abnormality of genes relating to neuronal nicotine receptors in schizophrenia (Leonard *et al.*, 2000). The release of different neuro-transmitters like, acetylcholine, dopamine, norepinephrine, serotonin (5-HT), glutamate, and aminobutyric acid (GABA), is affected by nicotine (George and Vessicchio, 2001). These neuro-transmitters have various effects and may play a role in some mental health disorders.

### *(b) Nicotine and depression*

Dopamine (and probably also norepinephrine and 5-HT) is used as a neuro-transmitter in reward pathways, therefore, it is speculated that the systems involved in these neuro-transmitters may be involved in depression in human beings. Antidepressants commonly increase dopamine, norepinephrine and 5-HT. Similarly, nicotine stimulates the release of these neuro-transmitters, thereby counteracting depression (Le Housezec, 1998). Nicotine administration is shown to improve depression in never-smoking depressed patients (Malpass, 2001). This explains the association between smoking cessation and major depression in depressed smokers (George and Vessicchio, 2001).

### *(c) Nicotine and schizophrenias*

There is some evidence that nicotine may have anti-schizophrenic properties. This includes increasing dopamine in the cortex, improving sensory gating, and improving smooth eye pursuit. The deficit of sensory gating in schizophrenia is best demonstrated by playing two auditory tones in rapid succession. Normal subjects have some inhibition for startle response on the second tone, but the schizophrenics and their first degree relatives do not show this inhibition. Nicotine corrects this in schizophrenics and their first degree relatives, but actually decreases inhibition in normal. Similarly when schizophrenics and their first degree relatives track a moving object with their eyes, their eye movements are not smooth compared with normal. Nicotine corrects this also.

Dysfunction of dopamine and other neuro-transmitters is associated with schizophrenia (Dalack *et al.*, 1998). Positive symptoms of schizophrenia are believed to be because of excess dopamine in substantia nigra, whereas negative symptoms are due to concurring deficits of dopamine in the cortex. Schizophrenics who smoke present more of positive symptoms of schizophrenia than nonsmokers (Goff *et al.*, 1992 and Ziedonis *et al.*, 1994). A recent study involved 101 patients with schizophrenia in which antipsychotic medication was discontinued. At baseline, smokers had more positive symptoms and were apparently more functionally impaired than nonsmokers. This difference was however no longer apparent after 30 day medication discontinuation period (Apud *et al.*, 2000). This suggests an interaction between the medication, smoking and positive symptoms of schizophrenia.

Findings for the negative symptoms have been contradictory with increased (Goff *et al.*, 1992), similar (Ziedonis *et al.*, 1994) or decreased (Beratis *et al.*, 2001) negative symptoms being observed in smokers compared with nonsmokers. Relationship between heavy smoking and positive and negative symptoms of schizophrenia has been studied and it is found that most positive symptoms and a significantly lower number of negative symptoms are associated with heavy smoking (25 or more cigarettes per day).

Smoking in schizophrenia could therefore be related to ameliorating positive symptoms. This self-medication is not only to ameliorate the positive symptoms but also to reduce the number of negative symptoms. It seems that smoking in schizophrenics is an attempt to self-medicate the symptoms of the illness, in particular the negative symptoms. Negative symptoms associated with schizophrenia may be related to a lowered activity of the systems involving dopamine. Smoking may reverse this effect by stimulating the release of dopamine.

*(d) Link between negative symptoms-P50 schizophrenia and other mental health problems.*

Patients with schizophrenia are generally unable to ignore distracting stimuli, for example, abnormal auditory filtering is found in patients with schizophrenia. The abnormal filtering is often referred to as an auditory sensory gating deficit. To measure this abnormal filtering, paired auditory stimuli are delivered half a second apart. The subjects with no schizophrenia inhibit the response to second stimulus. Schizophrenics show similar response to both stimuli. This is referred to as diminished suppression of auditory-evoked P50 response.

This deficit in schizophrenics may be related to the nicotine receptors in the brain. Nicotine and cigarette can transiently reverse these deficits. A typical medication may also normalize P50 deficits in schizophrenia.

Genetic evidence links nicotine function with the diminished P50 response as P50 is released to *alfa* nicotine receptors in the brains of the families affected with schizophrenia. Smoking also improves smooth pursuit eye movement in schizophrenics and it has been suggested that dysfunctional nicotine receptors may be involved (Olincy *et al.*, 1998).

*(e) Nicotine and adult attention deficit hyperactivity disorder*

Acute administration of nicotine in adults with attention deficit hyperactivity disorder showed improvement in the symptoms (Levin *et al.*, 1996 and Levin *et al.*, 2001). It is postulated that this may be due to nicotine receptors and neurotransmitters.

### (f) Nicotine and cognition

Many psychiatric patients continue smoking probably because nicotine improves their cognitive functioning or they get relief from incipient adverse withdrawal effects that have been wrongly labeled by them. Nevertheless there may be positive benefits, for example, there is some evidence of improved focusing of attention in smokers over non-smokers (Ernst *et al.*, 2001).

### (g) Interaction between nicotine and medication for treatment of schizophrenia

Generally, *anti-psychotic medication* blocks dopamine receptors in the brain and hence blocks the passage of nerve signals by dopamine. In so doing they reduce the symptoms of schizophrenia (Crocker, 2000). As the serotonin (5-HT) system interacts with the dopaminergic system, 5-HT may also be involved. Conventional anti-psychotics control positive symptoms more effectively than the negative symptoms while the newer anti-psychotics are effective in both positive and negative symptoms. The medication also causes side effects like dystonia, akathesia, and Parkinsonian movement disorders.

There is a relationship between cigarette *smoking and neuroleptics* prescription. Higher neuroleptic doses are prescribed to the schizophrenic smokers which might be due to the fact that smoking increases the metabolism of neuroleptic medication (Ziedonis *et al.*, 1994) although not all studies are consistent with this (Le Housezec, 1998). The choice of anti-psychotic medication influences the smoking behaviour. Clozapine is associated with a decrease in smoking and haloperidol is associated with an increase in smoking and nicotine blood levels (McEvoy *et al.*, 1995). Smokers show significantly greater therapeutic response to clozapine than non-smokers and smoked less when treated with clozapine than with conventional anti-psychotics.

This has been postulated that smoking may reduce the side effects of medication. It is known that anti-psychotic drugs block dopamine receptors and thus reduce pleasure. Nicotine counters this blockade of dopamine receptors.

Nicotine reverses some of the adverse side effects of haloperidol treatment and improved cognitive performance in schizophrenia (Levin Wilson and Rose, 1996). In one study, nicotine patches have been found to significantly reduce akathisia associated with anti-psychotic medication (Anfang and Pope, 1997). If the patients with schizophrenia smoke primarily to reverse the side effects of their anti-psychotic medications, then the chronic schizophrenics should smoke at a substantially high prevalence rates than first episode patients (McEvoy and Brown, 1999) but the studies reveal that there is no difference between the smoking behaviour of chronic and first episode schizophrenics indicating that it is not the treatment but the schizophrenia itself determines the smoking pattern.

A study has demonstrated that both social class and area level deprivation have independent association with mental health problems (Rasul *et al.*, 2001) and it is suggested that both personal disadvantage and the deprivation of the surrounding area are having an effect. Psychiatric patients smoke in a similar way to other deprived groups as a coping mechanism to deal with the stresses of their every day lives.

### 5. *Difficulties with Cessation and Withdrawal Effects*

Higher smoking rates in psychotic patients may be due to their experiencing greater difficulties with cessation and withdrawal effects when they try to stop. These difficulties vary according to the illness the person is suffering from. Exacerbation of symptoms of schizophrenia has not been detected on abstinence (Dalack *et al.,* 1999). Studies suggest that cessation rates for schizophrenics are considerably lower than among smokers than with other psychiatric diagnoses (Dalack and Meador-Woodruff, 1999).

New studies have shown that it is possible to treat smokers with schizophrenia for their tobacco dependence. The patients who were treated with atypical anti-psychotic medications (such as clozapine, risperidone, olanzapine, quetiapine) versus typical anti-psychotic medications (such as perphenazine, fluphenazine, haloperidol, chlorpromazine, thiothixene) along with trans-dermal nicotine patch reported high quit rates (George *et al.*, 2000). One possible reason for this high quit rate is that atypical anti-psychotics may mimic nicotine's effects on the central nervous system, thus minimizing the withdrawal symptoms (Ziedonis and George, 1997).

## The Impact of Smoking on Psychiatric Patients

### Economic Burden

Psychiatric patients spend a significant proportion of their income on smoking. Some schizophrenics spend up to one-third of their weekly income on cigarettes (Boyd and Lasser, 2001). According to McCreadie and Kelly (2000) there were at least 200,000 schizophrenics in the UK in 2000, 60% of whom were smoking an average of 26 cigarettes per day, spending 139 million Sterling Pounds per year on cigarettes. The costs of schizophrenia in the UK have been estimated to be between 397 and 714 million Sterling Pounds each year indicating that people with schizophrenia are, through their smoking, contributing substantially to the cost of their care. Money spent on cigarettes is not being spent on clothing, leisure pursuits and personal possessions, which could help to improve the quality of life of these patients (McDonald, 2000). No such data is available in Indian context however additional burden on patient care of the mentally ill smokers is quite evident.

Developing countries are the worst sufferers. Close to 60% of the 5,700 billion cigarettes smoked each year and 75% of the tobacco users are in the developing countries. Tobacco use and its associated burden of disease, tends to follow a gradient. It means that the poorer individuals tend to use tobacco products more than their wealthier counterparts. Similar patterns exist with respect to education and socio-economic status. The proportion of household expenditure used to purchase tobacco products is often very high in developing countries. For example, if two third of the money spent on cigarettes in Bangladesh were spent on food instead, it could save more than 10 million people from malnutrition. (10.4% of the total income was spent on tobacco products by the Bulgarian house-hold with at least one smoker in the year, 1995). Tobacco use in India is associated with worst nutrition and child-health outcomes. In China, smokers surveyed in Minhang district reported spending 17% of their household income on cigarettes (WHO, 2004).

## High Morbidity and Mortality

Psychiatric patients who smoke also suffer from the same smoking related diseases as those who are not psychiatric patients, however, the rate of affliction and mortality is twice as high among schizophrenia as in age-matched control population (Lader and Meltzer, 2001).

There may also be interaction between psychiatric illness and smoking. Depressed smokers have lower natural killer cell activity than control smokers and depressed and controlled non-smokers (Jung and Irwin, 1999). Dysfunctional natural killer cell activity may contribute to primary tumour development and metastatic cancer risk.

Recent studies indicate that smoking is a risk factor for dyskinesia independent of medication exposure (Dalack *et al.*, 1998). Tardive dyskinesia is linked to increased morbidity and mortality in those with chronic schizophrenia.

The patients with mental illness are often the least capable of coping with the devastating medical illnesses caused by smoking (Boyd and Lasser, 2001). Smoking is also a fire hazard, it causes many fires. In a study, 12% of fires involving care in the community patients over a two years period were due to careless disposal of smoke materials (Docherty, 1999).

## Smoking Cessation in Psychiatric Patients

Smoking cessation programme in psychiatric patients can be effective (Bobo *et al.*, 1998 and Ziedonis and George, 1997). Moreover, preliminary studies have shown that smoking-cessation treatment exacerbates the underlying co-morbid psychiatric conditions. Thus, while clinicians should exercise due caution, they should still treat patients for tobacco dependence. Smoking cessation programme in psychiatric patients can be viewed as follows:

1. Do psychiatric patients want to quit smoking?
2. Treatment for smokers with psychiatric illnesses.
    - (a) Effective smoking cessation treatments
    - (b) Brief opportunistic advice to quit
    - (c) Cognitive and behavioural therapy
    - (d) Group therapy and nicotine replacement therapy (NRT).
    - (e) Bupropion
    - (f) Offer smokers with mental health problems the best.
    - (g) Smoking reduction and nicotine replacement therapy.
3. Smoke-free policies
4. Smoking among mental health professionals.

### *1. Do Psychiatric Patients Want to Quit Smoking?*

Around half of the psychiatric patients smoking cigarettes express their desire to quit. Persons suffering from schizophrenia recognize that smoking is a problem and require help to quit it

(Addington *et al.*, 1997 and Ziedonis and George, 1997). However, there is no sufficient data on the effectiveness of a particular treatment in smokers with psychiatric problems.

## 2. Treatment for Smoking in Psychiatric Patients

### (a) Effective smoking cessation treatments

Evidence based and professionally endorsed smoking cessation guidelines of England emphasize an integrated smoking cessation strategy involving brief opportunistic advice to quit from mental health professionals (West, 2000), with a prescription of effective pharmacological treatments, backed up by intensive specialist cessation support for those smokers who need it. Two pharmacological treatments have proven efficacious for smoking cessation. *Nicotine replacement therapy* (NRT) is found to be effective in smoking cessation in various trials. NRT has excellent safety record and given that smokers are already inhaling nicotine there is no significant new risks involved when smokers use NRT. Currently, there are six products available as NRT: gum, patches, nasal spray, inhaler, sublingual tablet, and lozenges. There is little evidence of any difference in these products, and little scientific support for matching treatments to smokers except the 4-mg gum is better than the 2-mg gum for heavy smokers and the standard strength patch is more effective than the low dose patch for moderate to heavy smokers. There is also some evidence that combination of different types of NRT may be better than one alone (McNeill *et al.*, 2001).

*Bupropion* is used as a first line pharmacotherapy in tobacco management. However, it is contraindicated in current seizure disorder or any history of seizure, in patients with current or previous diagnosis of bulimia or anorexia nervosa and in patients with history of bipolar disorder. There are potential drug-interactions between bupropion and anti-depressants and anti-psychotics which also need to be taken into account before prescribing bupropion. Bupropion is therefore unsuitable for many patients taking concomitant medication. In US, Bupropion is licensed as an anti-depressant (not in the UK) and is used extensively in the patients with depression. Efficacy of bupropion for smoking cessation is independent of past history of depression and is not due to a reduction in depression following cessation (Hughes *et al.*, 2000).

In an eight week open label trial, bupropion, helped to decrease schizophrenic patients' cigarette consumption as measured by a decrease in expired air carbon monoxide (CO) levels. No worsening of positive symptoms or cognition or anxiety was observed (Hertzberg *et al.*, 2001). No change was found in suppression of P50 event-related potential, which might have been expected if nicotine intake decreased (McNeill, 2001).

*Brief opportunistic advice to quit is recommended by the* American Psychiatric Association (APA) Guidelines[2] for routine treatment of smoking for patients with psychiatric disorders. Surveys reveal that physicians identify the smoking status of such patients but do not provide any kind of therapeutic intervention to encourage and support smokers in stopping (Thorndike *et al.*, 2001).

---

2 Fiore M.C. (2000) United States, Tobacco Use and Dependence Guidelines Panel. Treating Tobacco Use and Dependence. Department of Health and Human Service, Public Health Service; Rockville, Maryland.

In Britain, National Service Framework for Mental Health states that people with severe mental illness should be physically assessed but there was little evidence that this was happening (Phelan *et al.*, 2001).

There is some suggestion that the mental health problems may undermine attempts at quitting rather than ability to stop. Therefore, it is critical that the mental health professionals who come in contact with smokers with psychiatric diagnoses routinely ask about smoking and advise their patients to stop smoking. Many smokers, however, need further support.

Finally, it is important not to offer treatment when mental illness is florid and very active (McNeill, 2001). A note can be made in patient's file, however, to intervene when the patient's condition stabilizes. Patient should be followed more closely to monitor anti-psychotic medication and as a precaution in case symptoms of the illness become exacerbated.

*(b) Cognitive and behaviour therapy*

Cigarette smokers, who had suffered from major depression in the past, were studied for effects of standard cognitive-behavioural smoking cessation treatment programme and cognitive-behaviour treatment along with this treatment for patients with depression. No pharmacological treatment was involved. Abstinence rates at one year were 25–33% and there was no difference between the treatments. However, the secondary analysis revealed that smokers with recurrent major depression and heavy smokers were significantly more likely to be abstinent if they received two treatment programmes rather than the standard treatment programme only. It is suggested that the additional programme for depression might provide benefits for some smokers with major depression (Brown *et al.*, 2001).

*(c) Group therapy and nicotine replacement therapy*

Group-therapy programmes have been reported to be successful in smoking cessation. In some studies nicotine patches have been used along with standardized group therapy with the continuation of pre-treatment anti-psychotic medication in schizophrenic patients. It enhanced the rate of smoking cessation significantly. Cessation rates were higher in those schizophrenics who were receiving a typical anti-psychotic. It is suggested that the medication targeting specific clinical symptoms and neurochemical aspects of schizophrenia could contribute in improving nicotine dependence (George *et al.*, 2000). In another study the patients preferred nicotine inhaler over the nicotine trans-dermal patch (D'Mello *et al.*, 2001).

*(d) Offer smokers with mental health problems the best*

Experts advise that if health professionals manage to encourage their smoking patients to make an attempt to quit, they should be offered the best treatment. Given that these patients tend to be heavier smokers, stronger dose of NRT may therefore be preferable and should be combined with specialist cessation support.

In addition, there is increasing evidence of effectiveness of using more than one NRT for treatment (McNeill, 2001). One study combining NRT with bupropion showed desirable results. Given the greater nicotine dependence in this population, combination therapy may increase the chances of successful stopping.

*(e) Smoking reduction and nicotine replacement therapy*

In the populations where there are lower rates of stopping and higher rates of smoking, a harm-reduction approach might be appropriate in parallel with encouraging cessation. Smoking related morbidity and mortality are dose (smoking) related, so that if cigarettes could be replaced with less harmful form of nicotine delivery, there might be overall benefit to smoker's health (McNeill, 2001). The potential downside to this approach is that it might discourage quit attempts. However, there is some evidence to suggest that by being able to control their smoking, using a less harmful form of nicotine delivery might actually encourage the smoker to quit. Smokers who are unwilling to quit should at least be given the choice of which form of nicotine delivery to use.

The studies, therefore, have examined the impact of NRT on *ad libitum* smoking in psychiatric patients and preliminary evidence suggests that this may be a useful approach.

### 3. *Smoke-free Policies*

Smoke-free policies reduce the harmful effects of second hand tobacco smoke, encourage smokers to quit, and help to make non-smoking the norm. Many psychiatric patients who are ex-smokers may relapse when hospitalized and vulnerable to constant smoking stimuli (Lawn *et al.*, 2002). Smoke-free policy produces significantly fewer adverse effects and the attitude of care-providers also becomes favourable.

Assessment of tobacco control policies in the NHS in the UK led to identify psychiatric units and long-stay units as posing particular challenges to successful policies limiting smoking. The emphasis of the report is on staff at all levels in the organization since staff is responsible for implementation of the policies. In India, hospitals are designated as smoke-free zones by law but effective implementation of this law is yet to come.

### *4. Smoking Among Mental Health Professional*

Smoking policy may also encourage psychiatric staff to stop smoking. There is a dearth of recent data on smoking among nurses (Rowe and Macleod Clark, 2000) and doctors. In an UK study, smoking prevalence in psychiatric nurses was found to be twice than other groups.

Psychiatric patients can be motivated to quit and successfully helped to stop smoking. Apart from the availability of successful treatment, approaches like harm-reduction should also be considered for unwilling to quit smokers. Smoke-free policies can be successfully introduced in psychiatric institutions to encourage smokers to quit. Mental health professionals have an important role to play in encouraging and supporting smokers' attempt to quit.

Although the studies discussed strengthen the case for treating tobacco dependence in patients with psychiatric co-morbidities, additional research is needed. Clinical culture and practice patterns need to change in order to ensure that all patients who use tobacco, including those with psychiatric co-morbidities, are identified and offered treatment. While smokers with co-morbid conditions have a greater risk of relapse, there is no evidence that patients relapse to their previous psychiatric condition while making a quit attempt. In fact, most evidence suggests that abstinence results in little adverse impact. Given the harmful nature of continued tobacco use and the existence of effective treatment, the guidelines recommended treating smokers with co-morbid psychiatric conditions with the same treatments identified as being efficacious for the general population.

## REFERENCES

Addington J., er-Guebaly N. and Addington D.: Readiness to Stop Smoking in Schizophrenia. *Canadian Journal of Psychiatry*, 42: 49-52, 1997.

Amering M., Benkier B. and Berger P.: Panic Disorder and Cigarette Smoking Behaviour. *Comprehensive Psychiatry*, 40:35–38. 1999.

Anda R.F., Williamson D.F., Escobedo L.G., Mast E.E., Govino G.A. and Remington P.L.: Depression and Dynamics of Smoking. *Journal of American Medical association*, 264:1541–1545, 1990.

Anfang M.K. and Pope H.G. Jr.: Treatment of Neuroleptic-induced Akathisia with Nicotine Patches. *Psychopharmacology*, 134: 153–156, 1997.

Apud J.A., Egan M.F. and Wyatt R.J.: Effect of Smoking During Anti-psychotic Withdrawal in Patients with Chronic Schizophrenia. *Schizophrenia Research*, 46:119–127, 2000.

Aubert I., Aurojo D.M., Cecyre D., Robitaille Y., Gothier S. and Quirion R..: 1992 Comparative Alterations of Nicotinic and Muscarinic Binding Sites in Alzheimer's and Parkinsonian Diseases. Journal of Neurochemistry, 58:529–541,

Beckham J.C., Roodman A.A., Shipley R.H.: Smoking in Vietnam Combat Veterans With Post-traumatic Stress Disorder. *Journal of Trauma & Stress*, 8: 461–472, 1995.

Beckham J.C., Kirby A.C. and Feldman M.E.: Prevalence and Correlates of Heavy Smoking in Vietnam Veterans With Chronic Post-traumatic Stress Disorder. *Addictive Behaviour*, 22:637–647, 1997.

Bell S.L., Taylor R.C., Singleton E.G., Henningfield J.E. and Heishman S.J.: Smoking After Nicotine Deprivation Enhancescognitive Performance and Decreases Tobacco Craving in Drug Abusers. *Nicotine and Tobacco Research*, 1:45–52, 1999.

Beratis S., Katrivanou A., Gourzis P.: Factors Affecting Smoking in Schizophrenia. *Comprehensive Psychiatry*, 45: 393–402, 2001.

Bobo J.K., McIlvain HE and Lando H.A.: Effect of Smoking Cessation Counseling on Recovery from Alcoholism: Findings from a Randomized Community Intervention Trial. *Addiction*, 93(6):877–887, 1998.

Borreli B., Bock B. and King T.: The Impact of Depression on Smoking Cessation in Women. *American Journal of Preventive Medicine*, 12(5):378–387, 1996.

Boyd J.W. and Lasser K.: Tobacco Madness. *Commentary, Psychiatric Times*, 17, 2001.

Breslau N., Kilbey M.M., and Andrewski P.: Nicotine Withdrawal Symptoms and Psychiatric Disorders: Findings of an Epidemiological Study of Young Adults. *American Journal of Psychiatry*, 149:464–469, 1992.

Breslau N., Peterson E.L. and Schultz L.R.: Major Depression and Stages of Smoking. A Longitudinal Investigation. *Archives of General Psychiatry*, 55:161–166, 1998.

Breslau N., and Klein D.F.: Smoking and Panic Attacks: an Epidemiological Investigation. *Archives of General Psychiatry*, 56:1141–1147, 1999.

Brown R.A., Kahler C.W. and Niaura R.: Cognitive–behaviour Treatment for Depression in Smoking Cessation. *Journal of Consulting and Clinical Psychology*, 1:762–767, 2001.

Brown S., Inskip H., Barraclough B.: Causes of Excessive Mortality in Schizophrenia. *British Journal of Psychiatry*, 177:212–217, 2000.

Budney A.J., Higgins S.T., Hughes J.R. and Bicken W.K.: Nicotine and Caffein use in Cocaine-dependent Individuals. *Journal of Substance Abuse*, 5(2): 117–130, 1993.

Campbell B.K., Wander N., Stark M.J. and Holbert T.: Treating Cigarette –Smoking in In Drug-abusing Clients. *Journal of Substance Abuse Treatment*,12(2): 89–94, 1995.

Chiles J.A., Cohen S. and Roland M.: Smoking and Schizophrenic Psychopathology. *American Journal of Addiction*, 2:215–219, 1993.

Chilcoat H.D. and Breslau, N.: Pathway from Adhd to Early Drug Use. *Journal of American Academy of Child and Adolescent Psychiatry*, 38:1347–1354, 1997.

Chong S.A. and Choo H.L.: Smoking Among Chinese Patients with Schizophrenia. *Australian and New Zealand Journal of Psychiatry*, 30:350–353, 1996.

Clarke P.B.S.: Tobacco Smoke, Genes and Dopamine. *Lancet*, 353:84–85, 1998.

Coger R.W., Moe K.L. and Serafetinides E.A.: Attention Deficit Disorder in Adults and Nicotine Dependence: Psychobiological Factors in Resistance to Recovery. *Journal of Psycho-active Drugs*, 28:229–240. 1996.

Colquhoun L.M. and Patrick J.W.: Pharmacology of Neuronal Nicotinic Acetylcholine Receptor Subtypes. Advances in Pharmacology,39: 191–220, 1997.

Combs D.R. and Advokat C.: Antipsychotic Medication and Smoking Prevalence in Acutely Hospitalized Patients With Chronic Schizophrenia. Schizophrenic Research, 46:129–137, 2000.

Covey L.S., Glassman A.H. and Stetner F.: Major Depression Following Smoking Cessation. *American Journal of Psychiatry*, 154:263–265, 1997.

Covey L.S., Glassman A.H. and Stetner F.: Cigarette Smoking and Major Depression. *Journal of Addictive Disorders*, 17:35–46, 1998.

Covin A., Mahomy E., O'Regan M.: Cigarette Smoking and Psychotic Symptoms in Bipolar Affective Disorder. *British Journal of Psychiatry*, 179:35–38, 2001.

Crocker A.: The Neuropharmacology of Tobacco Smoking. *Adelaide,* as Quoted in Smoking and Mental Health – A Review of the Literature (Ed) Mc Neill A, Smoke-free London Programme. Sflondon@Doh.gsi.gov.uk, 2000.

Dalack G.W., Brown L. and Hill E.: Nicotine Withdrawal and Psychiatric Symptoms in Cigatrette Smokers With Schizophrenia. *Neuropsychopharmacology,* 21 195–202, 1999.

Dalack G.W., Healy D.J., Meador-Woodruff J.H.: Nicotine Dependence in Schizophrenia and Laboratory Findings. *American Journal of Psychiatry,* 155:1490–1501, 1998.

Dalack G.W. and Meador-Woodruff J.H.: Smoking, Smoking Withdrawal and Schizophrenia: Case Report and a Review of Literature. Schizophreia Research,22:133–141, 1996.

Dalack G.W. and Meador Woodruff.: Acute Feasibility and Safety of a Smoking Reduction Strategy for Smokers With Schizophrenia. *Nicotine and Tobacco Research,* 1: 53–57, 1999.

Davranche K. and Audiffren M.: Effects of a Low Dose of Transdermal Nicotine on Information Processing. *Nicotine and Tobacco Research,* 4:275–285, 2002.

Dawe S., Gerada C. and Russell M.A.: Nicotine Intake in Smokers Increases Following a Single Dose of Haloperidol. *Psychopharmacology,* 117:110–115, 1995.

De Leon J.: Smoking and Vulnerability for Schizophrenia. *Schizophrenia Bulletin,* 22:405–409, 1996.

De Leon J., Dadvand M. and Canuso C.: Schizophrenia and Smoking: an Epidemiological Study in a Hospital. *American Journal of Psychiatry,* 152:453–455, 1995.

De Leon J., Becona E., Gurpegui M., Gonzalez-Pinto A. and Diaz F.J.: The Association Between High Nicotine Dependence and Severe Mental Illness May Be Consistent Across Countries. Journal of Clinical Psychiatry, 63: 812–816, 2002.

De Leon J. and Diaz F.J..: A Meta-analysis of Worldwide Studies Demonstrates an Association Between Schizophrenia and Tobacco Smoking Behaviour. Schizophrenia Research, 76:135–157, 2005.

D'Mello D.A., Bandlamudi G.R., and Colenda C.C.: Nicotine Replacement Methods on a Psychiatric Unit. *American Journal of Drug and Alcohol Abuse,* 27:525–527, 2001.

Docherty B.: Care in the community. *Fire Prevention,* 31726–27, 1999.

Ernst M., Heishman S.J., Spurgeon L. and London E.D.: Smoking History and Nicotine Effects on Cognitive Performance. *Neuropsychpharmacology,* 25:3113–3119, 2001.

Fiore M.C., Bailey W.C., and Cohen S.J.: Treating Tobacco Use and Dependence. Clinical Practice Guidelines. Rockville Md.: US Department of Health and Human Services, Public Health Service, 2000.

Freedman R., Coon H., Myles-Worsley M., Orr-Urtreger A., Olincy A., Davis A., Polymerpoulos M., Holik J., Hopkins J., Hoff M., Rosenthal J., Waldo M.C., Reimherr F., Wender P., Yaw J., Young D.A., Breese C.R., Adams C., Patterson D., Adler L.E., Kruglyak L., Leonard S. and Byerley W.: Linkage of Neurophysiological Deficit in Schizophrenia to a Chromosome 15 Locus. Proceedings of National Academy of Science, USA, 94: 587–592, 1997.

George T.P. and Vessicchio J.C.: Nicotine Addiction and Other Psychiatric Disorders. *Psychiatric Times,* Vol. Xviii, Issue 2, 2001.

George T.P., Ziedonis D.M., Feingold A.: Nicotine Transdermal Patch and Atypical Anti-psychotic Medications for Smoking Cessation in Schizophrenia. *American Journal of Psychiatry*, 157:1835–1842, 2000.

Gill B., Meltzer H., and Hinds K.: Psychiatric Morbidity Among Homeless People in Great Britain, *Report 7*. Hmso: London, 1996.

Glassman A.H., Stetner F. and Walsh B.T.: Heavy Smokers, Smoking Cessation, and Clonidine. Results of a Double-blind, Randomized Trial. *Journal of Academy of Medical Association* (Jama),259(19): 2863–2866, 1988.

Goff D.C., Handerson D.C. and Amico E.: Cigarette Smoking in Schizophrenia: Relationship of Psychopathology and Medication Side-effects. *American Journal of Psychiatry*, 149:11289–1194, 1992.

Gonzalez-Pinto, Gutierez M. and Ezcurra J.: Tobacco Smoking and Bipolar Disorder. *Journal of Clinical Psychiatry*, 59:225–228, 1998.

Gotti C., Fornasari D. and Clementi F.: Human Neuronal Nicotinic Receptors. *Progress in Neurobiology*, 53:199–237, 1997.

Gurpregue M., Martinez-Ortega J.M., Aguilar MC, Diaz F.J., Quintana H.M. and de Leon J.: Smoking Initiation and Schizophrenia: A Replication Study in a Spanish Sample. Schizophrenia Research, 2005.

Heishman S.J., Henningfield J.E. and Singleton E.G.: Tobacco, Nicotine and Human Cognition. *Nicotine and Tobacco Research*, 4:3–4, 2002.

Hertzberg M.A., Moore S.H., and Feldman M.E.: A Preliminary Study of Bupropion-sustained Release for Smoking–Cessation In-patients With Chronic Post-traumatic Stress Disorder. *Journal of Clinical Psychopharmacology*, 21:94–98, 2001.

Hughes J.R.: Co-morbidity and smoking: *Nicotine and Tobacco Research*, 1:S149–S152, 1999.

Hughes J.R.: Evidence for and Against the Self-medication Hypothesis for Smoking. International Journal of *Neuropsychopharmacology*, 3 (suppl. 1):S59. Abstract S.36.4, 2000.

Hughes J.R., Hatsukami J.K. and Mitchell J.E.: Prevalence of Smoking in Psychiatric Out Patients. *American Journal of Psychiatry*, 143:993–997, 1986.

Hughes J.R. Stead L.F. and Lancaster T.: Anti-depressants for Smoking Cessation. *Cochrane Database Systematic Review*, 2000.

Iversen L.L.: Smoking… harmful to the Brain, *Nature*, 382:206–207, 1996.

Jarvis M. and Wardle M.: Social Patterning of Health Behaviour: The Case of Cigarette Smoking. In: *Social Determinants of Health*. Eds.: Marmot M, Wilkinwon R Oup, Oxford, 1999.

Jung W. and Irwin M.: Reduction of Natural Killer Cytotoxic Activity in Major Depression and Cigarette Smoking. *Psychosomatic Medicine*, 61:263–270, 1999.

Kelly C. and McCreadie R.G.: Smoking Habits, Current Symptoms and Premorbid Characteristics of Schizophrenic Patients in Nithsdale Scotland. *American Journal of Psychiatry*, 156: 1751–1757, 1999.

Kelly C. and McCreadie R.G.: Cigarette Smoking and Schizophrenia. *Advances in Psychiatric Treatment*,6:327–341, 2000.

Knott V., Bosman M., Mahoney C., Livitsky V. and Quint K.: Trans-dermal Nicotine: Single Dose Effect on Mood, Eeg Performance, Event Related Performance. Pharmacology, Biochemistry and Behaviour, 63:253–261, 1999.

Knott V., Mohr E., Engeland C. and Livitsky V.: Effects of Acute Nicotine Administration on Cognitive Event-related Potentials With Alzheimer's Disease. Neuropsychobiology, 45:158–165, 2002.

Krammer TAM.: Psychiatric Co-morbidity in Smokers: Epidemiological Aspects. Xxii Congress of the Collegium Internationale Neuro-Psychopharmacologicum. http://www.medscape.com/, 2000.

Lader D. and Meltzer H.: Smoking Related Behaviours and Attitudes. ONS: London, 2001.

Lang B.C.: Treating Tobacco Dependence in Patients With Psychiatric Co-morbidities. *Psychiatric Times*,XVIII,9, 2004.

Lasser K., Wesley Boyd J., Woolhandle S.: Smoking and Mental Illness. A population Based Prevalence Study. *Journal of American Medical Association (JAMA)*, 284:2606–2610, 2000.

Lawn S.J., Pols R.G. and Barber J.G.: Smoking and Quitting: A Qualitative Study With Community-living Psychiatric Clients. *Social Siences and Medicine*, 54:93–104, 2002.

LeCrubier Y.: Psychiatric co-morbidity in Smokers: Epidemiological Aspects. *International Journal of Neuropsychopharmacology*, 3(suppl 1): S58. Abstract S.36.1, 2000.

LeHousezec J.L.: Nicotine: Abused Substance and Therapeutic Agent. *Journal of Psychiatry and Neurosciences*, 23:95–108, 1998.

Leonard S., and Bertrand D.: Neuronal Nicotine Receptors: from Structure to Function. *Nicotine and Tobacco Research*, 3:203–223, 2000.

Leonard S., Gault J., Hopkin J., Logel J., Vianzon R., Short M., Drebing C., Berger R., Venn D., Sirota P., Zerbe G., Olincy A., Rose R.G., Adler L.E. and Freedman R.: Association of Promoter Variants in the Alfa–7 Nicotine 'Acetylcholine Receptor Gene with an Inhibitory Deficit Found in Schizophrenia. Archives of General Psychiatry, 59: 1085–1096, 2002.

Leonard D., Breese C. and Adams C..: Smoking and Schizophrenia: Abnormal Nicotine Receptor Expression. *European Journal of Pharmacology*, 393: 237–242, 2000.

Levin E.D.: Nicotine Receptor Subtypes and Cognitive Function. Journal of Neurobiology, 53:633–640, 2002.

Levin E.D., Connors C.K. and Silva D.: Effects of Chronic Nicotine and Methylphenidate in Adults With Attention Deficit Hyperactivity Disorder. *Experimental Clinical Psychopharmacology*, 9:83–90, 2001.

Levin E.D., Connors C.K. and Sparrow E.: Nicotine Effects on Adults With Attention Deficit Hyperactivity Disorder. *Psychopharmacology*, 123: 55–63, 1996.

Levin E.D., Wilson W. and Rose J.E.: Nicotine Haloperidol Interaction and Cognitive Performance in Schizophrenics. *Neuropsychopharmacology*,15: 429–436, 1996.

Lohr J.B. and Flynn K.: Smoking and Schizophrenia, *Schizophrenia Research*, 8:93–102, 1992.

Lopes F.L., Nascimento I., Zin W.A., Valenca A.M., Figueira I. and Nardi A.E.: Smoking and Psychiatric Disorders. Brazilian Journal of Medical and Biological Research, 35:961–967,

Lukas R.J.: Neuronal Nicotine Acetylcholine Receptors. In: The Acetylcholine Receptor: Current Views and Future Trends. Springer Vertag: Berlin, 145–173, 1998.

Maier W. and Schwab S.: Molecular Genetics of Schizophrenia, *Current Opinion in Psychiatry*.11:19–25, 1998.

Malpass D.: Smoking and Mental Health Seminar Presentation, as Quoted in Smoking and Mental Health – A Review of the Literature (ed) McNeill A.: 2001 Smoke-free London Programme. sflondon@doh.gsi.gov.uk, 2001.

McCreadie R.G. and Kelly C.: Paients with Schizophrenia Who Smoke. Private Disaster, Public Resource. *British Journal of Psychiatry*, 176:109, 2000.

McDonald C.: Cigarette Smoking in Patients with Schizophrenia. *British Journal of Psychiatry*,176:596–597, 2000.

McEvoy J.P. and Brown S.R.N.: Smoking in First Episode Patients With Schizophrenia. *American Journal of Psychiatry*, 156:1120–1121, 1999.

McEvoy J.P., Freudenreich O. and Levin E.D.: Haloperidol Increases Smoking in Patients With Schizophrenia. *Psychopharmacology*, 119:124–126, 1995.

McEvoy J.P., Freudenreich O. and Wilson W.H.: Smoking and Therapeutic Response to Clozapine in Patients With Schizophrenia. Biological Psychiatry, 46:125–129, 1999.

McGehee D.S. and Role L.W.: Physiological Diversity of Nicotine Acetylcholine Receptors Expressed By Vertebrate Neurons. Annual Review of Physiology, 57:521–546, 1995.

Mc Neill A.: Smoking and Mental Health – A Review of the Literature. Action on Smoking and Health. Smoke free London Programme, *Regional NHS London*, 2001.

McNeill A., Foulds J. and Bates C.: Regulation of Nicotine Replacement Therapies (NRT). A critique of current practice. Addiction, 96:1757–1768, 2001.

Meltzer H., Gill B., Petticrew M.: Economic Activity and Social Functioning of Adults With Psychiatric Disorders (OPCS *Survey of Psychiatric Morbidity in Great Britain Report 3) HMSO, London*, 1995.

Menzza M.A., Grossman N. and Van Horn M.: Smoking and Movement Disorders in Psychiatric Patients. *Biological Psychiatry*.,30: 109–115, 1991.

Milberger S., Biederman J., Faraone S.V., Chen L., Jones J.: ADHD is Associated With Early Initiation of Cigarette Smoking in Children and Adolescents. *Journal of American Academy of Child and Adolescent Psychiatry*,36:37–44, 1997.

Milberger S., Biederman J., Faraone S.V., Chen L., and Jones J.: Further Evidence of an Association Between Maternal Smoking During Pregnancy and Attewntion Deficit Hyperactivity Disorder: Findings from a High Risk Sample of Siblings. Journal of Clinical Child Psychology,27: 352–358, 1998.

Morens D.M., Grandinetti A. and Reed D.: Cigarette Smoking and Protection from Parkinson's Disease: False Association Or Aetiological Clue? *American Academy of Neurology*, 45:1041–1051, 1995.

Mortensen P.B. and Juel K.: Mortality and Causes of Death in First Admitted Schizophrenic Patients. *British Journal of Psychiatry*, 163:183–189, 1993.

Newhouse P.A., Potter A., Corwin J. and Lenox R.: Acute Nicotine Blockade Produces Cognitive Impairment in Normal Humans. *Psychopharmacology'* 108:480–484, 1992.

Newhouse P.A., Sunderland T., Tariot P.N., Blumhard C.L., Weingartner H., Mellow A. and Murphy D.L.: Intravenous Nicotine in Alzheimer's Disease: A Pilot Study. *Psychopharmacology*. 95:171–175, 1988.

Nilsson A., Waller L., and Rosengren A.: Cigarette Smoking Is Associated With Involuntary Abnormal Movements in the General Male Population. *Biological Psychiatry*, 41:717–723. 1997.

Niaura R., Britt D.M. and Shadel W.G.: Symptoms of Depression and Survival Experience Among Three Samples of Smokers Trying to Quit. *Psychology of Addictive Behaviours*, 15:13–17, 2001.

Olincy A., Ross R.G., Young D.A., Roath M., and Freedman R.: Improvement in Smooth Pursuit Eye Movement After Smoking Cigarette in Schizophrenia Patients. *Neuropsychopharmacology*, 18:175–185, 1998.

Olincy A., Young D.A. and Freedman R.: Increased Levels of Nicotine Metabolite Cotinine in Schizophrenic Smokers Compared to Other Smokers. *Biological Psychiatry*, 42:1–5, 1997.

Overall J.E. and Gorham D.R.: The Brief Psychiatric Rating Scale. *Psychological Reports*, 10:799–812, 1962.

Patton G.C., Hibbert M. and Rosier M.J.: Is Smoking Associated With Depression and Anxiety in Teenagers? *American Journal of Public Health*, 86:225–230, 1996.

Petersen R.: Normal Aging, Mild Cogmitive Impairment, and Early Alzheimer's Disease. *Neurology*, 1:326–344, 1995.

Petersen R., Smith G., Waring S. and Ivnik R.: Mild Cognitive Impairment: clinical characterization and outcome. Archives of Neurology, 56:303–308, 1999.

Phelan M., Stradins L. and Morrison S.: Physical Health of People With Severe Mental Illness. *British Medical Journal*, 322: 443–444, 2001.

Pohl R., Yergani V.K. and BaLON r.: Smoking in Patients With Panic Disorder. *Psychiatric Research*, 43:253–262, 1992.

Pomerleau C.S., Ehrlich E., Tate J.C.: The Female Weight-control Smoker: A Profile. *Journal of Substance Abuse*,5: 391–400, 1993.

Pomerlau O.F., Downey K.K., and Stelson F.W.: Cigarette Smoking in Adult Patients Diagnosed With Attention Deficit Hyperactivity Disorder. *Journal of Substance Abuse*, 7:373–378, 1995.

Pontieri F.E., Tanda G. and Orzi F.: Effects of Nicotine on Nucleus Accumbens and Similarity to Those of Addictive Drugs. *Nature*, 382:255–256, 1996.

Procyshyn R.M., Ihsan N. and Thompson D.: A Comparison of Smoking Behaviour Between Patients Treated With Clozapine and Depot Neuroleptics. International Clinical Psychopharmacology, 16:291–295, 2001.

Provost SC and Woodward R.: Effects of Nicotine Gum on Repeated Administration of the Stroop Test. Psychopharmacology, 104:536–540. 1991.

Rasul F, Stansfeld SA, Davey–Smith G.: Sociodemographic Factors, Smoking and Common Mental Disorders in Renfew Pansley (MIDSPAN) Study. *Journal of Health Psychology*,6:149–158, 2001.

Riggs P.D., Mikulich S.K., Whitmore E.A. and Crowley T.J.: Relationship if ADHD, Depression and Non-tobacco Substance Use Disorder to Nicotine Dependence in Substance-dependent Delinquents. *Drug and Alcohol Dependence*, 54:195–205, 1999.

Rowe K. and Macleod-Clark J.: The Incidence of Smoking Among Nurses: A Review of the Literature. *Journal of Advanced Nursing*,31:1046–1053, 2000.

Salokangas R.K.R., Saarijarvi S. and Taiminen T.: Effect of Smoking on Neuroleptics in Schizophrenia. *Schizophrenia Research*, 23:55–60, 1997.

Slotkin T.A., Cho H., Whitmore W.L.: Effects of Prenatal Exposure on Neuronal Development. Selective Action on Central and Peripheral Catecholaminergic Pathways. *Brain Research Bulletin*,18:601–611, 1987.

Thorndike A.A.N., Stafford R.S. and Riggoti N.A.: US Physicians Treatment of Smoking in Outpatients With Psychiatric Diagnosis. *Nicotine and Tobacco Research*,3: 85–91, 2001.

Villafane G., Degos J.D., Lagrue G. and Cesaro P.: Long-term Nicotine Administration Can Improve Parkinson's Disease – *Report of a Case. Poster, SRNT Europe Conference Paris.* West R, McNeill a and Raw M.: 2000 Smoking Cessation Guidelines for Health Professionals: an update. *Thorax*, 55:987–999, 2001.

West R.: Nicotine as a Cognitive Enhancer: The Current State of the Evidence. Presentation At Srnt Europe Conference, Paris, 2001.

West R.J.: Signs and Symptoms During The Acute Phase of Smoking Cessation. International Journal of Neuropsychopharmacology, (SUPPL 1) Abstract S.36.4, 2000.

White H.K. and Levin E.D.: Four-week Nicotine Patch Treatment Effect on Cognitive Performance in Alzheimer's Disease. *Psychopharmacology*, 143:158–165. 1999.

White and Levin, 2005.

Whitehouse P., Hedreen J. and White C.: Basal Forebrain Neurons in Dementia of Parkinson's Disease. Annals of Neurology, 13:243–248, 1983.

Wilson A.L., Langley L.K., Monley J., Bauer T., Rottunda S., McFalls E., Kovera C. and McCarten J.R.: Nicotine Patches in Alzheimer's Disease: Pilot Study on Learning, Memory and Safety. Pharmacology, Biochemistry and Behaviour' %:509–514, 1995.

World Health Organization (WHO) *World No Tobacco Day*, Geneva, 2004.

Wu L-T and Anthony J.C.: Tobacco Smoking and Depressed Mood in Late Childhood and Early Adolescence. *American Journal of Public Health*, 89:1837–1840, 1999.

Yassan R., Lal S. and Korpassy A.: Nicotine Exposure and Tardive Dyskinesia. *Biological Psychiatry*, 22: 67–72, 1987.

Ziedonis D.M. and George T.P.: Schizophrenia and Nicotine Use: Report of a Pilot Smoking Cessation Programme and Review of Neuro-biological and Clinical Issues. Schizophrenia Bulletin,23: 247–254, 1997.

Ziedonis D.M., Kosten T.R. and Glazer W.M.: Nicotine Dependence and Schizophrenia. *Hospital and Community Psychiatry*, 45: 204–206, 1994.

# CHAPTER 10

# Smoking-cessation and Treatment of Tobacco Dependence

*Worldwide, 1.3 billion people smoke and, unless urgent action is taken, 650 million of them will die prematurely due to tobacco use. Current statistics indicate that it will not be possible to reduce tobacco-related deaths over the next 30-50 years, unless adult smokers are encouraged to quit.*

— World Health Organization, 2003

Tobacco smoking is one of the most common forms of tobacco consumption and a leading cause of preventable deaths all over the world. Nicotine in tobacco is a potent psycho-active drug that induces euphoria, serves as a re-inforcer for its use, and leads to withdrawal syndrome when absent from user's body. Nicotine use meets the criteria for a highly addictive drug comparable to other dependence producing drugs. However, till recently, much of the work done on dependence potential of nicotine was yet to see its clinical application in the treatment of tobacco users. In the last few decades, some progress has been made in the development of pharmacotherapies for tobacco use disorder.

It is known that both physical and psychological factors are responsible for initiation and maintenance of smoking behaviour and these factors become closely linked in a conditioning process in which smoking is associated with multiple cues. A highly dependent smoker, who presents for treatment, has even longer and more extensive history of nicotine self-administration than does an average smoker. Such learning is not seen with other types of drug-abuse. Similar to other drug-addictions, tobacco dependence is a chronic relapsing disorder, which often requires repeated treatments until long-term abstinence is achieved. US Public Health Service (PHS) recommends that all patients visiting a doctor should be asked about their tobacco use; those attempting to quit smoking should be prescribed at least one of the first-line pharmacotherapies in the absence of contraindications for these drugs (Fiore, 2000). These recommendations[1] are especially relevant for psychiatrists, given that individuals with a mental disorder are twice as likely to be smokers. These recommendations in the guideline generally apply to all tobacco users even though not all tobacco users meet dependence criteria. This is because most of the principles for treating nicotine dependence apply to non-dependent tobacco users as well. Psychiatrists should assess the smoking status of all their patients on a regular basis. Since many psychiatric patients are not ready to quit, the goal of assessment will often be to motivate patients to contemplate cessation by reviewing the benefits of quitting and offering support and treatment and identifying factors posing difficulties in smoking cessations. Intervention procedures for tobacco users who seek assistance should address to the addictive properties of tobacco and the ways that these can be overcome.

Most of the times, instead of being a planned and deliberate act, cigarette smoking becomes a spontaneous unconscious effort influenced by environmental factors which are otherwise seemingly insignificant. These factors act as cues to induce smoking in the smokers and help in maintaining smoking behaviour. Other than the environmental cues, there are individual factors in the smokers themselves which pose difficulty in the process of smoking cessation. All these factors play a significant role in smoking behaviour and need to be addressed in the management strategies of smoking cessation.

## Cues to Smoking

Generally there is a considerable regularity in the cigarette smoking frequency of smokers but it may not always be the case. Some people smoke when they work alone and others when they are in company. There are certain cues, which determine smoking frequency like ashtray, cigarette packet, sight of other person smoking and even the smell of smoke can elicit strong craving not only in current smokers and newly abstained smokers, but also in individuals who have achieved long term abstinence (Abrams, 1986). Some cues disappear quickly after cessation of smoking while others may persist especially in long-term dependent smokers. Those smokers who smoke more when they are angry, frustrated, or unhappy may be vulnerable to a crisis even when the crisis occurs after an extended period of abstinence (Pomerleau *et al.*, 1978). Infrequently encountered cues continue to elicit conditioned cravings over a longer period of time. Some smokers rely more heavily upon nicotine in regulating mood, especially negative affect, some use smoking as a means of sustaining attention while some others use it as an aid to relaxation (Ikard and Tompkind, 1973). Nicotine in cigarette smoke affects mood and performance that can become the source of addiction to tobacco (Hughes, Goldstein *et al.*, 1999). Physiological reactions (such as elevated heart rate) to smoking cues have been documented to persist for extended intervals. The combination

[1] Cigarette smoking among adults – United States, 2000. Morbidity, Mortality Weekly Report, 2002:51(29):642–645.

of tobacco pharmacology and users conditioning histories can help to explain cravings even after long periods of abstinence. In a study of smoking behaviour of 140 subjects, Glad and Adesso (1976) observed that the company of smokers significantly increases the incidence of smoking, though the effect is greater amongst subjects smoking fewer than ten cigarettes per day than among those smoking more than fifteen cigarettes. Light and heavy smokers of cigarette respond differently to the prominence with which cigarettes are displayed. Herman (1974), in an experiment involving two conditions, in which a cigarette pack was placed either directly under the main source of illumination in a room or in shadow and observed smokers' behaviour. He found that light smokers lit up in an average of five minutes when their attention was directed to the cigarettes by the 'obvious' external cue, but took fifteen minutes in not so obvious cue. On the other hand, heavy smokers, motivated more by the internal cues (such as need for nicotine) lit up cigarettes in six minutes in both conditions.

Most of former smokers who have quit smoking did so without formal treatment programme or smoking cessation devices (Fiore *et al.*, 2000). Not only the smokers but also other drug takers often discontinue the use of dependence producing drug outside the context of formal intervention. There are certain common factors operating to influence smokers to quit the drug such as response to social pressure, observed and anticipated health consequences, one's own determination to quit etc. However, the number of such quitters is very small in comparison to the number of new individuals who have been recruited to smoking.

## Barriers to Tobacco Cessation

Despite the well-known health hazards of smoking and the documented difficulties in quitting, few intensive treatment options are available. Tobacco dependence or addiction can be as intractable as any addictive disorder and there are considerable similarities in relapse processes between tobacco and other drugs of dependence. Cigarette smoking like any other form of drug dependence, involves both pharmacological and behavioural factors and therefore treatment approaches may also involve pharmacological agents, behavioural strategies, or a combination of both. Similarly, there are certain barriers which operate to affect the efficacy of these therapeutic modalities. These barriers are:

### 1. Addiction

The main barrier for tobacco use cessation is the physical addiction to nicotine (Kenkel and Chen, 2000). Information provided by the treating physician about the risk is often incomplete and poorly conveyed. Individual smokers often do not believe that they are at as much risk of becoming addicted as other smokers (Weinstein, 1998). Social and psychological associations attached to cigarette use are achieved with classical and secondary conditioning. It may be the intake of just four cigarettes that a person is exposed to the risk of becoming an addict (Russell, 1990). The first symptoms of nicotine addiction can appear within days to weeks of the onset of occasional use, often before the onset of daily smoking (DiFranza *et al.*, 2000). Addiction then becomes the main barrier for cigarette cessation. Withdrawal symptoms in adults and children include increased irritability, restlessness, depression, difficulty with concentration, hunger and craving (Shiffman, 1979). Physiological changes occur in brain, along with a drop in the heart rate and adrenal output, and a rise in skin temperature (Gilbert and Pope, 1982 and Mansvelder, 2000). Women are less confident about their ability to quit smoking as compared to men (Audrain *et al.*, 1997).

### 2. Fear of Weight Gain

Many girls and women dread being overweight or obese (Brownell, 1991). Sometimes girls and women tend to smoke as a method of weight control (Halek *et al.*, 1993). The relationship between body weight and cigarette smoking shows the adult cigarette smokers weigh lesser than their non-smoking counterparts but have a greater proportion of abdominal fat (Shimokata *et al.*, 1992). Evidence shows that cigarette smoking increases metabolic rate, which may fall with smoking cessation (Moffatt and Owens, 1991). Nicotine has been shown to increase the energy expenditure associated with light activity (Perkins *et al.*, 1989). Cigarette smoking may independently reduce serum leptin concentrations, rather than smokers having lower leptin levels just because they are leaner. Nicotine, through its various effects on the central nervous system (Williams *et al.*, 1994), may modify leptin sensitivity, resulting indirectly into reduced leptin levels and maintenance of a lower body weight. Many women start and continue to smoke to control appetite and reduce bodyweight (Pirie *et al.*, 1992) that may be an attempt to restrain post-puberty fatness (Crisp, 1985).

Women expect to gain weight when they quit smoking (Pirie, 1991) and it is observed that women gain more weight than men after cigarette smoking cessation in the proportion of 3.8 kg in women and 2.8 kg in men (Williamson *et al.*, 1992). Higher dose smokers tend to gain more weight during attempts to quit (Killen *et al.*, 1990). During the first month of cigarette smoking cessation, the average caloric intake increases by 300–400 calories per day (Perkins, 1992). Fear of weight gain leads to relapse after cessation. Weight control smoking occurs in 12 to 25 percent of males but up to 40 percent in females (Weekley *et al.*, 1993). Young women are three to four times as likely as men to report weight gain as a cause of smoking relapse (Gilbert and Pope, 1982).

### 3. Depression

Depression is twice as common among women as men (21.3 percent versus 12.7 percent) and can present as a barrier for smoking cessation in women (Blazer *et al.*, 1994). Childbirth (Pritchard, 1994) and menstrual cycle (Craig *et al.*, 1992) are associated with depression and may even serve as trigger for an episode of major depression (Borrelli *et al.*, 1996). Depression is also found to be four times more common among smokers than nonsmokers (60 percent versus 15 percent) (Glassman *et al.*, 1988). Hormones related to the reproductive cycle also influence depression and smoking behaviour. Women have reportedly used cigarette smoking not only for their mood management but also for coping with stressful situations (Ward *et al.*, 1997). Because nicotine in cigarettes can increase the feeling of well being and elevate mood, some smokers may self-medicate depressed moods with nicotine (Carmody, 1989). Nicotine in cigarette is a powerful pharmacologic agent with a wide variety of stimulant and depressant effects involving peripheral and central nervous system. A review of neurobiology of tobacco smoking provides examples of the mechanism for reinforcing tobacco use, including the enhancement of memory and treatment for depression with nicotine and MAO inhibiting chemicals in tobacco smoke (Gamberino and Gold, 1999). A history of depression and current symptoms of depression are independently associated with failure to quit smoking (Glassman *et al.*, 1990). Smoking cessation itself may provoke depression among smokers who may or may not have histories of major depression. When depressive symptoms emerge during withdrawal chances for both cessation failure and relapse are higher. Resumption of smoking can reverse depression symptoms (Glassman, 1993).

### 4. Stressors and Other Factors

Stress-inducing situations include family environment, social relations with classmates, schoolwork, peer pressure etc. may help to initiate, to continue and to restart smoking. Higher rates of smoking and relapse are found in the disadvantaged groups and minority communities of a society. In India, the erstwhile untouchables of the British India who were a socially deprived class, consumed excessive amounts of narcotics, alcohol and tobacco in order to relieve their stress in comparison to others (Briggs, 1920). Their smoking was intimately related to their life situations of poverty, isolation and care giving and tobacco smoking proved to be a mechanism for coping with the stress of their lives (Stewart *et al.*, 1996). Any attempt at quitting to smoke among these people was hindered by the factors mentioned below.

#### *Tobacco Related Factors*

- Withdrawal symptoms lead to feeling of discomfort or distress, reduce capacity to work or handle stressful situations, and heighten the urge to resume smoking.
- Tobacco use produces effects, which are perceived to be desirable by the user, thereby providing a strong incentive for continuation of cigarette smoking. Nicotine can enhance performance of smokers on certain attention and memory tasks. Nicotine also exerts an important role in the relationship between smoking and body weight, as already mentioned.
- For cigarette smokers, handling of cigarette, and the hand-oral manipulation may be important (Ikard *et al.*, 1969).

Absorption of nicotine from tobacco smoke provides a means of verification and quantization of tobacco consumption. Concentrations of nicotine and its metabolites (such as cotinine) and other chemicals associated with tobacco smoke present in biological fluids such as blood, saliva and urine are measured. These parameters provide information about the amount and the time of tobacco intake and thus help in therapeutic intervention. However, different measures vary in severity, specificity and difficulty of analysis.

## Biological Markers of Tobacco Intake

Absorption of nicotine from tobacco smoke provides a means of verification and quantization of tobacco consumption. Concentrations of nicotine and its metabolites (such as cotinine) and other chemicals associated with tobacco smoke present in biological fluids such as blood, saliva and urine are measured. These parameters provide information about the amount and the time of tobacco intake and thus help in therapeutic intervention. However, different measures vary in severity, specificity and difficulty of analysis.

### Treatment

Here are many similarities as well as many differences between nicotine and other drugs of dependence. For example, although nicotine dependence produces dramatic health problems, it does not produce significant interpersonal or financial problems. Before starting any treatment programme, a detailed assessment of history of smoking, level of addiction, current smoking status and motivation to leave smoking, physical and mental health status and co-morbidity need to be carried out. Environmental factors, possibly working as reinforcers need to be evaluated in details. Patient should be informed about the benefits of tobacco-cessation and the cessation process along with the possible withdrawal symptoms, which he/she may have to experience. Long-term abstinence is the ultimate goal of the treatment of nicotine dependence.

## Assessing Dependence

For assessment of the severity of nicotine dependence certain tests and questionnaires are used to provide individualized treatment plans.

### *i. CAGE Questionnaire*

The CAGE questionnaire is a simple and accurate tool for screening patients with addictive disorders (Crowe *et al.*, 1997 and Morton and Jones, 1996). Its revised version is used for smokers (Lairson *et al.*, 1992) and can be included in clinical interview. The questionnaire has four components: (a) Cut down (b) Annoyed (c) Guilt and (d) Eye opener. These components are framed in a questionnaire. Two or more "yes" responses qualify a person to be dependent on tobacco and need to be included for treatment.

*Table 1: CAGE questionnaire*

| | |
|---|---|
| a. | Have you ever felt a need to cut down or control your smoking, but have difficulty doing so? |
| b. | Do you ever get annoyed or angry with people who criticize your smoking or tell you that you ought to quit? |
| c. | Have you ever felt *guilty* about your smoking or about you did while smoking? |
| d. | Do you ever smoke within half an hour of waking up (eye opener)? |

**Modified smoking behaviour. Lairson DR; Harrist R; Martin DW; Ramby R; Rustin TA; Swint JM (1992) Screening for patients with alcohol problems: severity of patents identified by the CAGE. Journal of Drug Education; 22:337-352.*

### *ii. Four Cs Test*

Experts engaged in addiction treatment rely on either DSM-IV or ICD-10 criteria to diagnose substance dependence. These criteria are applicable to all addictive disorders and can be grouped into four categories that conveniently begin with the letter "C"

**a. Compulsion** is the intensity with which the desire to use a chemical overwhelms the patient's thoughts, feelings and judgment.

**b. Control** is the degree to which patients can (or can not) control their chemical use once they have started using.

**c. Cutting down** is the effects of reducing chemical intake; withdrawal.

**d. Consequences** is denial or acceptance of the damage caused by the chemical. The four "Cs" test can be used to assess a patient's dependence on nicotine (Table 2)

### *iii. Fagerstrom Test*

Patients who quit smoking and relapse within two or three weeks usually do so to relieve withdrawal symptoms due to their physical dependence on nicotine. The Fagerstrom test for Nicotine Dependence is a standard instrument for assessing the intensity of this physical addiction (Heatherton *et al.,* 1991). The higher the Fagerstrom score, the more intense is the patient's physical dependence. Higher scores indicate that treatment of withdrawal symptoms, usually with nicotine replacement therapy, will be an important factor in the patient's plan of care.

*Table 2: Assessing nicotine addiction using the "4 Cs" test*

| | |
|---|---|
| *a.* | *Compulsion* Do you ever smoke more than you intend? Have you ever neglected a responsibility because you were smoking, or so you could smoke? |
| *b.* | *Control* Have you felt the need to control how much you smoke but were unable to do so easily? Have you ever promised that you would quit smoking and brought a pack of cigarettes that same day? |
| *c.* | *Cutting down* (and withdrawal symptoms) Have you ever tried to stop smoking? How many times? For how long? Have you ever had any of the following symptoms when you were for a while without a |

*Contd...*

cigarette: agitation, difficulty concentrating, irritability, mood swings? If so, did the symptoms go away after you smoked a cigarette?

*d.* *Consequences* How long have you known that smoking was hurting your body? If you continue to smoke, how long do you expect to live? If you were able to quit smoking today and never start again, how long do you think you might live?

***Source:*** *Assessing Nicotine Dependence. American Academy of Family Physicians; 62(3) 2000*

***Table 3: Modified Fagerstrom test for nicotine dependence***

1. How soon after you wake up do you smoke your first cigarette?
   (i) Within 5 minutes (3 points)
   (ii) 5 to 30 minutes (2 points)
   (iii) 31 to 60 minutes (1 point)

*After 60 minutes (0 point)*

2. Do you find it difficult not to smoke in the places where you should not, such as in church, or school, in a movie, at the library, on a bus, in court or in a hospital?
   (i) Yes (1 point)
   (ii) No (0 point).
3. Which cigarette would you most hate to give up; which cigarette do you treasure the most?
   (i) The first cigarette in the morning (1 point)
   (ii) Any other one (0 point)
4. How many cigarettes do you smoke each day?
   (i) 10 or fewer (0 point)
   (ii) 11 to 20 (1 point)
   (iii) 21 to 30 (2 points)
   (iv) 31 or more (3 points)
5. Do you smoke more during the first few hours after waking up than during the rest of the day?
   (i) Yes (1 point)
   (ii) No (0 point)
6. Do you still smoke if you are so sick that you are in bed most of the day, or if you have a cold or the flu and have trouble breathing?
   (i) Yes (1 point)
   (ii) No (0 point)

***Scoring:*** *7 to 10 points = high dependence; 4 to 6 points = moderate dependence; less than 4 points = minimal Dependence.*

*. *Adapted with permission from Heatherton TF; Kozlowski LT; Frecker RC, Fagerstrom KO (1991) The Fagerstrom Test for Nicotine Dependence: a revision of Fagerstrom Tolerance Questionnaire; British Journal of Addiction; 86:1119-1127.*

## Assessing Reinforcement

Patients who quit smoking but relapse more than six weeks later are not smoking to relieve withdrawal symptoms; their relapses are caused by a desire to smoke (craving) induced by internal or external events (cues). Assessing how each patient's smoking serves as a reinforcer can help the therapist identify potential relapse triggers for that person. Why are cigarettes so reinforcing to a smoker? Following questions help to identify the reinforcing aspects of smoking behaviour:

### *i. Sensory Reward*

Many smokers enjoy the feeling of a cigarette between their fingers; many enjoy puffing of smoke and warmth of cigarette, what about you?

### *ii. Rituals*

Some smokers like the way they handle the cigarette pack, the way they light the cigarette... what about you?

### *iii. Images*

What sort of people are they who smoke your brand? Smoker identifies himself/herself with the ad model or the persons smoking his/her brand.

### *iv. Emotional Relief*

Many smokers believe that cigarettes help them dealing with stressful feelings such as anger, frustration and boredom; do you also get relief from such feelings?

A smoker's profile can be assessed with the help of available questionnaires (Table 4). These questions are generally asked in the clinical interview to understand the nature of reinforcing situations in the patient. These factors need to be considered while outlining the treatment plan.

## Assessing Readiness to Change

Patient's needs to quit smoking are assessed by administering any of the above mentioned tools. However, these tools do not assess the patient's readiness to make a serious attempt to quit smoking. It is necessary to know patient's cognitive set to success in quitting smoking. Advice and treatment must match the patient's cognitive stage to be effective.

The Trans-theoretical Model of Change (Rustin and Tata, 1993) is a model based on discrete stages along the continuum of change in cigarette smoking behaviour. These stages are (Table 5):

| | |
|---|---|
| i | Pre-contemplation: response is non-ambiguous, with no intention to change |
| ii | Contemplation: indecisive response, not sure of change |
| iii | Preparation when resolved to decide for change |
| iv | Action when actually change occurs, patient leaves smoking. |
| v | Maintenance when person continues with the change stays abstinent |
| vi | Relapse: lack of adequate support brings person back to the previous stage. |

**The two major treatment approaches employed in the treatment of nicotine dependence are, pharmacological and behavioural.**

Possible cessation techniques should be discussed in detail with the patient including physician counseling, pharmacological management, behavioural training, group therapy, hypnosis and quitting. The treating physician needs to select one strategy that best fits patient's requirement.

*Table: 4: Smoker's profile*

| |
|---|
| *Stress relief* |
| (i) When you are frustrated or angry, do you automatically think of smoking a cigarette? |
| (ii) If you are upset or scared, does a cigarette help you calm down? |
| (iii) Do you rely on cigarettes when you are under stress? |
| (iv) Recall a time when you stopped smoking for a while. After you stopped smoking, did you want a cigarette more whenever you got upset or angry? |
| (v) Did you miss cigarettes more when you were under lot of stress or tension? |
| *Conditioned responses* |
| (i) How often do you smoke while driving a car or drinking a cup of coffee? |
| (ii) If you are with someone who is smoking, do you automatically smoke, too? |
| (iii) Do you usually smoke a cigarette during or after a meal? |
| (iv) Recall a time when you stopped smoking for a while. Did being around smokers make it hard to not smoke? Were there certain people, places or things that made you want to smoke? |
| *Relief of withdrawal symptoms* |
| (i) When do you smoke your first cigarette of the day? |
| (ii) Do you get irritable if you have to go more than 2 hours without a cigarette? |
| (iii) Do you have trouble concentrating if you are not smoking? |
| (iv) Recall a time when you stopped smoking for a while. Did you get irritable or moody during the first few days after you stopped? |
| (v) Did you have trouble concentrating during the first few days after you stopped smoking? |
| *Elevation of depressed mood* |
| (i) Recall the time when you stopped smoking for a while. Did you become more depressed? |
| (ii) When you woke up in the morning, did you feel that you could spend all day in bed? |
| (iii) How was your energy level after you stopped smoking? |

***Source:*** *Assessing Nicotine Dependence. American Academy of Family Physicians 62(3), 2000.*

## Pharmacological Approches

According to Public Health Service (PHS) Guideline all smokers trying to quit should receive pharmacotherapy except in the presence of contraindication. Five first-line pharmacotherapies for smoking cessation have been identified by the PHS guidelines. These are sustained release (SR) bupropion, nicotine gum, nicotine patch, nicotine inhaler and nicotine nasal spray. Other medications used are clonidine, nortriptyline and others as second line treatment (Table 6).

Pharmacotherapy for tobacco-cessation can be broadly classified into:

1. Nicotine Replacement Therapy
2. Other Pharmacological Therapies

**Table 5: Counseling based on stages of change**

| *Stages of change* | *Patient's response to feelings of quitting smoking* | *Goal of intervention* | *Typical physician thoughts and intervention* |
|---|---|---|---|
| Pre-contemplation | "I like to smoke." | Introduce ambivalence | "Your emphysema will improve after you have quit smoking" |
| Contemplation | "I like to smoke but better | Resolve ambivalence I know I need to quit." | "How will your life be after you have quit smoking?" |
| Preparation | "I am ready to quit." | Identify successful strategies | "Choose a 'quit day' and let us make plans for it." |
| Action | "I am not smoking, but I still think about smoking from time to time." | Provide solutions to specific relapse triggers | "How can you deal with your desire to smoke in those situations?" |
| Maintenance | "I used to smoke." | Solidify patient's commitment to a smoke-free life | "This would be a good time to share your experiences with other people." |

**Source:** *Assessing Nicotine Dependence. American Academy of Family Physicians. 62(3) 2000.*

**Table 6: Medications for smoking cessation**

| *Medication* | *Dosage* | *Administration* |
|---|---|---|
| First-line Treatment | | |
| 1. Bupropion Hydrochloride SR (Zuban) | 150 mg | 150 mg per day for 3 days, then 150 mg twice a day for 7–12 weeks (smoking quit date 1–2 weeks after beginning medication) |
| 2. Nicotine polacrilex gum (Nicorette) | 2 mg/piece if, 25 cigarettes /day 4 mg/day if> 25 cigarettes/day | 1 piece every 1–2 hrs for 6 weeks, then 1 piece every 2– 4 hours for 2 weeks, then 1 piece every 4–8 hrs for 2 weeks, maximum 24 pieces per day. |

*Contd...*

| | | |
|---|---|---|
| 3. Trans-dermal nicotine (Nicodern CQ) | 21 mg /24 hrs, 14 mg/24 hrs and 7 mg/24 hrs | If >10 cigarettes per day, 21 mg for 6 weeks, then 14 mg for 2 weeks, then 7 mg for 2 weeks. If < 10 cigarettes per day, 14 mg for 6 weeks, then 7 mg for 2 weeks. |
| 4. Nicotine Lozenge | 2 mg/piece if 25 cigarettes per day, 4 mg if>25 cigarettes per day | 1 piece every 1–2 hour for 6 weeks, then 1 piece every 4 hours for 2 weeks and the 1 piece every 4–8 hours for 2 weeks, maximum 24 pieces per day. |
| 5. Nicotine nasal spray (Nicotrol NS) | 1-mg dose=1-spray each nostril | 1–2 doses per hour with maximum of 40 doses per day and maximum 3 months' use. |
| Nicotine Inhaler | 6 to 16 cartridges | 4 mg metered spray |
| Second-line treatment | | |
| 1. Clonidine | 0.15 to 075 mg/day | 0.1, 0.2 and 0.3 mg tablets |
| 2. Nortriptyline | 75 to 100 mg /day | 10, 25, 50 and 75 mg tablets |

***Source:*** *Sofuoglu M and Costen TR (2004) Pharmacological Management of Relapse Prevention in Addictive Disorders. Psychiatric Clinics of North America; 27: 627-648.*

## Nicotine Replacement Therapy

The general principle of replacement therapies is to present the patient with a safer and more therapeutically manageable form of the drug that directly alleviates the signs and symptoms of withdrawal and craving (Jaffe, 1985). Nicotine replacement therapy is modeled after those originally developed to treat dependence on heroin and other opiates (Henningfield and Jasinski, 1988). A variety of non-tobacco-based delivery systems provide potentially effective means for nicotine replacement.

Although guidelines for selecting different NRT have not been established, clinicians should individualize the treatment based on patient characteristics and adverse effect profile of each product. NRT attenuates the tobacco withdrawal symptoms and approximately doubles the success rate of quitting smoking relative to smoking. Nicotine polacrilex chewing gum (2 mg pieces) is the only one form of nicotine replacement strategy approved by the Food and Drug Administration (FDA) of United States. However, there are three other nicotine delivery systems available, and these are (1) Transdermal patches for delivery of nicotine through the skin. (2) Nasal nicotine solution and (3) Nicotine vapour inhalers (smokeless tobacco). Nicotine lozenge and sub-lingual tablets are also available as a form of nicotine replacement therapy. These devices increase quitting rates by approximately 1.5 to 2 times, regardless of setting. Recently, there has been considerable interest in nicotine replacement therapy (NRT) for smoking cessation, because:

- Nicotine is the critical dependence-producing component in tobacco.
- Treatment outcome data on the efficacy of first nicotine replacement therapy are encouraging.
- Other forms of nicotine substitution may hold further potential for more effective treatment.

Nicotine-specific withdrawal symptoms, which interfere with successful cessation, are prevented or attenuated by nicotine replacement. This therapy promotes cessation as well as prevents relapse (Grabowski and Hall, 1985). Various forms of nicotine replacement therapy are as follows:

(i) Nicotine injection (not in use in clinical practice)
(ii) Nicotine Polacrilex gum
(iii) Nicotine lozenge
(iv) Nicotine trans-dermal patch
(v) Nasal nicotine solution
(vi) Nicotine aerosols and Nicotine sublingual tablets.

*(i) Nicotine injection*

Johnston Lennox (1942), a Wallace general practitioner, reported for the first time the systematic use of nicotine replacement to help people quit smoking by intravenous administration of nicotine. He injected himself and other subjects with 1/7500 and 1/500 of a grain of nicotine, which he claimed was the amount that produced sensations equivalent to those following one deep inhalation from a cigarette. Non-smokers found the sensations queer, but the smokers found them pleasant and, after repeated injections, did not feel inclined to smoke for a while afterwards. This showed that the injected nicotine could substitute for sensations that were normally derived from smoking. However, both Johnston and his patients knew what was being injected and the result of the experiment was therefore, not free from the possible influence of conscious and unconscious expectations. In another experiment smokers receiving a slow intravenous infusion of either nicotine solution or saline water solution, were subjected to perform a variety of psychological tests such as reaction time, and time estimation. At the same time their blood pressure and the electrocardiogram were also measured. Smokers were allowed to smoke as and when they wished without being aware that their smoking behaviour was being studied. The injection of 6 mg of nicotine over six hours produced no significant effect, but the injection of 22 mg of nicotine (equivalent to the nicotine delivery of 22 medium-strength cigarettes) was accompanied by a 30% drop in the number of cigarettes smoked. There was also a significant increase in the amount of tobacco left un-smoked, showing that the cigarettes which were consumed were being consumed less fully. However, this approach is not clinically viable since the nicotine half-life is short and repeated administration of tobacco can lead to toxicity.

*(ii) Nicotine polacrilex Gum*

The next systematic approach was the development of nicotine polacrilex gum by Ferno, Lichtneckert, and Lundgren (1973). The weaning from nicotine actually begins with the switch from cigarette to gum in that nicotine polacrilex (a) produces slower-rising plasma nicotine levels than cigarette and (b) reduces the inhaled nicotine bolus effect believed to contribute to nicotine's addictive potential in smoke (Russell and Feyerabend, 1978). The same mechanism applies to other replacement approaches (Russell, 1986) including nicotine trans-dermal delivery, nasal nicotine solution, and smoke-free nicotine cigarettes. The different forms allow variation in delivery (dose and speed), which may influence effectiveness, relief of withdrawal, patient acceptance, and outcome.

"Nicotine resin complex" also commonly referred to as nicotine gum, is a nicotine delivery system in which the nicotine is incorporated into an ion exchange resin base, which permits release of nicotine in the proper environment (i.e. saliva in the mouth) when appropriate physical pressure (i.e. chewing) is applied. Twenty to thirty minutes of proper chewing results in the release of approximately 90 percent of nicotine (Ferno and Lichtneckert, Lundgren, 1973), although there are multiple determinants of how much nicotine actually is absorbed. 10 to 15 minutes of chewing results in the release of approximately 50 to 60 percent of nicotine in a piece of gum. Variability exists both within and across subjects. Swallowed nicotine is approximately 70 percent detoxified because of its first pass through the liver (Benowitz *et al.*, 1987).

Nicotine gum does not fully replace the nicotine provided by cigarette smoking. Russell *et al* (1983) reported that 4-mg nicotine gum produced plasma nicotine level approximating that of a 1.2 mg-nicotine-yield cigarette. Benowitz *et al* (1987) found only 50 percent replacement of nicotine with 4-mg gum. They reported that chewing of 10 pieces of 2-mg gum on an hourly schedule resulted in blood levels of nicotine that were one-third of those achieved while smoking. Therefore, ad libitum chewing of the 2-mg nicotine polacrilex gum probably results in even lower nicotine levels. When nicotine polacrilex gum is chewed, drug levels of plasma rise slowly and peak in around 20-30 minutes, while 4-mg gum replaces nicotine more completely. However, effective nicotine replacement strategies may not require the same range of nicotine *blood* levels as those produced by cigarette smoking. Perhaps because of this, only the 2-mg dose has been approved for use in United States. The 2-mg nicotine polacrilex gum increased nicotine cessation rates significantly in several placebo-controlled studies (Table 7). Nicotine gum is quickly absorbed and closely approximates the course of plasma nicotine levels observed after cigarette smoking.

**Withdrawal Symptom Relief**

Many short-term trials (8 hours to 5 days) have found that nicotine polacrilex gum reduces symptoms of withdrawal in comparison to placebo controls (Schneider *et al.*, 1984; West *et al.*, 1984). Jarvis (1982) reported relief of several symptoms for a six-week period. Expectancy may also play a role in withdrawal symptom relief. Irritability was consistently relieved in all studies, while other symptoms such as hunger, depression, anxiety, difficulty in concentration, restlessness, annoyance, hostility and somatic complaints were reduced in some, but not others. The degree to which most symptoms are relieved is directly related to the dose of nicotine that is actually obtained when the polacrilex gum is used (Henningfield and Jasinski, 1988). The urge to smoke (craving) is not reliably decreased by nicotine replacement (West and Schneider, 1987).

Ad libitum administration of the 2-mg gum replacement used in above mentioned studies might be insufficient to reverse some of the symptoms of nicotine withdrawal; 4-mg dose of gum is found to show more complete reversal of withdrawal (Henningfield *et al.*, 1986). Different withdrawal symptoms require different levels of nicotine replacement and there can be inter-subject as well as intra-subject variability in chewing, which can affect the amount of nicotine reaching the circulation (Benowitz *et al.*, 1983).

There is some evidence that weight gain, a significant problem in cessation, can be reduced by nicotine replacement (Fagerstrom, 1987). A 2-mg nicotine gum dose has been found to produce significantly less weight gain over a 10-week period compared with a placebo (Stitzer and Gross, 1988).

***Table 7: Efficacy trials for nicotine polacrilex gum follow-up abstinence rates (percentages) (placebo controlled studies)***

| *Study* | *Number* | *Active Gum* | *Placebo* | *Follow-up* | *P* |
|---|---|---|---|---|---|
| Puska *et al.*, 1987 | 160 | 35 | 28 | 6 months | **N.S.** |
| Malcom *et al.*, 1980 | 210 | 23 | 5 | 6 months | **P<0.05** |
| Fee and Stewart, 1982 | 352 | 13 | 9 | 1year | **N.S.** |
| Jarvis *et al.*, 1982 | 116 | 47 | 21 | 1 year | **P<0.01** |
| British Thoracic Society, 1983 | 802 | 10 | 14 | 1 year | **N.S.** |
| Schneider *et al.*, 1983 | 60 | 30 | 20 | 1 year | **N.S.** |
| Hjalmarson 1984 | 205 | 29 | 16 | 1 year | **P<0.05** |
| Jamrozic *et al.*, 1984 | 200 | 10 | 8 | 6 months | **N.S.** |
| Campbell *et al.*, 1987 | 985 | 3 | 2 | 1 year | **N.S.** |
| Hall *et al.*, 1987 | 139 | 44 | 21 | 1 year | **P<0.01** |

***Source :** Modeled after Fagerstrom (1988).*

### *Craving-urge-desire*

Definitions of craving have proven elusive and it is often described as an increase in the urge or desire to use a drug. It is the strength of an urge to use a drug. In the tobacco abstinence studies, craving generally was not relieved by nicotine replacement. However, to some extent, relief of craving has been reported with 2-mg nicotine polacrilex gum compared with placebo controls in an outcome trial (Hjalmarson, 1984). Craving should not be viewed simply as a symptom of a negative withdrawal state. Smokers clearly seek desired effects of nicotine in addition to relief from withdrawal. Nicotine polacrilex gum may reduce negative withdrawal symptoms without providing other effects.

### *Efficacy trials*

Earlier studies only assessed the capacity of nicotine in polacrilex gum to replace nicotine in cigarette, hence testing the "nicotine regulation hypothesis." Now, the studies have demonstrated that cigarette smoking can be decreased in laboratory subjects by replacement of the nicotine, which is normally obtained by smoking with nicotine delivered by gum (Nemeth-Coslett and Henningfield, 1986). In placebo-controlled clinical trials nicotine polacrilex gum significantly increased success rates for as long as 6 months in some studies (Schneider *et al.*, 1983). Other treatment procedures (such as group therapy) were applied in addition to nicotine gum or placebo. Nicotine polacrilex gum plus an intensive beaviour contact treatment (14 sessions over an 8 weeks period) was compared with nicotine polacrilex gum plus low-contact behaviour treatment (4 sessions over three weeks' period) and intensive behaviour treatment alone. The combination of intensive behaviour treatment and nicotine polacrilex gum was significantly superior to the other interventions through 6 months of follow-up. However, physicians' trials have resulted in lower overall success rates for all groups and some equivocal findings. This low success rate could be because of selection bias.

Differences in outcome comparing the clinic setting versus physician offices have been interpreted as indicating the requirement for support treatment with nicotine polacrilex gum. For a good outcome, follow-up is important. Another variable affecting the outcome is the duration of nicotine polacrilex gum use. Six months to one year use gives good results, however, use remains an unresolved issue.

### *Dose and patient relationship*

In various studies, 2- and 4- mg nicotine polacrilex gum has been used (Kortnitzer *et al.*, 1987). 4-mg nicotine polacrilex gum improved success rate for more highly dependent tobacco smokers, whereas 2-mg nicotine polacrilex gum was superior in less dependent smokers. The smokers who have a greater degree of dependence on nicotine may require treatment with higher doses than those required by less dependent smokers. Hall *et al* (1985) reported a positive correlation between smokers with high re-quit cotinine levels and abstinence with nicotine polacrilex gums. Jarvik and Schneider (1984) reported that the individuals scoring high on the Fagerstrom Tolerance Scale had greater success with replacement therapy. Physical health of the patient also plays an important role in the outcome of the treatment. Physically healthy nicotine dependents had better outcome at one year (45%) as compared to those who were suffering from chronic bronchitis (16.2%) (Tonnesen, 1985).

Generally 2 mg gum pieces are used for consumers who use less than 25 cigarettes per day and 4 mg gum pieces for those who smoke more than 25 cigarettes per day. The usual dose is one gum piece every 1–2 hour for the first 6 weeks and then one piece every 2–4 hours for 2 weeks (seventh to ninth week) and then one piece every 4–8 hours for another 2 weeks (Table 6). Nicotine polacrilex gum is available over the counter. Nicotine from the gum is absorbed through the buccal mucosa, with peak nicotine plasma concentration reached within 15 to 30 minutes, as compared with 1 to 2 minutes after smoking a cigarette (Benowitz 1996). Acidic beverages like coffee and juices should be avoided before and after the use of nicotine gum, because they decrease the absorption of nicotine. Nicotine gum also provides substitute oral activity during tobacco abstinence.

### *(iii) Nicotine Lozenge*

Similar to nicotine gum, the nicotine polacrilex lozenge is available over-the- counter as an aid for smoking cessation in 2 mg and 4 mg doses of nicotine. The 4 mg dose is preferred for highly dependent smokers – those who smoke within 30 minutes of awakening (Shiffman *et al.,* 2002). The nicotine lozenge delivers 25% more nicotine than nicotine gum, because some nicotine is retained in the gum, and nicotine is dissolved completely in lozenge (Choi *et al.,* 2003). The lozenge may have better patient acceptability, especially those who cannot use the gum because of dentures, temporomandibular joint pain or for those who do not prefer chewing gum.

### *(iv) Nicotine Trans-dermal Patch*

In a short term (hours) laboratory trials, a decrease in craving and nicotine preference in subjects using nicotine patch versus a placebo patch has been reported. A trans-dermal delivery system can eliminate some of the compliance and chewing problems associated with nicotine polacrilex gum. Steady-state administration expected from such a system may be more effective in preventing withdrawal symptoms. Since the patch does not allow for self-administration in response to the smoking urge, it could potentially be used in combination with the other rapidly absorbed forms of nicotine replacement. Nicotine trans-dermal system acts better when used in conjunction with a support programme such as counseling, group therapy or behaviour therapy.

The four trans-dermal formulations take advantage of ready absorption of nicotine across the skin (Silagy *et al.,* 1994). Three of these patches are for 24-hours use and one is for 16-hours (waking) use. For the 24-hours delivery system the recommended dose of trans-dermal patch for those who smoke more than 10 cigarettes per day, 21 mg patch is used every day for the first 6 weeks, then 14 mg every day for the next 2 weeks and then 7 mg patch every day for another 2 weeks. If the cigarette consumption is lesser than 10 cigarettes a day, 14 mg patch per day for first 6 weeks and then 7 mg patch per day for another two weeks is used (Table 6). For the 16-hour delivery system, where the patch is taken off before going to sleep, the recommended dose is 15 mg per day for 6 weeks. A meta-analysis shows no benefit of using nicotine patch longer than 8 weeks (Fiore *et al.,* 1994) With the nicotine patch, nicotine is absorbed slowly, with peak levels reaching 4 to 8 hours after application, and nicotine levels are about half those obtained through smoking. The nicotine patch is easy to administer, requires less frequent dosing, with fewer adverse effects and better compliance. The disadvantage of patch is the lack of acute (rescue) dosing for craving episodes, which can be provided with other NRTs (Hurt *et al.,* 1998). In fact, the nicotine patch may be combined with other NRTs to increase its efficacy in treatment resistant cases (Sweeney *et al.,* 2001).

The use of nicotine chewing gum or trans-dermal nicotine patches during smoking cessation delayed weight gain until nicotine replacement therapy was stopped (Hajek, Jackson, and Belcher, 1988). However, neither nicotine gum nor the patch combined with smoking cessation provides any long-term benefit of attenuating weight gain (Perkin *et al.,* 1997).

### *(v) Nasal Nicotine Solution (NNS)*

Nicotine replacement in the form of NNS, wherein a gel-like droplet of nicotine is squeezed into the nose from a small vial, has been investigated by Russell, Jarvis and colleagues (1983) and they found rapid and efficient absorption of nicotine than is possible with the nicotine polacrilex gum. In the United States nicotine nasal spray is available on prescription. It achieves peak venous nicotine levels within 4 to 15 minutes, faster than any other NRT. Because of the fast nicotine delivery, nicotine spray may have some abuse liability (patients continue to use spray even after quitting smoking) (West *et al.,* 2000).

One dose of nicotine nasal spray is equal to two sprays (0.5 mg per spray). The usual recommended dose is one to two doses per hour for 8 weeks, with a minimum of 8 doses per day and maximum of 40 doses per day and maximum 3 months use (Table 6). Between weeks 9 and 14, a gradual taper is recommended. The main disadvantage of nasal spray is the initial local irritation and for some patients stigma of its use.

### *(vi) Nicotine Aerosols (inhaler)*

The nicotine inhaler is available by prescription only in the United States. With nicotine inhaler, the nicotine is absorbed through the buccal mucosa in contrast to the absorption through the lungs with cigarette smoking. On inhalation with inhaler, peak plasma nicotine concentrations are typically achieved within 15 minutes (Schneider *et al.,* 2001). The recommended dose of nicotine inhaler is 6 to 16 cartridges per day for 12 weeks, with a gradual weaning over 6 to 12 weeks. Each cartridge contains 10 mg of nicotine and delivers a maximum of 4 mg of nicotine. One cartridge provides 20 minutes of active puffing.

## Comparison of Preparations

All nicotine replacement products produce side effects. Nicotine polacrilex gum may produce mouth sores, gastric upset, and hiccups. NNS produces runny nose and irritation, whereas trans-dermal devices can result in skin irritation. Trans-dermal devices have the advantage of better patient compliance with treatment and steady-state drug levels, whereas NNS and nicotine polacrilex gum have the advantage of ad libitum access to replacement. Because trigger to smoke can appear at any time, the flexibility offered by the latter may be essential. A combination of preparations may be most useful to control symptoms as well as to allow instant responses to smoking urges.

**Dependence on Nicotine Replacement**

Withdrawal symptoms upon abrupt cessation of nicotine polacrilex gum have been reported which indicate that nicotine polacrilex gum produces physical dependence. Some workers point out that it could be the part of continued dependence on nicotine that originated with smoking and is bound to transfer during weaning.

Since nicotine can increase a baby's heart rate, a pregnant woman or a nursing mother should seek the advice of a health professional before using a nicotine replacement therapy. Moreover, these products should not be used by anyone below 18 years of age or who continues to use any other product that contains nicotine. Side effects and complications associated with these products are similar to those found when smoking cigarettes and include irregular or rapid heart beat, palpitation, nausea, vomiting, dizziness and weakness. Persons with heart disease, recent myocardial infarction and hypertension, and gastric ulcer, insulin treatment for diabetes mellitus and prescription drugs for depression or asthma should consult a physician prior to use (Schuh *et al.*, 1997).

The original concept of nicotine replacement therapy was to supply nicotine to prevent withdrawal symptoms that occur after smoking cessation. Clinical trials have confirmed that nicotine replacement therapy (NRT) does reduce withdrawal symptoms, although some symptoms are reduced partially. Hunger and body weight gain may be suppressed to some extent, once nicotine is stopped, body weight increases to the same degree that occurs in the smoker who quits without nicotine replacement therapy (NRT). How much should be the length of treatment with nicotine replacement devices, is still not clear. Many abstinent smokers are unable to discontinue nicotine polacrilex gum use.

Nicotine replacement therapies are generally well tolerated and smoking-cessation rates are higher with long-term usage. Long-term nicotine exposure, as occurs with regard to tobacco use, is associated with desensitization of some (but not all) subtypes of nicotine cholinergic receptors. Nicotine induced desensitization of nicotine cholinergic receptors could result in a state in which noradrenaline release that would normally be stimulated by endogenous acetylcholine would be impaired. The same phenomenon could occur for the effects of nicotine on other neurotransmitter systems. Nicotine replacement therapy with sustained release properties, such as trans-dermal nicotine, would also be expected to desensitize nicotine receptors, producing a desirable state in the abstinent smoker either by desensitization *per se* and/or by blunting the reinforcing effects of any cigarette that might be smoked during a cessation slip. Smoking cessation rates are maximum when NRT products are used as part of combination intervention including behavioural intervention (Sutherland, 2002).

Criteria for the determination of successful outcome in nicotine replacement studies are ambiguous. It is unclear how to interpret the results in which nicotine replacement is significantly more effective than a placebo at six months, but not at one year (Fagerstrom, 1982). Nicotine replacement may be effective in facilitating cessation and in developing early resistance to relapse but may not have residual effects that prevent relapse (Piper; Fox and Fiore, 2001).

Overall, the outcome of experimental and clinical trials of nicotine polacrilex gum is modestly encouraging, at least for short-term results. In the vast majority of these trials, however, nicotine polacrilex gum has been combined with additional treatment components.

The combination of low doses (with the 2-mg gum), poorly defined criteria for self-administration, compliance problems, and variable absorption of polacrilex gum is part of the rationale for the development of alternative replacement strategies (Pomerleau *et al.,* 1988). Availability of a 4-mg preparation might be useful for highly tobacco-dependent individuals.

## Other Pharmacological (Non-nicotine) Therapies

Non-nicotine medications may work in a variety of ways, including nicotine cholinergic receptor agonism (lobeline), nicotine like effects on neurotransmitter systems (anti-depressants, clonidine), nicotine cholinergic receptor antagonism (mecamylamine) and sensory stimulation/ aversion (citric or ascorbic acid inhalants or sprays, silver acetate). These drugs can be classified as follows:

(i) Non-specific Pharmacotherapies

(ii) Symptomatic Treatment,

(iii) Nicotine Blockade Therapy, in which the behaviour controlling effects of the dependence producing drug are blocked by pre-treatment with an antagonist; and

(iv) Deterrent Therapy in which the administration of the treatment drug results in the occurrence of aversive consequences.

### *(i) Non-specific Pharmacotherapy*

Administration and withdrawal from nicotine produces a number of neurohormonal and other physiological effects and these effects mediate the various actions of tobacco. Because several such effects are functional in maintenance of cigarette smoking and in relapse, it is generally assumed that addressing such factors would enhance treatment programmes. Such strategies are also an integral part of many interventions for drug addiction in general.

There is a long history of generally unsuccessful pharmacologic treatment of smoking cessation. Experimentation with ***lobeline sulfate*** as a smoking substitute dates back to early 1900s. *Lobeline* is a plant alkaloid which acts in some of the same ways as nicotine. It is extracted from the herb and seeds of *Lobelia inflate,* (Indian tobacco).The chemical formula of *lobeline* is $C_{22} H_{27} NO_2$ for a molecular mass of 337.47. *Lobeline* is a partial nicotine agonist (that is, it blocks the effects of nicotine), which has been used in a variety of commercially available preparations to help stop smoking. The rationale for its use in tobacco cessation is that it may block the rewarding effect of nicotine and thus reducing the urge for smoke. However, *Lobeline* appears to be no more effective than a placebo in facilitating abstinence. *Bupropion, nortriptyline doxepine* are other **Anti-depressants** of particular interest in the treatment of smoking cessation.

**Bupropion**

It is available in the US since 1989 (FDA approved) as an antidepressant in a sustained release form with its action as a neuronal reuptake inhibitor of dopamine and noradrenalin. It also decreases the firing of the locus ceruleus (Cooper *et al.*, 1994). It is observed that the depressives treated with bupropion spontaneously stopped smoking. The dopaminergic and noradrenergic properties of bupropion hydrochloride provide a theoretical benefit in smoking cessation, in treating the neurochemical changes resulting from nicotine addiction and withdrawal. Bupropion hydrochloride has the benefit of being an oral non-nicotine therapy. After two large, multi-centric clinical trials demonstrated the efficacy of *Bupropion* Sustained Release (SR) for the treatment of tobacco dependence (Hurt *et al.*, 1997) and the US regulatory approval in May,1997. It is recommended as a first-line treatment for tobacco cessation. *Bupropion* alone (30%) or in the combination of nicotine patch (35%) has been demonstrated to be significantly more effective at 1-year follow-up than the nicotine patch alone (16%) or placebo (16%). *Bupropion* is equally effective in smokers with or without a history of depression; however, this drug could be a better choice in the smokers with the history of depression. The depressives already being treated with some anti-depressants and wish to quit smoking can be given *bupropion* additionally.

*Bupropion* is chemically unrelated to nicotine or other agents currently used in the treatment of tobacco dependence. It is an aminoketone, structurally related to phenothylamines and resembling the anorectic drug diethylpropion.

*Mechanism of action:* Bupropion is a weak but selective inhibitor of the neuronal reuptake of dopamine and noradrenalin, with a very minimal effect on serotonin, and does not inhibit monoamine-oxidase. Abstaining effect of bupropion is presumably related to its dopaminergic and/or adrenergic properties and to involve the two pathways in the brain that are important in the addiction process. It is hypothesized that dopaminergic activity of bupropion affects the area implicated in the reinforcing properties of the addictive drug and the development of dependence – the reward pathway, or mesolimbic system – while its noradrenergic activity in the locus ceruleus plays a role in withdrawal from nicotine.

*Bupropion* increases the levels of extracellular dopamine in the nucleus accumbens and enhances dopaminergic activity in the ventral tegmental area (VTA) of the midbrain via inhibition of reuptake. These effects of dopamine are responsible for overcoming the dependence on nicotine and helping to reduce the craving associated with nicotine dependence.

*Bupropion* decreases the firing rate of noradrenergic neurons in the locus ceruleus; enhances noradrenergic activity, which account for the reduction in nicotine withdrawal symptoms. Bupropion also produces an acute functional blockade of human nicotine receptors

***Dose and Administration:*** Bupropion is started while the patient is still smoking and a target date to stop smoking is fixed within two weeks of onset of therapy. This is done to allow the time for plasma levels of bupropion to reach steady state and, hence, for the drug to start working effectively. The initial dose should be 150 mg daily for 3 days, increasing to 150 mg twice daily to a remainder of two months course (Maximum length of treatment 9–12 weeks). However, some authors recommend treatment duration to be up to 6 months (Miller and Brady, 2004). The length of treatment for tobacco use cessation depends upon many factors, including addiction to nicotine level and the presence or absence of co-morbidities. It is important that the patients complete the full treatment course prescribed in order to maximize the likelihood of long-term abstinence from smoking and so that any patient who fails to quit smoking on their 'stop date' can set a new one with the possibility of quitting later in the treatment course (Johnston *et al.*, 1999). There should be an interval of at least 8 hours between successive doses. Maximum single dose should not exceed 150 mg and the total daily dose should not exceed 300 mg.

Similar to other antidepressants, bupropion also lowers seizure threshold and should not be used in those with history of seizure disorder, serious head trauma, eating disorders (bulimia or anorexia nervosa), and in those who receive other medications that may lower seizure threshold.

### Nortriptyline

Nortriptyline is a tricyclic antidepressant (TCA) medication that demonstrated efficacy in for smoking cessation in two clinical trials (Prochazka *et al.*, 1998 and Hall *et al.*, 1998). It increases noradrenaline levels by blocking reuptake and decreases firing in locus ceruleus. Unlike bupropion, nortriptyline blocks serotonin reuptake, does not block dopamine reuptake, has anticholinergic effects and may be sedating. Efficacy for smoking cessation is independent of depression history. It is recommended as a second-line medication for tobacco cessation (Fiore, 2000) in the dosage of 75 to 100 mg per day for a period of 8 to 12 weeks.

### Doxepine

It is another tricyclic anti-depressant studied for tobacco cessation. 150 mg of the drug per day for three weeks before cessation and four weeks after the quit date, was found to be effective. Point Prevalence cessation at nine weeks was significantly greater in doxepine group (78%) compared with placebo group (10%). Anti-depressants such as **fluoxetine** and other serotonin-specific reuptake inhibitors (SSRIs) have also been tried in tobacco-cessation, however, there are not enough follow-up reports. **Moclobemide** a reversible MAO-A inhibitor, has been studied for smoking cessation.

### Clonidine

Another pharmacological agent used to aid smoking cessation, was originally approved to lower blood pressure. *Clonidine*, an anti-hypertensives agent, is an alfa-2-adrenergic receptor agonist and imidazoline receptor agonist that decreases central sympathetic activity. Via its alfa-2 agonist effects, clonidine inhibits the release of noradrenaline and inhibits the firing of locus ceruleus leading to sedation and anxiolysis. It acts on the central nervous system and may reduce withdrawal symptoms associated with tobacco cessation. It was one of the first non-nicotine prescription medications evaluated for smoking cessation. In a Cochrane Review (Gourlay *et al.*, 1999) randomized controlled trials of *clonidine* versus placebo, clonidine was found to be more effective. Glassman and colleagues (1988) reported a clinical intervention study with *clonidine* in a sample of 71 smokers who consumed at least one pack/day and who had made at least one previous unsuccessful quit attempt. Each smoker began taking one 50-ug-tablet *clonidine* (N=33) or a matched placebo (N=38) at least three days prior to smoking quit date. Dosage was increased by one tablet every day until subjects were taking four tablets by the quit date. Subjects were seen weekly for the next four weeks. After four weeks of treatment, *clonidine* was gradually withdrawn (50-ug every three days over an average of 12 days). Success rates, both at the end of 4 weeks on *clonidine* or placebo and follow-up 6 months after discontinuation of medication favoured *clonidine*. At 6-month follow-up, 27 percent of the subjects receiving *clonidine* and 5 percent of those on placebo reported abstinence. Potentially hazardous side effects of *clonidine* should be considered before starting it as an adjunct therapy for tobacco cessation. Abrupt cessation of *clonidine* in some cases has led to severe hypertension and in rare cases to hypertensive encephalopathy and even death. More common is sedation and one should not use it while driving or under similar situations.

Although *clonidine* is effective for smoking cessation, its clinical use is limited by significant adverse effects, like sedation, dizziness and dry mouth. *Clonidine* appears to be more effective in female smokers and it is a second-line option for smoking cessation pharmacotherapy (Fiore, 2000).

Medications intended to reduce withdrawal symptoms (***anticholinergics, sympathomimetics, and anticonvulsants***) also have failed to improve outcome relative to placebo. There is little evidence of effectiveness of anxiolytics, benzodiazepines, in improving smoking cessation (Hurt *et al.*, 1997).

### *(ii) Symptomatic Treatment*

The signs and symptoms of tobacco withdrawal vary in nature and severity among individuals. Symptoms can be treated independently of their origin; symptomatic therapeutic approach might be useful in alleviation of tobacco abstinence-associated discomfort. Glassman and his colleagues (1984) used this approach in a study in which *alprazolam* (1 mg orally) and *clonidine* (0.2 mg orally) were compared with placebo for heavy cigarette smokers on the days when they abstained from tobacco. The subjects were exposed to one of the medication conditions on each of the three smoking abstinent study days, which were separated by at least 3 days of normal smoking. *Alprazolam* and clonidine were more effective than the placebo in reducing the craving for a cigarette.

*Buspiron,* a non-benzodiazepine anxiolytic, is believed to work primarily as a serotonin 5-HT[1-A] receptor partial agonist, but also increases firing rates of dopaminergic and nonadrenergic neurons. In various clinical trials of tobacco-cessation *buspiron* has been implicated to reduce the anxiety and other dysphoric aspects of nicotine withdrawal, while being non-sedating and having a relatively low abuse potential.

Nicotine may serve as a regulator of mood, selective use of minor tranquilizers, antidepressants, or even psychomotor stimulants may be beneficial in preventing relapse. Stressful situations lead to increased smoking and that smoking may reduce smoker distress responses to stressful stimuli and enhance reported mood (Glasgow *et al.,* 1986). Relapse to cigarette smoking generally occur in response to stressful situations.

### *(iii) Nicotine Blockade Therapy*

The goal of both replacement therapy and symptomatic treatment is to relieve withdrawal by mimicking effects of the drug. Blockade therapy provides no such potentially rewarding or therapeutic effect. The goal of blockade therapy is to reduce or eliminate any rewarding pharmacological effects, should the person attempt to resume the drug use. The prototype blockade therapy is that used in treatment of opioid dependence (Jaffe, 1985). The long-acting opiate antagonist naltrexone can be given on a daily basis to opiate abusers to prevent them from experiencing the reinforcing effects of agonists.

Pharmacological antagonists of nicotine, which diminish a variety of responses to nicotine, have been known for several decades (Domino, 1979). Those antagonists, which act both centrally and peripherally (mecamylamine), but not those that only act peripherally (*pentolinium* and *hexamethonium*), appear to have functional effects on pattern of cigarette smoking in humans. Certain antagonists also alter the behavioural effects of nicotine (including self-administration) in animals (Stolerman, 1986).

**Mecamylamine** could be used as an antagonist to block the nicotine-mediated reinforcing consequences of cigarette smoking. The following findings are of particular relevance: (a) *Mecamylamine* pretreatment produces a dose-related blockade of the ability of animals and humans to discriminate nicotine from a placebo (*mecamylamine* is injected in animals and administered orally in humans), (b) *Mecamylamine* pretreatment diminishes the reinforcing efficacy of intravenous nicotine administration in animals (Goldberg *et al.,* 1983) and possibly in human beings (Henningfield and Goldberg, 1983), (c) *Mecamylamine* pretreatment increases the preference for high-nicotine-delivering cigarette smoke (apparently by reducing its nicotine effects) when subjects are tested with a device which blends smoke from high and low nicotine-delivering cigarettes (Rose *et al.,* 1985), (d) *Mecamylamine* pretreatment increases various measures of cigarette smoking behaviour and tobacco smoke intake when subjects are allowed to freely smoke.

In heavy cigarette smokers, *mecamylamine* combined with counseling, reduced craving for smoking and helped 50 percent of the subjects quit smoking within two weeks of initiation of treatment. The mean dose of *mecamylamine* at the time of quitting was 26.7 mg/day. Because *mecamylamine* blocks the effects of nicotine, it precipitates withdrawal and hence is not of help in acute cessation (Tennant, Traver and Rawson, 1984).

The difficulties to this treatment approach are the ganglionic blocking and anti-hypertensive effects of *mecamylamine* the strong likelihood of considerable difficulty of obtaining adequate therapeutic compliance, and conditioned and non-nicotine mediated reinforce of tobacco use which may be powerful enough to sustain urges to smoke even when they are no longer associated with the pharmacological effects of nicotine.

### *(iv) Deterrent Therapy*

This therapy is based on the premise that pretreatment with an agent may transform smoking from a rewarding to an aversive behaviour. Disulfiram treatment of alcoholism provides the pharmacologic analogy for this form of treatment. With regard to cigarette smoking, the main analog to disulfiram treatment is the administration of *silver acetate*. The physiological basis of the approach is that sulfide salts are produced when *silver acetate* contacts the sulfides in tobacco smoke. The resulting silver sulfides are extremely distasteful for most people. This approach is not specific to nicotine intake, but rather to sulfide-containing smoke. Most recently, a gum preparation of *silver acetate* has been tested as a mean to maintaining abstinence from tobacco smoking (Malcolm *et al.*, 1986). The gum must be chewed upon awakening and then repeatedly during the day to assist in abstinence, because a single piece of gum is apparently only effective for a few hours.

An Arab pharmaceutical company has developed and tested a mouth wash preparation for use as an aid to tobacco cessation (Zmeili *et al.*, 1999). 74 Jordanian healthy male smokers were given the A.S. mouthwash (active ingredient 0.5 percent *silver nitrate*) and 63 male smokers received a placebo solution in a double blind fashion. Mouthwash solutions were administered three times daily for two weeks; gargling lasting for duration of one minute. When compared to the placebo, the smokers treated with A.S. mouthwash showed a significant ($p<0.05$) reduction in the number of cigarettes smoked.

***Varenicline***, a partial agonist at alfa-4, beta-2 nicotine receptor site weakly mimicking the action of nicotine replacement with treatment such as nicotine gum or patch, has recently been introduced in the market for treatment of tobacco dependence. The partial agonism of varenicline is also responsible for the release of dopamine in the mesolimbic system; this mimics the benefits of treatments such as bupropion. Due to the receptor occupation, the physiological effects of exogenous nicotine are attenuated or blocked by the drug (Foulds, 2006). Therefore, it is a new class of approved treatments for nicotine dependence, one that is different from nicotine replacement therapy and bupropion. It has been approved for smoking cessation by the Food and Drug Administration (FDA), USA in May 2006 (FDA 2006).

12 weeks of treatment with varenicline for tobacco-cessation was found to be superior with either bupropin or placebo (Gonzales *et al.*, 2006 and Jorenby *et al.*, 2006). Varenicline is safe and well tolerated across 24 weeks of continuous treatment; however, it does not prevent the weight gain that accompanies abstinence from smoking. Side-effect profile of the drug includes: nausea (33%), insomnia (20%) and headache (12%).

Unlike other drugs, relapse is preventable for a longer period of time with varenicline. In fact, more than half of those treated with bupropion or NRT and achieved abstinence relapse within a year. Smokers who achieve abstinence for a least one week at the end of 12 weeks of varenicline treatment (dose 1 mg twice daily) are likely to remain continuously abstinent during a further 12 weeks of varenicline treatment, and during a subsequent treatment-free period of 28 weeks. In other words, 24 weeks of varenicline treatment improves the prospects of a year of abstinence from smoking.

## Behavioural Treatment

Pharmacological strategies have a useful role in alleviating withdrawal symptoms or in blocking gratification typically derived from smoking, but these agents do not address conditioned cues and re-inforcers or social context of the tobacco use. For effective treatment behavioural intervention is needed in addition to pharmacological agents. Pharmacological intervention is more effective when applied in a context that includes social support and skills training. Behavioural intervention may also be useful in increasing adherence to pharmacologic treatment procedures (Epstein and Cluss, 1982). Behaviour interventions include physician intervention, community trials, and worksite smoking programmes. The vast majority of smokers who have quit to date have done so in the absence of formal treatment.

### *1. Aversion Therapy*

Aversion procedures involve pairing of smoking with unpleasant imagery scripts (covert sensitization), with electric shock, or with the unpleasant effects produced by smoking itself. These techniques are designed to create aversions to cigarette smoke-effective reactions characterized by distaste, disgust, fear, or displeasure. Such reactions reduce the incentive to smoke, which include satiation, rapid smoking, and focused smoking.

### *2. Satiation*

In satiation cigarette smoking is dramatically increased prior to attempted abstinence. Smokers typically are asked to at least double their smoking intake. Satiation has been used in multi-component programmes (Best *et al.,* 1978) in which its contribution to outcomes has been difficult to ascertain. It has been suggested that satiation represents a plausible preparation strategy for quitting. However, there is little evidence that satiation results in an aversion to cigarette (Tiffany *et al.,* 1986).

### *3. Rapid Smoking*

Rapid smoking requires smokers to inhale cigarette smoke every 6 seconds until they reach the point that they would become ill if they were to continue. Standardized regimes include six to eight sessions (Hall, Rugg *et al.,* 1984). Multi-component programmes including rapid smoking generally yield good outcomes, but when used by itself, rapid smoking continues to yield variable results. Hall and associates have consistently obtained high rates of success using rapid smoking alone, both with normal volunteers as well as medical patients.

Hall, Sachs and colleagues (1984) observed that, in contrast to many recent applications of rapid smoking, their procedure was similar to that of early, successful-rapid smoking interventions (Lichtenstein *et al.*, 1973). Their procedure involved

(i) A single client format.

(ii) A warm client-therapist relationship.

(iii) Positive expectations of success

(iv) Individualized scheduling

(v) Office rather than home treatment.

(vi) Warnings against smoking outside of therapy sessions (Danaher, 1977).

### 4. Reduced Aversion Techniques

Relaxation training or progressive relaxation is a popular treatment for anxiety-related disorders. As noted previously, smokers often resort to smoking to cope with anxiety and stress. A large proportion of smoking relapses occurs during negative emotional states (Shiffman *et al.*, 1982). Relaxation training should provide smokers with means other than smoking for coping with stress and negative emotion. At present, relaxation technique is used into multi-component behavioural skills training programmes (Tiffany *et al.*, 1986) and it may best be conceptualized as one of many possible stress-coping skills taught to clients. However, studies show that relaxation training does not improve the outcome of a rapid-smoking treatment. Seventy-five subjects were assigned to rapid smoking only; rapid smoking and relaxation training; rapid smoking, relaxation and contingency contracting; or contingent rapid smoking. In none of these conditions did 1-year abstinence exceed 25 percent.

### 5. Contingency Contracting

To treat tobacco smokers, the operant conditioning i.e. reward and punishment strategies is employed. The usual procedure is to collect monetary deposits from the clients early in treatment with periodic repayments contingent on client achievement of abstinence goals. Variations include having the client pledge to donate money to a disliked organization or an individual for every cigarette smoked, or contracting for non-monetary rewards and punishments based on smoking status. The rational behind this technique is that they may bolster commitment to abstinence by providing contingent concrete rewards. Contracts are in effect until withdrawal has abated and the individual has had an opportunity to begin alternative non-smoking activities that may be rewarding. Stitzer and Bigelow (1982) provided contingent payments of \$5 to subjects for reducing carbon monoxide (CO) levels by 50 percent. Other attempts to increase effectiveness of contingency contracts by manipulating the length, frequency or amount of deposit have largely been unsuccessful (Paxton, 1983).

### 6. Social Support

Hamilton and Bornstein (1979) developed a package that included a buddy system among group members and public announcements of client successes at quitting smoking. When this package was combined with behavioural treatment programme, it significantly increase abstinence rates compared with those for behavioural treatment alone. Spouses of the smokers are also included in smoking cessation programme to teach them how to be supportive of clients' quitting programme. Outcome of such a programme is far better than the outcome of the programme where spouses did not participate in the programme. However the worksite-controlled smoking programme was affected by encouraging the social support of quitting co-workers.

### *7. Coping Skills Training*

Smokers who use cognitive and /or behavioural coping responses when they are tempted to smoke reduce their likelihood of relapsing. The rationale for coping skills training of tobacco-dependent individuals is similar to that for such training in other forms of drug dependence. Alternative behavioural repertoires are developed that help to maintain comfortable, satisfactory functioning in the absence of drugs. Behavioural coping responses may include distracting activities, escape from a stressor, relaxation and physical activity. Cognitive coping may involve reminding oneself of benefits of quitting or negative consequences of smoking or simply telling oneself that smoking is not an option. Coping responses may be directed either at the smoking temptation/urge itself or at a precipitating stressor (Wills and Shiffman, 1985). Coping skills training appears to be effective in enhancing short-term outcomes, especially when combined with an aversive-smoking procedure. The long-term effects are less clear.

### *8. Stimulus Control*

*Stimulus control* treatments are based on the assumption that a wide variety of environmental cues are associated with and serve to trigger smoking. A gradual reduction in smoking is accompanied by having clients progressively eliminate situations in which they smoke. In some cases, temporal, rather than situational, constraints upon smoking are instituted. A gradual reduction in smoking should result in a weaker and more manageable withdrawal syndrome. Stimulus control procedures generally have produced weak transient results when used alone and have been of questionable value when combined with other self-management techniques (Lando, 1978). Some studies have used stimulus control primarily as an element in multi-component programmes in which its effectiveness is difficult to ascertain (Rabkin *et al.,* 1984).

Some workers have used stimulus control component designed to maximize client self-efficacy (Bandura, 1977) to a nicotine fading treatment. The combined treatment produced a 5-month abstinence rate of over 50 percent—twice than that of the fading procedure alone. This level of success is unusual in the research on stimulus control techniques and may be due to the self-efficacy manipulation rather than stimulus control *per se.*

### 9. Nicotine Fading

Nicotine fading (or brand switching) is based upon a simple pharmacological logic rationale that the intensity of withdrawal syndrome can be reduced when the dependence-producing drug is gradually withdrawn. The process involves smokers monitoring their nicotine consumption while switching (in 3–6 stages) to cigarette brands with progressively lower rated tar and nicotine deliveries, and then quitting completely. Non-abstinent nicotine fading subjects would benefit from continued smoking of low tar and low nicotine brands. This treatment strategy is based primarily on the idea that the gradual phase out of smoking will minimize nicotine withdrawal symptoms. It is an alternative to "cold turkey" quitting. Nicotine fading should be differentiated from gradual reduction procedures in which smokers are instructed to progressively reduce the number of cigarettes. Smokers typically report that the remaining cigarettes are more reinforcing and they often reach a "Stuck point" beyond which additional reduction does not occur.

### 10. Relaxation Training

Relaxation therapy is a popular treatment for anxiety related disorders (Haugen, Dixon, Dickel, 1958). Smokers often tend to smoke more when they are tense and anxious. A large number of smoking relapses occur during negative emotional states (Brandon *et al.,* 1986). Theoretically, relaxation training should be helpful to avoid smoking in anxious and tense individuals; however, relaxation is rarely used as a sole treatment and is instead incorporated into multi-component behavioural skills training programmes (Hall *et al.,* 1985). It is one of many possible stress-coping skills.

### 11. Controlled Smoking

To treat smokers who are unable or unwilling to quit completely, controlled smoking is used and is based on the assumption that reduced smoking will be associated with diminished health hazards. The prototypical programme attempts to decrease risk by reducing cigarette consumption, altering smoking inhalation patterns (number of puffs, duration of puff, CO intake), and minimizing the tar and nicotine content of cigarettes (fading). Stimulus control procedures may also be used (Glassgow, Klesgres, Vasey, 1983). In addition, clients may be taught coping skills to use as substitutes for smoking.

The basic premise of the controlled smoking approach – that it reduces health risk-remains to be validated. However, possible risk reduction is not the only rationale for this type of approach. Controlled smoking interventions may appeal to a large cross-section of smokers, may have a positive impact upon self-efficacy, and may facilitate subsequent progress toward complete abstinence.

### 12. Multi-component Programmes

Smoking is a multi-determined and relatively invulnerable to any single therapeutic intervention (Schwartz, 1987). The most effective multi-component programmes yield almost universal short-term abstinence and long-term abstinence rates that approach or exceed 50 percent (Tiffany *et al.,* 1986). These results are extremely encouraging and are rarely matched in trials that place exclusive emphasis upon pharmacologic intervention.

## Other Treatment Strategies

### 1. Hypnotherapy

*Hypnotherapy* is used to weaken the desire to smoke or strengthen the will to stop. The usual intent of hypnosis is to increase client's motivation or ability to quit smoking through post-hypnotic suggestions. The most common suggestions (Spiegel, 1970) are:

i. Smoking is a poison to your body.
ii. You need your body to live.
iii. You owe your body this respect and protection.

Suggestions may also involve problem-solving techniques (Frank *et al.,* 1986), desensitization to environmental cues (Wagner *et al.,* 1983), review of client's smoking history (Javel, 1980), and an assortment of other elements (Katz, 1980). Hypnosis might be applied most usefully to the small percentage of population that is highly susceptible to hypnotic induction.

In the Cochrane Review (Abbot *et al.,* 1999) randomized trials of *hypnotherapy* reporting smoking cessation rates at least six months after the beginning of treatment were evaluated. There was significant heterogeneity between the results of the individual studies, with conflicting results for the effectiveness of *hypnotherapy* compared to no therapy or to advice.

### 2. Acupuncture

*Acupuncture* involves the use of needles or staple like attachments and commonly is given at the ear either by press needle or staple puncture. *Acupuncture* has been used as an intervention for tobacco cessation. In Cochrane Review (White and Rampes, 1999), 16 randomized controlled trials comparing sham acupuncture another intervention or no intervention, for smoking cessation were evaluated. Abstinence from smoking after twelve weeks, at six months, and at one-year follow-up in patients smoking compared at baseline was assessed. Meta-analysis was used when appropriate. Acupuncture was found to be not superior to sham acupuncture in smoking cessation at any point of time.

## Efficacy Outcome Measures

Smoking abstinence is defined as:

(a) *Point prevalence abstinence rate*: no smoking for a consecutive 7-day period, usually in the 7 days prior to a clinic visit.

(b) *Continuous abstinence rate*: no smoking during a continuous period from the stop date (usually a day 8) through to the end of treatment and then to specified time points during the follow-up period.

Abstinence is determined by the patients' self-reported smoking status, and biochemically confirmed at clinic visits by carbon monoxide levels 10 ppm in expired air.

*Point prevalence* abstinence includes patients who have not smoked during the previous 7 days but who might have had few cigarettes prior to that. It is accepted that some patients may have occasional lapses after their stop date without truly relapsing and, therefore, may better represent 'real life' success.

*Continuous abstinence and point prevalence abstinence:* continuous abstinence is an extremely rigorous measure of outcome. It requires patients not to have had any cigarette at all – not even a single puff - since the day they stopped smoking. As nicotine dependence is increasingly recognized as a chronic, relapsing condition, it may be unrealistic to expect that the average smoker will maintain this level of abstinence over a prolonged period of time.

*Secondary outcome*: Other efficacy outcome measures include severity of nicotine withdrawal symptoms, cigarette-craving or urge-to-smoke scores, consumption, scores on Beck Depressive Inventory (BDI), and changes in weight. Patients may keep diary cards documenting the number of cigarettes smoked per day and their daily rating of cravings, and withdrawal symptoms (on a 5 point scale).

## Treating the Former Tobacco Users

Preventing Relapse to Tobacco Use. Effective relapse prevention treatment to all patients who have recently quit tobacco use needs to be provided. With the extraordinary high rate of relapse to smoking, patient's decision to quit needs to be reinforced, benefits of quitting are reviewed, and the residual problems arising out of quitting need to be resolved. Minimal relapse prevention consists of congratulating success, encouraging continued abstinence, and discussing with the patient the benefits of quitting, the problems encountered during quitting and the anticipated challenges to staying abstinent (such as depression, weight gain, alcohol etc.). Some patients report feeling of lack of support for their cessation attempt. In response to this concern, the physician can schedule follow-up visits or telephone calls, help patient identify sources of support within environment and work to increase extra treatment social support. If the patient reports negative mood or depression it needs to be addressed to. In case of extended or severe withdrawal, appropriate medication needs to be started.

Weight gain is a common concern among smokers who are trying to quit. In such smokers, emphasize the importance of a healthy diet and physical exercise. If the patient shows flagging motivation, and feeling of deprivation, he should be reassured that these feelings are common and short lasting.

Although most relapse occurs early in the quitting process, some relapse occurs months or even years after the quit date. Therefore, physicians should continue to engage in relapse prevention intervention even with former tobacco users who no longer consider themselves actively engaged in quitting process.

## Guideline Strategies Treating Patients Who are Unwilling to Quit

There are some tobacco users who are unwilling to quit; they need to be motivated to quit. The PHS Guidelines suggest using a strategy based upon the 5 R's: relevance, risks, rewards, roadblocks, and repetition.

### *Relevance*

Relevance of quitting smoking should be conveyed to the patient and should be motivated to quit taking various factors in account like health status, children, current disease condition etc.

### *Risks*

Patient should be asked to identify potential negative consequences of tobacco use. Acute risks include:

- shortness of breath,
- exacerbation of asthma,
- harm to pregnancy,
- impotence, and
- increased serum carbon monoxide.

Long-term risks include:

- heart attacks and strokes,
- cancer of lungs, larynx, oral cavity, pharynx, oesophagus, pancreas, bladder, cervix,
- chronic bronchitis,
- emphysema etc.

Environmental risks include:

- increased risk of lung cancer and heart disease in spouses,
- higher rates of smoking by children of tobacco users,
- increased risk for low birth weight,
- sudden infant death syndrome (SIDS),
- asthma,
- middle ear disease, and
- respiratory infections in the children of smokers.

### *Rewards*

Patient should be asked to identify potential benefits of stopping smoking and their relevance in the patient's case should be emphasized like, improved health, improved sense of smell; improved self-esteem, money saving, a good example for children etc.

### Roadblocks

Patient should identify the barriers or the impediments that prevent him from quitting smoking. Typical barriers might include withdrawal syndrome, fear of failure, weight gain, lack of support, depression and enjoyment of tobacco.

### Repetition

Motivational interventions should be repeated every time an unmotivated patient visits the clinic.

### Treating Tobacco Use and Dependence in Specific Population

PHS Guidelines address to the need of treatment in specific populations using tobacco. Generally, the same treatments are found to be effective in all populations.

**Women:** Same treatment interventions can be used in both men and women; however, women may face different stressors and barriers to quitting they may be addressed in the treatment. These include greater likelihood of depression, greater weight control concerns, hormonal cycles and others. Women may benefit from tobacco dependence treatment that addresses these topics.

### Pregnant Women

Because smoking during pregnancy imparts risks to both the woman and the foetus, women are motivated to quit during pregnancy, and the health-care professionals can take advantage of this motivation by reinforcing the knowledge that cessation will reduce health risks to the foetus and that there are post-partum benefits for both the mother and the child. Quitting smoking prior to conception or early in the pregnancy is most beneficial, but health benefits result from abstinence at any stage. The PHS Guidelines recommend that whenever possible, pregnant smokers should be offered extended or augmented psychosocial intervention that exceeds minimum advice to quit.

### Hospitalized Smokers

Smoking may interfere with the recovery by negatively affecting bone and wound healing. Among cardiac patients, second heart attack is more common in those who continue to smoke. Patients who are successfully treated for cancer of the lungs or head and neck but who continue to smoke are at elevated risk for second cancer. The PHS Guidelines reveal that provision of augmented treatment to the hospitalized smokers significantly increases abstinent rates. Patients in long-term care facilities should also receive tobacco dependence interventions identified to be effective.

### Smokers with Psychiatric Co-morbidity

Psychiatric co-morbidity places smokers at increased risk for relapse; such smokers can be helped by smoking cessation treatments. Currently there is insufficient data to determine whether smokers with psychiatric co-morbidity benefit more from specialized or tailored cessation treatments or than from standard treatments. Because bupropion SR and nortriptyline are effective at treating depression and are efficacious smoking medications, they should be especially considered for use in depressed patients.

Some smokers may experience exacerbation of a co-morbid condition upon quitting smoking, but most evidence suggests that abstinence entails little adverse impact. It is important to note that stopping smoking may affect pharmacokinetics of certain psychiatric medications. Treating psychiatrist should monitor closely the side effects, action etc. of the medication.

The treatment of tobacco dependence can be provided concurrently with treatment for other chemical dependencies. With regard to patients in treatment for drug-dependence, there is little evidence that the patients with other drug dependencies relapse to other drug use when they stop smoking. However, such patients should be followed closely after they stop smoking.

### *Children and Adolescents*

PHS Guidelines recommend the physicians screen pediatric and adolescent patients and their parents for tobacco use and provide a strong message about totally abstaining from tobacco use. Children and adolescents may benefit from community- and school-based intervention activities. The treating physician should reinforce the message delivered by these programmes. The Guideline further recommends that clinicians in a pediatric setting offer stop-smoking advice to parents to limit children's exposure to second-hand smoke.

Tobacco presents a serious health risk to all smokers. A brief three-minute intervention by a physician has been shown to have an impact on helping smokers to quit and stay abstinent. Smoking cessation is an important goal for all smokers, and physicians can facilitate this difficult task.

## Relapse

As already discussed, the process of smoking cessation involves several discrete stages which may include pre-contemplation, contemplation, decision, action, and maintenance (Wilcox *et al.,* 1985) and there are many factors related to successful maintenance of nonsmoking once initial cessation has been achieved during the action stage. However, many patients slip into smoking again even after achieving cessation of smoking. Long-term studies indicate that relapse is far more common than maintenance of nonsmoking (Hunt, Barnett and Branch, 1971). The National Working Conference on Smoking Relapse recommends duration of 24 hours of continuous tobacco abstinence to define initial cessation. A slip is defined as a "period of not more than 6 consecutive days of smoking following 24 hours of abstinence" (Ossip-Klein *et al.,* 1986). Smoking beyond 6 consecutive days is then defined as a relapse. However, many investigators consider longer period of initial abstinence (48 hours or 1 week) for a quit episode and regard even a few smoking occasions as a relapse rather than a slip.

An individual's relapse or successful maintenance depends upon a number of factors which include individual characteristics and the environment that make the individual more or less vulnerable.

Social learning theory explains the effects of environmental and behavioural elements on maintenance of nonsmoking that are mediated by the factors such as prior experience with smoking cessation and beliefs about the cessation process. In addition, personal demography, smoking and quitting history, social support, smoking cues in the social environment, stress, cognitive factors such as self-efficacy, outcome attributions, and perceptions about the consequences of quitting smoking, also play an important role.

Initial smoking following a period of abstinence is likely to occur in certain types of high-risk situations that include intra-personal factors such as negative affect and severe withdrawal symptoms following a long history of heavy smoking. Failure to cope in the situation coupled with the positive expectations about the effects of smoking can lead to an initial slip.

## Predisposing Factors

### *Demographics*

Although men and women may be equally likely to relapse, data suggest that their return to smoking is precipitated by different factors. Strong craving and alcohol intake are the two main reasons for restarting smoking in men while a negative affect and influence of other smokers may cause relapse in women (Hirvonen, 1983).

### *Smoking and Quitting History*

The length of a person's smoking history influences the process of initial cessation (Coppotelli and Orleans, 1985). The time between waking up and smoking the first cigarette is a good predictor of outcome (Kabat and Wynder, 1987)

Those who smoke to control their negative affect and those who experience craving when emotionally upset, are more likely to relapse after smoking cessation. There is a positive relationship between the number of previous quit attempts and success in quitting smoking (Tiffany *et al.,* 1986).

### *Withdrawal and Dependence*

Withdrawal symptoms, whether elicited by acute deprivation or by conditioned stimuli, are hypothesized to be the link between dependence and relapse (Baker, Morse and Sherman, 1987). The symptoms include craving for cigarette, irritability, anxiety, difficulty in concentrating, restlessness and increased appetite. Some physical signs are also commonly reported, but with the possible exception of bradycardia, these appear to be less consistent (Hughes and Hatsukami, 1986). The syndrome has a rapid onset and generally declines within 2 weeks.

### *Cognitive Factors*

Quitting smoking often results in weight gain (Grunberg, 1986) which may be due to decreased metabolism, increased food consumption, and increased preference for sweet-tasting, high-caloric foods. Highly dependent smokers and those who tend to eat in response to specific emotional and environmental cues appear to be at greatest risk of gaining weight following smoking cessation (Emont and Cummings, 1987). Smoker perceptions concerning weight gain may be critical. For some individuals, gain of one or two kilograms may be viewed as a cause of great concern.

Marlatt's theory specifies that people's ability to resist the use of a substance (such as a cigarette) in a high-risk situation depends on, among other factors, their self efficacy levels (Marlatt and Gordon, 1980). If people have expectations that they can cope with a smoking urge without smoking, they are less likely to relapse. Moreover, people who successfully resist temptation should experience an increase in self-efficacy. The theory also states that self-efficacy is a determinant of whether people who experience an initial lapse are able to prevent escalation to full relapse.

### *Social Factors*

Most exposure to smoking-specific cues is socially mediated, like watching others smoking. Such exposures have been labeled "social contagion" (Shiffman and Jarvik, 1987). Social support can serve as a buffer to reduce the negative psychological effects of stressors (Cohen *et al.,* 1986). The level of perceived social support is related to smoking cessation and maintenance. General social support from spouses, as well as smoking-specific spousal support, has been related to smoking treatment outcome. Greater perceived support predicts maintenance.

### *Stress*

Stress and coping theories of smoking imply that deficiencies in personal resources for coping with stress may enhance the risk of relapse. Those who can cope with the life stresses adequately after smoking cessation are more likely to remain abstinent for longer periods.

## Precipitating Factors

### *High-Risk Situations*

Initial smoking following cessation tends to occur in specific types of high-risk situations. Craving/withdrawal, intrapersonal negative emotional states (e.g. frustration, boredom and anxiety), interpersonal conflict situation, and social pressure, both direct and indirect are common types of high-risk situations. Relapse is commonly seen under these situations. Other smokers serve not only as cues for smoking but also source of cigarettes thus create high-risk situation. 50% of all relapse episodes, another smoker provide the cigarettes that are smoked. This does not imply that the smokers exert social pressure to smoke; in most cases, the ex-smoker specifically asks for a cigarette (Brandon *et al.,* 1986). Relapse can also be cued by other stimuli or activities that have become associated with smoking through contiguity, for instant food, drink or relaxation (Ossip-Klein *et al.,* 1986).

### *Coping Strategies*

Coping strategies can be used both to prevent (anticipatory coping) and to directly respond to (immediate coping) high-risk situations. In either case, the strategies used can be behavioural, consisting of responses that are outwardly visible (leaving the party where others are smoking, engaging in physical activities), or cognitive, consisting of internal responses such as thoughts or images. One of the most commonly anticipatory coping strategies is the stimulus control – the avoidance of stimuli associated with smoking. However, it is better to use both cognitive and behavioural coping strategies when faced with a risk situation (Curry *et al.,* 1987).

### *Abstinence Violation Effects*

Abstinence Violation Effect (AVE) is an attributional construct that mediates the transition from an initial lapse to a full-blown relapse. Curry *et al* (1987) found that individuals who smoked but did not return to regular smoking reported significantly greater AVEs than those who relapsed following an initial slip.

## Indian Experience with Tobacco Cessation

With the establishment of National Tobacco Control Cell as a part of World Health Organization (WHO) and Government of India initiative on tobacco control, tobacco cessation services are among the areas that have to be addressed as per the Framework Convention on Tobacco Control (FCTC). 13 clinics were started on a pilot basis for tobacco cessation in 2002. World Health Organization (WHO) supported the setting up of 12 tobacco cessation clinics (TCCs) in diverse settings to help people stop tobacco use. All these clinicss are provided with trained staff including clinical psychologists and social workers in addition to the treating physicians. Cotinine test kits and bupropion tablets are also provided. An algorithm consisting of initial assessment, three steps of intervention and evaluation at regular intervals, preferably with urinary cotinine estimation as an objective measure of cessation is provided. The 13$^{th}$ clinic was added later, which is located in a chest diseases institute.

All the centres where these clinics are situated organize community intervention programmes to attract patients who present with co-morbidities and then refer them to these clinics. Periodic monitoring of these clinics is carried out and mid-course corrections are introduced as required.

In the first year of inception of these clinics, self-help tips and behavioural-change counseling modules were developed for effective therapeutic intervention. Counseling the most common form of intervention is supplemented by bupropion at some centres.

During these four years of existence of these clinics, they have gathered large number of patients. Therapeutic interventions are grouped into counseling alone and counseling and pharmacotherapy. The outcome of the intervention is ascertained at 6 weeks classified as complete abstinence or reduced to more than 50% of the initial use. The initial results show that the overall quit rate at 6 weeks was around 16%. The addition of pharmacotherapy improved the quit rates. Counseling is cost-effective and can be the preferred option for expanding the services while pharmacotherapy may be limited to services which have good clinical support.

## REFERENCES


Abbot N.C., Stead L.F., White A.R., Barnes J., Ernst E.: Hypnotherapy for Smoking Cessation (Cochrane Review). In: The Cochrane Library, Issue1Oxford: Update Software. *(http://www.cochrane.org/cochrane/revabstr/ab001008.htm)*, 1999.

Abrams D.B.,: Roles of Psychosocial Stress, Smoking Cues and Coping in Smoking Relapse Prevention. *Health Psychology*. 5(supplement): 91 – 92, 1986.

American Academy of Family Physicians, Vol. 62(3) 2000.

Audrain J., Gomez-Caminero A., Robertson A.R.: Gender and Ethnic Differences in Readiness to Chang Smoking Behaviour. *Women's Health*, 3:139 – 150, 1997.

Baker T.B., Morse E. and Sherman J.E.: The Motivation to Take Drugs: A Psychobiological Analysis of Urges. In: Rivers C (Eds) Nebraska *Symposium on Motivation*. University of Nebraska Press: Lincoln, Nebraska, 1987.

Bandura, A.: Self-efficacy: Toward a Unifying Theory of Behavioural Change. *Psychological Review*. 84:191 – 215, 1977. 1996.

Benowitz N.L.: Pharmacology of nicotine: Addiction and Therapeutics. *Annual Review of Pharmacology and Toxicology*, 36: 597–613.

Benowitz, N.L., Hall, S.M., Herning, R.I., Jacob, P III., Jones, R.T., Osman, A.L.: Smokers of Low Yield Cigarettes do Not Consume Less Nicotine. *New England Journal of Medicine*. 309(3): 129 – 142, 1983.

Benowitz, N.L., Jacob, PIII., Savanapridi, C: Determinants of Nicotine Intake While Chewing Nicotine Polacrilex Gum. *Clinical Pharmacology and Therapeutics*. 41: 467 – 473, 1987.

Best, J.A., Owen, L.E., Trentadue, L.: Comparison of Striation and Rapid Smoking in Self-managed Smoking Cessation. *Addictive Behaviour* 3(2): 71 –78, 1978.

Blazer D., Kessler R., McGonagle K., Swartz S.: The Prevalence and Distribution of Major Depression in A National Community Sample: the National Comorbidity Survey. *American Journal of Psychiatry*, 151: 979 – 986, 1994.

Borrelli B., Bock B., King T., Pinto B., Marcus B.H.: The Impact of Depression on Smoking Cessation in Women *American Journal of Preventive Medicine*, 12: 378 – 387, 1996.

Brandon T.H., Tiffany S.T. and Baker T.B.: The Process of Smoking Relapse. In: Tim FM., Leukefeld CG (Eds) Relapse and Recovery in Drug-abuse. NIDA Research Monograph 72. US Department of Health and Human Services. Alcohol, Drug-Abuse and Mental Health Administration. National Institute of Drug Abuse DHHS Publication No (ADM) 86–1473, 1986.

Briggs G.W.: The Chamars: Religious Life of India. *Association Press, Calcutta*, 1920.

British Thoracic Society: Comparison of Four Methods of Smoking Withdrawal in Patients With Smoking Related Diseases. *British Medical Journal* 286(6366):995–997, 1983.

Brownell K.D.: Dieting and the Search for the Perfect Body: Where Physiology and Culture Collide. *Behaviour Therapy*, 22:1 – 12, 1991.

Carmody T.P.: Affect Regulation, Nicotine Addiction, and Smoking Cessation. *Journal of Psychoactive Drugs*, 21:331–342, 1989.

Campbell I.A., Lyons E., and Prescott R.: Stopping Smoking: Do Nicotine Chewing Gum and Postal Encourage Add to Doctors' Advice? *Practioner*, 231:114–117, 1987.

Choi J.H., Dresler C.M., Norton M.R. and Strahs K.R.: Pharmacokinetics of a Nicotine Polacrilex Lozenge. *Nicotine Tobacco Research*, 5(5): 635–644, 2003.

Cohen S., Sherrod D.R. and Clark M.S.: Social Skills and Stress-protective Role of Social Support. *Journal of Personality and Social Psychology*, 50:963–974, 1986.

Cooper *et al*,1994.

Coppotelli H.C. and Orleans C.T.: Partner Support and Other Determinants of Smoking Cessation Maintenance Among Women. *Journal of Consulting and Clinical Psychology*, 53(4):455–466, 1985.

Craig D., Parrott A., Coomber J: Smoking Cessation Among Women: Effects on the Menstrual Cycle. *International Journal of Addiction*. 27: 697 – 706, 1992.

Crisp AH: Regulation of the Self in Adolescence With Particular Reference to Anorexia Nervosa. *Transcultural Medical Sociology*, 100: 67 – 74, 1985.

Crowe R.R., Krammer JR., Hesselbroch V., Manos G and Bucholz KK: 1997. The Utility of the Brief MAST and the CAGE in Identifying Alcohol Problems: Results from National High-risk and Community Samples. *Archieves of Family Medicine*, 6: 477–483, 1985.

Curry S., Marlatt G.A., and Gordon J.R.: Abstinence Violation Effect: Validation of An Attributional Construct With Smoking Cessation. *Journal of Consulting and Clinical Psychology*, 55(2): 145–149, 1987.

DiFranza J.R. Rigotti N.A., McNeill A.D., Ockene J.K., Savageau J.A., St Cyr D., Coleman M: 2000. Initial Symptoms of Nicotine Dependence in Adolescence. *Tobacco Control*, 9:313 –319. 1987.

Domino, E.F.: Behavioural, Electrophysiological, Endocrine and Skeletal Muscle Action of Nicotinr and Tobacco Smoking. In: Remond, A, Izard, C. (eds.) Electrophysiological Effects of Nicotine. Amsterdam: Elsevier? North Holland Biomedical Press, pp 133 – 146, 1979.

Emont S.L. and Cummings K.M.: Weight Gain Following Smoking Cessation: A Possible Role for Nicotine Replacement in Weight Management. *Addictive Behaviour*, 12: 152–155, 1987.

Epstein, L.H. and Cluss, P.A.: A Behavioural Medicine Perspective on Adherence Long-term Medical Regimens. *Journal of Consulting and Clinical Psychology*. 50(6): 950 – 971, 1982.

Fagerstrom K.O.: Effects of a Nicotine-enriched Cigarette on Nicotine Titration, Daily Cigarette Consumption, and Levels of Carbon Monoxide and Nicotine. *Psychopharmacology*, 77(2):164–167, 1982.

Fagerstrom, K.O.: Reducing the Weight Gain After Stopping Smoking. *Addictive Behaviour*. 12:91 – 93, 1987.

FDA. www.fda.gov/bbs/topics/NEWS/2006/NEW01370.html. Accessed on August 24, 2006.

Fee W.M. and Stewart M.J.: A Controlled Trial of Nicotine Chewing Gum in a Amoking Withdrawal Clinic. *Practioner*, 226(1363):148–151, 1982.

Ferno, O., Lichtneckert, S. and Lundgreen, C.A.: A Substitute for Tobacco Smoking. *Psychopharmacologia*. 31:301 – 304, 1973.

Fiore M.C.: Tobacco Use and Dependence Guideline Panel. Treating Tobacco Use and Dependence. US Department of Health and Human Services, Public Health service, Rockville (Maryland), 2000.

Fiore M.C., Bailey W.C., Cohen S.J.: Treating Tobacco Use and Dependence. A Clinical Practice Guideline. US Department of Health and Human Services. Rockville MD, 2000.

Fiore M.C., Smith S.S., Jorenby D.E. and Baker T.B.: The Effectiveness of Nicotine Patch for Smoking Cessation. A Meta-analysis. *Journal of American Medical Association*, 271(24): 1940–1947, 1994.

Foulds J: The Neurobiological Basis for Partial Agonist Treatment of Nicotine Dependence: Varenicline. International Journal of Clinical Practice, 60:571–576, 2006.

Frank R.G., Umlauf R.L., Wonderlich S.A., Ashkanazi, G.S.: Hypnosis and Behavioural Treatment in A Worksite Smoking Cessation Programme. *Addictive Behaviours*. 11: 59 – 62, 1986.

Gamberino W.C., Gold M.S.: Neurobiology of Tobacco Smoking and Other Addictive Disorders. *Psychiatric Clinics of North America*, 22: 301 – 312, 1999.

Gilbert R.M., Pope M.A.: Early Effects of Quitting Smoking. *Psychopharmacology*, 78:121 – 127, 1982.

Glad W. and Adesso V.J.: The Relative Importance of Socially Induced Tension and Behavioural Contagion for Smoking Behaviour. *Journal of Abnormal Psychology*. 85, 119 – 121. 1976.

Glasgow R.E.: Klesgres R.C., and Vasey M.W.: Controlling Smoking for Chronic Smokers: An Extension and Replication. *Addictive Behaviour*, 8(2):143–150, 1983.

Glasgow R.E., Lando H. and Rand: Pharmacological Treatment of Tobacco Dependence: Proceedings of the World Congress. *Health Psychology* (suppl.) 5:53–68, 1986.

Glassman A.H.: Cigarette Smoking: Implications for Psychiatric Illness. *JAMA*, 150: 546 – 553, 1993.

Glassman A.H., Helzer J.E., Covey L.S., Cottler L.B., Stetner F., Tipp J.E., Johnson J.: Smoking, Smoking Cessation and Major Depression. *JAMA*, 264: 1546 – 1549, 1990.

Glassman, A.H., Jackson W.K., Walsh, T., Roose, S.P., Rosenfield, B.,: Cigarette craving, Smoking withdrawal and Clonidine. *Science*. 226:864 – 866, 1984.

Glassman A.H., Stetner F., Walsh B.T., Raizman P.S., Fleiss J.L., Cooper T.B. and Covey L.S.: Heavy Smokers, Smoking Cessation and Clonidine: Results of A Double Blind, Randomized Trial. *Journal of the American Medical Association*. 259(19):2863–2866, 1988.

Goldberg, S.R., Spealman, R.D., Risner, M.E., Henningfield, J.E.: Control of Behaviour By Intravenous Injections in Laboratory Animals. *Pharmacology, Biochemistry and Behaviour.* 19(6): 1011 –1020, 1983.

Gonzales D., Rennard S.I., Nides M., Oncken C., Azoulay S. and Billing C.B.: Varenicline, an alfas-4, beta-2 Nicotine Acetylcholine Receptor Partial Agonist, Vs Sustained Release Bupropin and Placebo for Smoking Cessation: A Randomized Controlled Trial. *Journal of American Medical Association* (JAMA),296:47–55, 2006.

Gourlay S.G., Stead L.F., Benowitz N.L.: Clonidine for Smoking Cessation (Cochrane Review) In: Cochrane Library, Issue 1Oxfors: Update Software. *(http://www.cochrane.org/cochrane/revabstr/ab000058.htm)*, 1999.

Grabowski J.G. and Hall S.M.: Pharmacological Adjuncts in Smoking Cessation. NIDA Research Monograph 53. US Department of Health and Human Services, Publication Health service, Alcohol, Drug Abuse, and Mental Health Administration. National Institute on Drug Abuse, DHHS Publication No (ADM) 85–1333, 1985.

Grunberg N.E.: Behavioural and Biological Factors in the Relationship Between Body Weight and Tobacco Use. in Katkin ES, Manuck SB (Eds) *Advances in behavioural Medicine.* Vol. 2: JAI Press Inc: Greenwich, Connecticut, 1986.

Hajek P. Jackson P. Belcher M.: Long-term Use of Nicotine Chewing Gum: Occurrence, determinants, and effect of weight gain. *JAMA,* 260:1593 – 1596, 1988.

Halek C., Kerry S., Humphrey H., Crisp A.H. and Hughes J.M.: Relationship Between Smoking, Weight and Attitudes to Weight in Adolescent School Girls. *Postgraduate Medical Journal,* 69:100–106, 1993.

Hall, S.M., Rugg, D., Tunstall, C., and Jones, R.T.: Preventing Relapse of Cigarettes Smoking By Behavioural Skill Training. *Journal of Cinsulting and Clinical Psychology.* 52(3): 372 – 382, 1984.

Hall, R.G., Sachs, D.P.L., Hall, S.M., Benowitz, N.L.: Two Year Efficacies and Safety of Rapid Smoking Therapy in Patients With Cardiac and Pulmonary Disease. *Journal of Consulting and Clinical Psychology.* 52(4): 574 – 581. 1984.

Hall S.M., Tunstall C., Rugg D., Jones R.T. and Benowitz N.L.: Nicotine Gum and Behavioural Treatment in Smoking Cessation. *Journal of Counseling and Clinical Psychology,* 53(2): 256–258, 1985.

Hall S.M., Tunstall C., Ginsberg D., Benowitz N.L. and Jones T.R.: Nicotine Gum and Behaviour Treatment: A Placebo Controlled Trial, *Journal of Consulting and Clinical Psychology,* 55(4):603–605, 1987.

Hall, Reus V.I. and Munoz R.F.: Nor-triptyline and Cognitive-behaviour Therapy in the Treatment of Cigarette Smoking. *Archieves of General Psychiatry,* 55(8): 683–690, 1998.

Hamilton S.B., Bornstein P.H.: Broad-spectrum Behavioural Approach to Smoking Cessation: Effects of Social Support and Paraprofessional Training on the Maintenance of Treatment Effects. *Journal of Consulting and Clinical Psychology.* 47(3): 598 – 600, 1979.

Heatherton T.F., Kozlowski L.T., Frecker R.C. and Fagerstrom K.O.: The Fagerstrom Test for Nicotine dependence: a Revision of Fagerstrom Tolerance Questionnaire. *British Journal of Addiction.* 86:1119–1127, 1991.

Henningfield, JE, and Goldberg, SR: Control of Behaviour by Intravenous Nicotine Injections in Human Subjects. *Pharmacology, Biochemistry and Behaviour*. 19(6): 1021 – 1026, 1983.

Henningfield, J.E, Sampson, A., Nemeth-Coslett, R.: Effect of Nicotine replacement in tobacco withdrawal. Presented at the *American Psychological Convention*, Washington DC, 1986.

Henningfield J.E., and Jasinki D.R.: Pharmacological Basis for Nicotine Replacement. In: Pomerleau, O.F, Pomerleau C.S, Fagerstrom K.O, Henningfield J.E,Hughjes J.R (eds) Nicotine Replacement: A Critical Evaluation. Alan R Liss: New York, 1988.

Herman C.P.: External and Internal Cues As Determinants of the Smoking Behaviour of Light and Heavy Smokers. *Journal of Personality and Abnormal Psychology*. 30:664 – 672, 1974.

Hirvonen L.: Premises and Results of Smoking Withdrawal. In: forbes W.F., Frecker R.C., and Nostbakken D. (Eds) Proceedings of the Fifth world Conference on Smoking and Health. Canada Council on Smoking and Health, Winnipeg. Vol 2 pp 215–220.

Hjalmarson A.I.M.: Effect of Nicotine Chewing Gum in Smoking Cessation. A Randomized, Placebo-controlled, Double-blind Study. *Journal of the American Medical Association*, 252(20): 2835–2838, 1984.

Hughes, J.R., Goldstein, M.G., Hurt R.D., and Hoffman S: Recent Advances in the Pharmacotherapy of Smoking. *Journal of American Medical Association*, 281 72 – 76, 1999.

Hughes J.R. and Hatsukami D.: Signs and Aymptoms of Tobacco Withdrawal. *Archieves of General Psychiatry*, 43(3): 289–294, 1986.

Hunt W.A., Barnett L.W., and Branch L.G.: Relapse Rates in Addiction Programmes. *Journal of Clinical Psychology*, 27(4): 455–456, 1971.

Hurt R.D., of ford K.P. and Croughan I.T.: Temporal Effects of Nicotine Nasal Spray and Gum on Nicotine Withdrawal Symptoms. Psychopharmacology, 140(1): 98–104, 1998.

Hurt R.D., Sachs D.R., Glover E.D., of ford R.P., Johnston J.A.: dale L.C.: A Comparison of Sustained Release Bupropion and Placebo, for Smoking Cessation. *New England Journal of Medicine*. 337: 1195 – 1202, 1997.

Ikard, F.F., Green, D.E., Horn D.: A Scale to Differentiate Between Types of Smoking As Related to the Management of Affect. *International Journal of Addictions*.4 (4):649 – 659, 1969.

Ikard, F.F., and Tompkind, S.: The Experience of Affect As A Determinant of Smoking Behaviour: A Series of Validity Studies. *Journal of Abnormal Psychology*. 81(2): 172 – 181, 1973.

Jaffe J.H.: Drug addiction and Drug abuse. In: Gilman AG and Goodman LS, Rail TW, Murad F (Eds) Goodman and Gilman's the Pharmacologic Basis of Therapeutics. 7th edition, McMillan: New York, 1985.

Jamrozic K., Fowler G., Vessey M. and Wald N.: Placebo Controlled Trial of Nicotine Chewing Gum in General Practice. British Medical Journal, 289(6448): 794–797, 1984.

Jarvik, M.E. and Schneider, N.G.: Degree of Addiction and Effectiveness of Nicotine Gum Therapy for Smoking. *American Journal of Psychiatry*. 141(6):790 – 791, 1984.

Jarvis M.J.: Nasal Nicotine solution: Its Potential in Smoking Cessation and As A Research Tool. In: Ockne Jk (Eds) the Pharmacologic Treatment of Tobacco Dependence. Proceedings of the World Congress. Institute for the Study of Smoking Behaviour and Policy: Cambridge Massachusetts, 1982.

Jarvis M.J., Raw M., Russell M.A.H. and Feyerabend C.: Randomized Controlled Trial of Nicotine Chewing-gum. British Medical Journal, 258(6341):537–540, 1982.

Javel A.F.: One-session Hypnotherapy for Smoking. A Controlled Study. *Psychological Reports.* 46(part 1): 895 – 899. 1980.

Johnston J.A., Hughes A.R. and Ascher J.A.: Evaluation of Safety and Tolerability of Bupropion Sr As An Ad to Smoking Cessation. Poster Presentation at the 5th Annual Meeting of *the Society for Research on Nicotine and Tobacco.* San Diego CA, 1999.

Johnston, Leonox M: Tobacco smoking and Nicotine. *Lancet.* 2:242, 1942.

Jorenby D.E., Hays J.T., Rigotti N.A., Azoulay S., Wastsky E.J. and Williams K.E.: Efficacy of Varenicline, an alfa-4, beta-2 Nicotine Acetylcholine Receptor Partial Agonist, Vs Placebo Or Sustained Release Bupropion for Smoking Cessation: A Randomized Controlled Trial. *Journal of American Medical Association* (JAMA),296:56–63, 2006.

Kabat G.C. and Wynder E.L.: Determinants of Quitting Smoking. *American Journal of Public Health,* 77:1301–1305, 1987.

Katz N.W.: Hypnosis and the Addiction: a Critical Review. *Addictive Behaviours.* 5(1): 41 – 47, 1980.

Kenkel, D., Chen, L.: Consumer Information and Tobacco Use. In: Jha, P., Chaloupka, FJ, eds.*Tobacco Control in Developing Countries.* Oxford University Press: Oxford. 177 – 214, 2000.

Killen J.D., fortmann S.P., Newman B.: Weight Change Among Participants in A Large Sample Minimal Contact Smoking Relapse Prevention Trial. *Addictive Behaviour,* 15: 323 – 332, 1990.

Kornitzer, M., Kittel, F., Dramaix, M., Bourdoux, P.: A Double Blind Study of 2 Mg Vs 4 Mg Nicotine Chewing Gum in An Industrial Setting. *Journal of Psychosomatic Research.* 31(2):171 – 176, 1987.

Lando H.A.: Stimulus Control Rapid Smoking and Contractual Management in the Maintenance of Nonsmoking. *Behaviour Therapy.* 9: 962 – 963, 1978.

Lairson D.R., Harrist R., Martin D.W., Ramby R., Rustin T.A. and Swint J.M.: Screening for Patients With Alcohol Problem: Severity of Patients Identified with CAGE. *Journal of Drug Education,* 22:337–352, 1992.

Leventhal, H., and Cleary, P.D.: The Smoking problem: a Review of Research and Theory in Behavioural Risk Modification. *Psychological Bulletin.* 88(2): 370 – 405, 1980.

Lichtenstein, E., Harris, D.E., Birchler, G.R., Wahi, J.M., Schmahal, D.P.: Comparison of Rapid Smoking, Warm, Smoky Air, and Attention Placebo in the Modification of Smoking Behaviour. *Journal of Consulting and Clinical Psychology.* 40(1): 92 – 98, 1973.

Malcom R.E., Sillett R.W., Turner J.A.M. and Ball K.P.: The Use of Nicotine Chewing Gum As An Aid to Stopping Smoking. *Psychopharmacology.*70:295–296, 1980.

Malcolm, R., Currey, H.S., Mitchell, M.A. and Keil, T.: Silver Acetate Gum As A Deterrent to Smoking. *Chest* 90(1): 107 – 111, 1986.

Mansvelder H.D., McGehee D.S.: Long-term Potentiation of Excitatory Inputs to Brain Reward Areas By Nicotine. *Neuron,* 27:349 – 357, 2000.

Marlatt G.A. and Gordon J.R.: Determinants of Relapse: Implications for the Maintenance of Behaviour Change. In: Davidson PO and Davidson SM (Eds) Behavioural Medicine: Changing Health Life-style Brunner Mazel, New York, 410–452, 1980.

Miller N.S. and Brady K.T.: Addictive Disorders. *Psychiatric Clinics of North America*, 2727(4): 627–648, 2004.

Moffatt P.M., Owens S.G.: Cessation from Cigarette Smoking: Changes in Body Weight, Body Composition, Resting Metabolism and Energy Consumption. *Metabolism*, 40: 465 – 470, 1991.

Morton J.L., Jones T.V. and Manganaro M.A.: Performace of Alcoholism Screening Questionnaire in Elderly Veterans. *American Journal of Medicine*, 101: 153–159, 1996.

Nemeth-Coslett, R., and Henningfield, J.E.: Effects of Nicotine Chewing Gum on Cigarette Smoking and Subjective and Physiological Effect. *Clinical Pharmacology and Therapeutics*. 39(6): 625 – 630, 1986.

Ossip-Klein D.J., Giovino G.A., Black P., Shulman E., Bonnani A.M. and Seidman R.: Determinants of Smoking Relapse and Predictors of Outcome. Presented at the Meeting of the Society of Behavioural Medicine, San Francisco, California, 1986.

Paxton R.: Prolonging the Effects of Deposit Contracts With Smokers. *Behavioural Research and Therapy*. 21(4): 425 – 433, 1983.

Perkins K.A.: Effects of Tobacco Smoking on Caloric Intake. *British Journal of Addiction*, 87: 193 – 205, 1992.

Perkins K.A., Epstein L.H., Marks B.L., Stiller R.L., Jacob R.G.: The Effect of Nicotine on Energy Expenditure During Light Physical Activity. *New England Journal of Medicine*, 320: 898 – 903, 1989.

Perkin K.A., Levine M.D., Marcus M.D., Shiffman S.: Addressing Women's Concern About Weight Gain Due to Smoking Cessation. *Journal of Substance Abuse Treatment*. 14: 173 – 182, 1997.

Pirie P.L., McBride C.M., Hellersteidt W., Jeffery R.W., Hatsukami D., Allen S., Lando H.: Smoking Cessation in Women Concerned About Weight. *American Journal of Public Health*, 82: 1238 – 1243, 1992.

Pirie P.L., Murray D.M., Luepker, R.V.: Smoking and Quitting in A Cohort of Young Adults. *American Journal of Public Health*, 81: 324 – 327, 1991.

Piper M.E., Fox B.J. and Fiore M.C.: Strategies for Smoking Cessation, *American College of Chest Physicians*, Lesson 13 volume 15, 2001.

Pomerleau, O.F., Adkins, D., Pertschuk, M.: Predictors of Outcome and Recidivism in Smoking Cessation Treatment. *Addictive Behaviour*. 3(2): 65 – 70, 1978.

Pomerleau, O.F., Pomerleau, C.S., Fagerstrom, K.O., Henningfield, J.E., Hughes, J.R.: Nicotine Replacement: A Critical Evaluation, Alan R Liss Inc, New York, 1988.

Pritchard C.W.: Depression and Smoking in Pregnancy in Scotland. *Journal of Epidemiology and Community Health*. 484: 377 – 382, 1994.

Prochazka A.V., Weaver M.J., Keller R.T., Fryer G.E., Licari P.A. and Lofaso D.: A Randomized Trial of Nortriptyline for Smoking Cessation. *Archieves of International Medicine*, 158(18): 2035–2039, 1998.

Puska P., Bjorkqvist S. and Koskela K.: Nicotine Containing Chewing Gum in Smoking Cessation: A Double Blind Trial With Half Year Follow Up. *Addictive Behaviour* 4(2): 141–146, 1987.

Rabkin S.W. Boyko E., Shane F. and Kaufert J.: A Randomized Trial Comparing Smoking Cessation Programme Utilizing Behaviour Modification, Health Education and Hypnosis. *Addictive Behaviour*, 9(2): 157–173, 1984.

Raw M., McNeill A., West R.: Smoking Cessation: Evidence Based Recommendations for the Health-care System. *British Medical Journal*. 318: 182 – 185, 1999.

Rose J.E., Sampson A. and Henningfield J.E.: Blocking of Smoking Satisfaction with Mecamylamine. Paper Presented to American Psychological Association' Los Angeles (CA). 1985.

Russell M.A.H.: Conceptual Framework for Nicotine Substitution. In: Ockne JK (Eds)The Pharmacologic Treatment of Tobacco Dependence: Proceedings of World Congress, Institute for Study of Smoking Behaviour and Policy. Cambridge, Massachusetts. 1986.

Russell, M.A.H.: The Nicotine Addiction Trap: A Four-year Sentence for Four Cigarettes. *British Journal of Addiction*. 85:293 – 300, 1990.

Russell M.A.H. and Feyerabend C.: Cigarette Smoking: A Dependence on High-nicotine Boli. *Drug Metabolis Review*, 8(1): 29–57, 1978.

Russell M.A.H., Jarvis M.J. Feyerabend C. and Ferno O.: Nasal Nicotine Solution: A Potential Aid to Giving Up Smoking. *British Medical Journal*, 286(366): 683–684, 1983.

Rustin T.A. and Tata J.C.: Measuring the Stages of Change in Cigarette Smokers. Journal of *Substance Abuse Treatment*, 10:209–220, 1993.

Schneider N.G., Jarvik M.E., forsythe A.B., Read L.L., Eliott M.L., Schweiger A.: A Nicotine Gum in Smoking Cessation: A Placebo Controlled Double Blind Trial. *Addictive Behaviour* 8(3): 256 – 261, 1983.

Schneider N.G., Jarvik, M.E., forsythe A.B.: Nicotine Versus Placebo Gum in the Alleviating the Withdrawal During Smoking Cessation. *Addictive Behaviour* 9(2): 149 – 156, 1984.

Schneider N.G., Olmstead R.E., Franzon M.A. and Lunell E.: The Nicotine Inhaler: Clinical Pharmacokinetics and Comparison With Other Nicotine Treatments. *Clinical Pharmacokinetics*, 40(9):661–684, 2001.

Schuh K.J., Schuh L.M., Henningfield J.E., Stitzer, M.L.,: Nicotine Nasal Spray and Vapor Inhaler: Abuse Liability Assessment. *Psychopharmacology*. 130: 352 – 365, 1997.

Schwartz J.L.: Review and Evaluation of Smoking Cessation Methods: United Public Health Service, National Institute of Healt NIH. Publication No 87, 2940, 1987.

Shiffman S.M.: The Tobacco Withdrawal Syndrome. In: Krasnegor NA (Ed) Cigarette Smoking as a Dependence Process. *NIDA Research Monograph*, 23:158 – 184, 1979.

Shiffman S., Dresler C.M., Hajek P., Gilburt S.J., Targett D.A. and Strahs K.R.: Efficacy of a Nicotine Lozenge for Smoking Cessation. *Archieves of Internal Medicine*, 162(11): 1267–1276, 2002.

Shiffman S.M. and Jarvik M.E.: Situational Determinants of Coping in Smoking Relapse Crises. *Journal of Applied Social Psychology* 17(1): 3–15, 1987.

Shiffman, S., Maltese, J., Jarvik, M.E.: Coping Skill and Coping Style in the Maintenance of Nonsmoking. A symposium conducted at the meeting of the *American Psychological Association*. Washington DC, 1982.

Shimokata H., Muller D.C., andres R.,: Studies in the Distribution of Fat: Effects of Cigarette Smoking. *Journal of American Medical Association*, 261:1169 – 1173, 1992.

Silagy C., Mant D., Fowler G. and Lodge M.: Meta-analysis on Efficacy of Nicotine Replacement Therapies in Smoking Cessation. Lancet, 343:139–142, 1994.

Sofuoglu M. and Kosten T.R.: Pharmacological Management of Relapse Prevention in Addictive Disorders. *Psychiatric Clinics of North America*, 27,627–648, 2004.

Spiegel H.: A Single-treatment Method to Stop Smoking Using Ancillary Self-hypnosis. International *Journal of Clinical and Experimental Hypnosis*. 18(4): 235 – 250. 1970.

Stewart M.J., Bosky G., Gillis A., Jackson S., Johnston G., Kirkland S., Leigh G., Pawliw-Fry B.A., Persud V., Rootman I.: Disadvantaged Women and Smoking. *Canadian Journal of Public Health*, 87: 257 – 260, 1996.

Stitzer M.L. and Bigelow G.E.: Contigent Re-inforcement for Reduced Carbon Monoxide Levels in Cigarette Smokers. *Addictive Behaviours*. 7:403 – 412, 1982.

Stitzer, M.L. and Gross, J.: Smoking Relapses: The Role of Pharmacological and Behavioural Factors. In: Pomerleau, OF, Pomerleau, CS, Fagerstrom, KO, Henningfield, JE, Hughes, JR (Eds.) *Nicotine Replacement: a Critical Evaluation*. New York: Alan R Liss Inc, 1988.

Stolerman, I.P.: Discriminative Stimulus Properties in Nicotine: Correlations with Nicotine Binding. Proceedings of the International Symposium on *Tobacco Smoking and Health: A Neuro-biologic Approach*, 1986.

Sutherland Gay: Current approaches to the Management of Smoking Cessation. *Drugs*. 62(Suppl) 2: 53–61, 2002.

Sweeney C.T., Fant R.V., Fagerstrom K.O., McGovern J.F. and Henningfield J.E.: Combination Nicotine Replacement Therapy for Smoking Cessation: Rationale Efficacy and Tolerability. CNS Drugs, 15(6)453–467, 2001.

Tennant F.S., Traver A.L., Rawson R.A.: Clinical Evaluation of Mecamylamine for Withdrawal From Nicotine Dependence. In: Harrison LS (Ed) Problems of Drug-dependence 1983 NIDA. Research Monograph 49 UD Department of Health and Human Services, 1984.

Tiffany, S.T., Martin, E.M., Baker, T.B.: Treatments for Cgarette Smoking: An Evaluation of the Contributions of Aversion and Counseling Procedures. *Behavour, Research and Therapy*.24 (4): 437 – 452, 1986.

Tonnessen, P: International Update on Nicotine, In: Ockene, JK (ends) the Pharmacologic Treatment of Tobacco Dependence: Proceedings of the World Congress. Cambridge, Massachusetts: Institute for the *Study of Smoking Behaviour and Policy*. 1985.

Wagner T.J., Hindi-Alexander M., Horwitz M.B.,: A One Year Follow-up Study of the Damon Group Hypnosis Smoking Cessation Programme. *Journal of the Oklahoma State Medical Association*. 76(12), 414 – 416, 1983.

Ward K.D., Klessges R.C., Zbikowski, S.M., Bliss, R.E., Garvey A.J.: Gender differences in the outcome of an unaided smoking cessation attempt. *Addiction Behaviour*. 19:159 – 173. 1997.

Weekley C.K., Klesges R.C., Relyea G.: Smoking as a Weight Control Strategy and Its Relationship to Smoking Status. *Addictive Behaviour*, 17: 259 – 271, 1993.

Weinstein N.D.: Accuracy of Smokers' Risk Perception. *Annals of Behavioural Medicine.* 20:135 – 140, 1998.

West R.J., Hajek P., Foulds J., Nilsson F., May S. and Meadow A.: A Comparison of the Abuse Liability and Dependence Potential of Nicotine Patch, Gum, Spray and Inhaler. Psychopharmacology, 149(3): 198–202, 2000.

West R.J., Jarvis M.J., Russell M.A.H., Feyerabend C.: Plasma Nicotine Concentrations From Repeated Doses of Nasal Nicotine Solution. *British Journal of Addiction.* 79: 443 – 445, 1984.

West R.J. and Schneider N.: Craving for Cigarettes. *British Journal of Addiction.* 82: 407 – 415, 1987.

White A.R., Rampes H.: Acupuncture for Smoking Cessation. (Cochrane Review). In: The Cochrane Library, Issue 1 Oxford: Update Software. (http://www.cochrane.org/cochrane/revabtr/ab000009.htm), 1999.

Wilcox N.S., Prochaska J.O., Velicer W.F. and Diclemente C.C.: Subject Characteristics as Predictors of Self Change in Smoking. *Addictive Behaviour.* 10:407–412, 1985.

Williams M., Sullivan J.P., Arneric S.P.: Neuronal Nicpotinr Acetylcholine Receptors. *Drug News and Perspective.* 7: 205 – 223, 1994.

Williomson *et al*, 1991.

Wills T.A., Shiffman S.: Coping and Substance Use: A Conceptual Framework, In: Shiffman S, Wills TA (eds.) *Coping and Substance Use.* Academic Press, Orlando, 3 – 24, 1985.

World Health Organization, Policy Recommendations for Smoking Cessation and Treatment of Tobacco Dependence, http://www.who.int/tobacco/resources/publications/tobacco_dependence/en. 2003.

Zmeili S., Salhab A., Shubair K., Gharaibeh M., Suliman N., Al-Kayed A., Shubair M., Abu Hijleh N., Abu Jbara M.: Clinical Evaluation of A New A.s. Mouthwash 881010 As An Antismoking Agent: A Placebo-controlled Double Blind Trial. *International Journal of Clinical Pharmacology and Therapeutics.* 37: 41 – 50, 1999.

CHAPTER

# 11 Tobacco Control in India

*Tobacco use has an adverse impact on health, environment, education ... and leads to poverty, malnutrition. Consequently, tobacco control has to be recognized as a key component of efforts to reduce poverty, improve development and progress towards the Millennium Development Goals.*

— UN Secretary General's Report on Tobacco Control, 2004.

Since the introduction of tobacco cultivation in Jamestown, Virginia in 1613, tobacco has assumed major social, industrial, economic and medical importance in the world history. Tobacco rapidly became the mainstream commodity of the Maryland and Virginia economics and in the early 18$^{th}$ century it served as the currency of Virginia (Morison, 1994). Consequently, cultivation, production, sale and consumption of tobacco have witnessed a varied range of regulations and legislation throughout the world. For nearly 400 years now, these regulations have been effected to control or influence its production, sale and to a lesser extent, its use. Even before its introduction on commercial scales in Jamestown, the attempt to impose regulatory control on tobacco use was made by King James I of England in 1604 by imposing a heavy tax on its import so that only rich people could afford it. However, his fulminations against tobacco use could do little to check its proliferation when he discovered tobacco to be a rich source of revenue. Unlike James I of England, King Luis XIV (1643–1715) of France never attacked tobacco but his dislike for it was well known. However, when he came to know the financial gains from tobacco trade, it was used as a source of much needed revenues. In Italy, Pope Innocent X, forbade tobacco use in St Peter's basilica under penalty of excommunication in 1650, however, tobacco use continued due to similar reasons. Evidently, the economics of tobacco were most seductive in all European countries.

While the Western European governments with initial resistance finally became flexible towards tobacco production and use, Russia and Turkey prohibited it with severest of punishments. The Turkish attitude was based on religious and lay opposition. Most of the crusades by anti-tobacconists, from the very beginning were notably their intolerance; their ignorance and more often than not their complacent stupidity[1]. Tobacco regulations devised to curb the prevalence of

---

[1] Brooks Jerome E (1952) The Mighty Leaf: Tobacco through the Centuries. Little Brown & Company: Boston.

tobacco use only helped further the prosperity of the industry to make it available everywhere by seventeenth century. Subsequent years of global availability of tobacco permitted the concerned governments to experiment with prohibitions and permissions from time to time and country to country but there has never been a time when tobacco was prohibited throughout the world. The campaign inaugurated at the end of nineteenth century, and resumed prior to World War I, was the most venomous and acrimonious of all. The spectacular growth of cigarette consumption immediately following the war infuriated opponents of smoking habit and inspired them to intensify efforts for further regulations. These regulations meant to prohibit cigarette use, only served as a lure and helped to raise revenue. The dynamics of taxation played a part in the acceptance of tobacco products especially the cigarettes. Some lawmakers favoured taxation because they considered it to be a restrictive measure[2].

Experiences show, however, that smokers, though they might grumble, would pay whatever taxes were assessed. By the time this acquiescence is generally conceded, the fast growth of revenue to governments raises cigarette taxes to a place of importance in government budgets

No doubt, though tobacco offers bountiful revenue to the governments, provides employment to many, and helps societies with several other economic "benefits," anti-tobacconists opposed its cultivation and use for various reasons.

Between 1895 and 1909 twelve American states banned cigarettes totally, but every ban had to be repealed by 1927 (Brooks, 1952). Opposition to tobacco was based on moral and aesthetic principles with little emphasis on the health consequences. On the other hand, proponents of the leaf stressed its social benefits and its economic and industrial significance. Some enthusiasts even endorsed its alleged medical and psychological benefits. Opposed were those who were convinced of its immorality.

A feature of the present situation, however, is that antismoking sentiment is firmly anchored in widely accepted medical evidence. Reports on adverse effects of smoking started pouring in from the first quarter of the 20th century and today, it is proved beyond doubt that tobacco consumption is a major cause of morbidity and mortality and imposes considerable costs, including the direct costs of health care and indirect costs of lost productivity. It is clearly evident that tobacco use is harmful for health, and in course of time, can lead to grave health hazards in the form of lung cancer, chronic bronchitis, heart and artery diseases and cancers of various other organs.

Tobacco may cause property loss through fires, raise the cost of fire protection, and may lead to deforestation because of extensive use of wood for flue curing of tobacco. Equally important are the real costs entailed in looking after the smokers during their illness, the loss of production and lower productivity, on account of avoidable tobacco-related diseases and mortality, higher overall health and welfare spending, opportunity cost foregone by its consumption[3].

---

2. Wagner Susan (1971) Cigarette Country: Tobacco in American History and Politics. Praeger: New York.
3 Warner KE (1998) Economics of Tobacco and Health: An overview. In: Abedien I, *et al.*, (eds.) Proceedings of the Conference on Economics of Tobacco Control; towards an optimal policy mix. Applied Fiscal Research Centre, University of Cape Town: Cape Town.

While the governments and health agencies of the developed countries have met with considerable success in their campaign to reduce prevalence of cigarette smoking, the position in the developing countries is reversed (Taha and Ball, 1980).

The expanding market for the cigarettes in the developing countries is supplied primarily by imports. The number and variety of individuals, cigarette companies and governments vitally interested in continued growing, trading and manufacturing, pose serious hurdles in the process of tobacco control.

Global cooperation is crucial to the success of efforts to prevent health hazards of smoking by controlling its use. Trends affecting tobacco consumption are increasingly cross-border. While tobacco consumption in the industrialized world has declined in the last twenty years, it has steadily increased in the developing countries especially the South Asian countries.

The status of tobacco control has varied widely among countries in South Asian Region that is the target of major companies. Some countries totally lacked or had very minimal tobacco control laws, while other countries having much better control measures. The need for tobacco control in this region becomes necessary because in addition to causing health problems, tobacco causes individual economic hardship. Among very poor people, expenditures on tobacco often occur in lieu of expenditures on other essential items. Political commitment to tobacco control in the region, till recently, has remained rather weak, and advocacy efforts in this direction were nearly non-existent. Initiative by the WHO to curb the menace of tobacco is an important step in this direction.

## The W.H.O. Framework Convention on Tobacco Control (FCTC)

As an UN organization, the WHO has a constitutional mandate to initiate the development and facilitate the adoption of international treatise, such as a framework convention. A framework convention is an international legal instrument that contemplates progressive development of international law by establishing a general system of governance for a specific issue. It lays down general requirements for countries (member states of WHO), with respect to the measures they need to take in the area covered by the convention. It is expected that the member states would modify existing laws or develop new national laws that would reflect the commitments they have undertaken. At the international level, more specific commitments and institutional arrangements for implementing them would be developed and adopted through specific protocols that cover some of the key areas identified by the convention. Follow-up action is taken both at national and international levels. For tobacco control, WHO's 39$^{th}$ World Health Assembly meeting on 15$^{th}$ May, 1986 urged the member states to implement the measures to ensure that effective protection was provided to non-smokers from involuntary exposure to tobacco smoke and to protect children and young people from being addicted to the use of tobacco. WHO reiterated its concern in meeting held on the 17th May, 1990 and urged the member states to consider in their tobacco control strategies for legislation and other effective measures for protecting their citizens with special attention to risk groups such as pregnant women and children from involuntary exposure to tobacco smoke and to discourage the use of tobacco and impose progressive restrictions and take concerted action to eventually eliminate all direct and indirect advertising, promotion and sponsorship concerning tobacco. In May, 1999, WHO's Framework Convention on Tobacco Control (FCTC) provided the basic tool for the countries to enact comprehensive tobacco control legislation and take on the powerful tobacco industry. The treaty commits nations to ban all tobacco advertising, promotion, and sponsorship (with an exception of constitutional constraints) and to require large warning labels covering at least 30% of the display area of the cigarette pack.

In May, 2003 the World Health Organization (WHO) completed five years of work that brought scientific certainty and political will around a set of global rules for tobacco sales, promotion and consumption. The Organization's 192 member states unanimously adopted the Framework Convention on Tobacco Control (FCTC). While supporting the resolution the WHO member countries called for an international attempt to regulate tobacco use; a record breaking 50 countries out of 192 pledged financial and political support. In adopting and signing the treaty, the WHO's member states expressed their firm commitment to tackle the public health challenges posed by tobacco and resolved to address such key issues as price and tax measures, tobacco related issues, cross-border smuggling, tobacco advertising and promotion, and people's right to clean indoor air. Following are the actions to be taken by the member states and international cooperation measures taken at convention level (Table 1).

***Table 1: Framework for national action and international cooperation****

| *Framework for national action* | *Framework for international cooperation* |
|---|---|
| • Comprehensive ban on advertising<br>• Protection against secondary smoke<br>• Prohibition of youth access<br>• Prominent health warnings<br>• Testing and regulation of contents<br>• Increase in tobacco taxes<br>• Cessation programmes<br>• Alternative crops<br>• Surveillance | • Ban on cross-border advertising<br>• Prevention of illicit trade<br>• Scientific and legal cooperation<br>• Technical assistance<br>• Financial support for FCTC implementation (bilateral and multilateral channels)<br>• Monitoring |
| Requires partnership within countries | Requires partnership among countries. |

**Report on Tobacco Control in India (1964) Government of India Publication, 2004*

The WHO has been encouraging the adoption of national laws and regulations for tobacco control for a long time, the FCTC is the first ever-international public health treaty of any kind. FCTC has designed the fundamental matrix of measures essential for tobacco control, while the protocols would be negotiated later on specific issues such as cross-border advertising, promotion and sponsorship of tobacco product regulation, illicit trade in tobacco, and liability. The final text of the FCTC is developed and approved by the International Negotiating Body (INB). The FCTC sets out guidelines for various national and international measures that would encourage smokers to quit and restrain non-smokers from taking to the habit. It promotes smoke-free environment policies, banning of advertisements, increase in taxes, reduced youth access to tobacco products as well as education and media campaigns to increase awareness about the health hazards of tobacco consumption and the health benefits of tobacco cessation. It envisages international co-operation, including promotion and transfer of technical, scientific and legal expertise, and technology, in assisting the development of a strong legislative foundation and technical programmes for protection from exposure to tobacco smoke and other tobacco products. Each member country is expected to implement these provisions, in accordance with its capacity and constitution. However, there is large degree of operational flexibility in implementing the measures recommended by the FCTC, though it explicitly encourages countries to implement measures that are stronger than the minimum standard required by the treaty.

India has advocated strong provisions that would favour effective tobacco control, has provided leadership to the Southeast Asian countries. To achieve the objective of the Convention and to implement its provisions, certain guiding principles are elaborated which emphasize the need for: informing people of the health hazards of tobacco; strong political commitment on tobacco control; international cooperation; multi-sectoral tobacco policies; liability as a tobacco control strategy; technical and financial assistance for economies adversely affected by tobacco control programmes; and the participation of civil society in tobacco control efforts. General obligations on the part of the Member States are to develop and periodically update and review comprehensive multi-sectoral national tobacco control strategies, plans and programmes in accordance with the Convention.

To achieve the objective, FCTC recommends demand reduction measures, supply reduction measures and measures to establish and enhance international cooperation (Table 2). The FCTC is without the mandated provision for a voluntary global fund. The COP is to review the existing and potential sources. However, the Treaty became international law on 27th February, 2005 when it completed 40 ratifications which was the minimum requirement for the FCTC to enter into force. FCTC is an international legal instrument to control the devastating health, social, environmental and economic consequences of tobacco consumption worldwide. On 26th May, 2006, of the 168 signatories of FCTC 128 countries have ratified it.

Recent legislation enactment and Framework Convention on Tobacco Control (FCTC) ratification by India are the steps towards beginning of a major national effort to deal with the threat posed by tobacco effectively. A comprehensive multi-component strategy implemented through coordinated multi-sectoral measures is required. The strategy should combine measures for demand reduction and reduction of supply. Demand reduction usually leads to reduction in supply, it may not be completely true in case of tobacco because of its addictive properties. Such measures involve interventions at multiple levels:

The Indian government has been pursuing a proactive and bold strategy for tobacco control. Although the Indian Tobacco Act (2003) goes beyond the obligations set out in the FCTC in many respects, there is a need for some additional measures to be taken, to ensure full conformity with the FCTC.

*Table 2: FCTC Recommendations*

***Taxation and Duty-free sale***

Tax policies should aim to help tobacco control.

- Tax and price policies to promote tobacco control recommended for national-level action. Duty-free sales are discouraged.
- Countries may prohibit/restrict duty-free sales and importation.

***Second hand smoking (Article 8)***

Non-smokers must be protected from exposure to tobacco smoke. Such protection must extend to :

Indoor workplaces.

- Public transport.
- Indoor public places.
- Other public places, as appropriate.

***Product Regulation and ingredient disclosure (Article 9 and 10)***

Tobacco products are to be regulated.

- COP shall propose guidelines for testing and measuring the contents and emission.
- Countries shall adopt and implement measures for such testing, measuring and regulation. Ingredients are to be disclosed.
- Manufacturers and importers shall disclose, to the governmental authorities, information on content and emission.
- Measures for public disclosure of information about toxic constituents and emissions.

***Packaging and Labeling (Article 11)***

Large health warning labels are required.

- Rotating warnings.
- Large, Clear, Visible and Legible.
- Should be 50% or more of the principal display area (should not be less than 30%).
- May be in the form of or include pictures/pictograms. Deceptive labels must be prohibited.
- False/misleading term, descriptor, trademark or any other sign shall be prohibited (e.g. mild, low tar, light).

*Contd...*

*Education, Communication, Trading and Public Awareness (Article 12)*

Each party shall promote and strengthen public awareness of tobacco control issues.

- Broad excess to effective and comprehensive educational and public awareness programmes on:-
  — Health risks of tobacco consumption
  — Risks of exposure to tobacco smoke
  — Risk of addiction
  — Benefits of tobacco-cessation
- Public access to a range of information on the tobacco industry.
- Training or sensitization and awareness programmes to various stakeholder groups.
- Public awareness and access to information on the health, economic and environmental consequences of tobacco production and consumption.

*Advertising, Promotion and Sponsorship (Article 13)*

A comprehensive ban is required. Restriction regime is permitted only for countries with constitutional barriers.

- Restriction regime is permitted only for countries with constitutional barriers.
- Minimum package of measures prescribed.
- Direct and indirect advertising and promotion covered.
- Cross-border advertising subject to ban and penalty.
- Protocol on cross-border advertising recommended.

*Tobacco dependence and Cessation (Article 14)*

Parties shall take effective measures to promote cessation of tobacco use and adequate treatment of tobacco dependence.

- Design and implement effective tobacco cessation programmes in such locations as educational institutions, health-care facilities, workplace and sporting environments.
- Include diagnosis and treatment to tobacco dependence and counseling services on tobacco cessation on national health and educational programmes, plans and strategies.
- Establish tobacco cessation programmes in health care facilities and rehabilitation centres.
- Facilitate accessibility and affordability for treatment of tobacco dependence including pharmaceutical products.

*Smuggling (Article 15)*

Action is required to eliminate tobacco smuggling.

- Origin and final destination must be indicated on packaging.
- Develop a practical tracking/tracing regime.
- Confiscate products and proceeds of illicit trade.
- Cooperate with one-another in anti-smuggling, law enforcement, and litigation efforts.

*Sale to and by Minors (Article 16)*

- Parties shall prohibit the sale of tobacco products under the age set by national law or eighteen years of age.

*Contd...*

- Parties shall prohibit or promote the prohibition of the distribution of the free tobacco products.
- Curb on or prohibition of tobacco vending machines.
- Prohibition of sale by minors, as per national law.

***Financing (Article 26)***

Parties have committed themselves to promote funding for global tobacco control.

- Mobilize financial assistance from all available sources for developing countries and economies in transition.
- Encourage regional and international intergovernmental organizations to contribute.
- Strengthen existing mechanisms for bilateral and multilateral contributions.
- COP will consider proposals for a global fund.

***Scope for economically viable alternatives (Article 17)***

Parties shall promote, as appropriate, economically viable alternatives for tobacco control.

***Liability (Article 19)***

Legal action is encouraged as a tobacco control strategy.

***National Coordination Mechanism (Article 5)***

Each party shall establish or reinforce and finance a national coordinating mechanism or focal point for tobacco control.

***Participation of Non-governmental Organizations (Article 12 and 20)***

Parties shall promote awareness and participation of non-governmental organizations, not affiliated with tobacco industry, in developing and implementing inter-sectoral programmes and strategies for tobacco control (Article 12) and cooperate with non-governmental agencies in regional and global tobacco surveillance and exchange of information (Article 20)

***Treaty Oversight (Article 23)***

A COP will oversee the implementation of the treaty.

*Secretariat (Article 24):* COP will designate a permanent secretariat. WHO will act as the interim secretariat.

***Settlement of Disputes (Article 27):*** Parties shall settle disputes through negotiation, mediation, or conciliation failing which arbitration will be restored to as prescribed by the COP.

***Source:*** *Report on Tobacco Control in India (2004) Government of India, Centres for Disease Control and Prevention USA and the WHO Publication.*

## Tobacco Control in India

In the initial decades of independent India, tobacco was considered as a source of revenue from taxes and exports rather than a harmful commodity. Even as the knowledge of tobacco's ill-effects grew, it was believed in most countries including India, that the taxes paid and other economic benefits flowing from tobacco related activities in terms of output, employment, exports, reduced pension and social benefits availed of by tobacco users, etc. easily offset the putative direct and indirect, pecuniary, costs arising from tobacco consumption(Kenneth, 1998).

Effective tobacco control in other parts of the world has been achieved via multi-pronged strategies focusing on reducing the demand for tobacco products (Jha *et al,* 2000). These strategies include the activities such as raising taxes; publishing and disseminating information about the adverse health effects of tobacco, including prominent health warning labels to products; imposing comprehensive bans on advertising and promotion; restricting smoking in workplaces and public places; and extending access to nicotine replacement alternatives and other cessation therapies.

## Legislative Control

The demand reduction strategies are typically accomplished through national legislation. Legislation provides for effective tobacco control and also the legal foundation to the control programme. It also helps to integrate the diverse components of a multifaceted programme, ensures continuity and retains a steady focus on sustained and concerted effort, as opposed to sporadic interventions by the governmental agencies. Legislation achieves two broader objectives. First, it is a means of raising awareness and a means of social mobilization. It helps to raise public awareness and builds popular consensus for pro-public health measures. Second, legislation is seen more fundamentally, as the most solemn expression and formal articulation of societal values.

India has a short history of tobacco-related legislation. Legislation for tobacco control in India started evolving in the mid-1970s. This was in response to increasing scientific evidence of tobacco being a major cause of mortality and morbidity in the world, growing awareness of the adverse health effects of tobacco consumption in India and rising demand for tobacco control elsewhere in the world.

## Tobacco Board Act, 1975

Through this Act, the Tobacco Board develops better varieties of tobacco seeds; runs seed banks and liaise with financial institutions to secure loans for farmers. It facilitates the regulation of production and curing of tobacco, fixed minimum prices and provides subsidies to tobacco growers; sets up and monitors trade in tobacco leaf at the selling platforms and ensures that tobacco farmers get fair prices. It also recommends support prices of tobacco crops to prop up the produce of the farmers. The Act also aims at facilitating research, marketing, warehousing, publicity and promotion abroad, and extension of market intelligence in competing countries. The Act focuses on establishing a single authority that could deal with various aspects of tobacco industry in an integrated and efficient manner and also provides for registration of Virginia tobacco growers. The objective was to develop India's tobacco market and make the industry export competitive (John, 2001). This Act is still in force.

However, Tobacco Board Act, 1975 brought tobacco under a single jurisdiction (the Central Government) and this fact was later utilized to expand the provisions of Tobacco Control Bill of 2003 to encompass all tobacco products whether under state or central government.

## Tobacco Cess Act, 1975

This Act was enacted to collect duty on tobacco for the development of tobacco industry (John, 2001).

These Acts reflect a contradictory public policy in operation. On one hand, smoking was discouraged and on the other tobacco itself was seen as a major source of public revenue.

## Cigarette (Regulation of Production, Supply and Distribution) Act, 1975*

India's first national level anti-tobacco legislation was the single-faceted Cigarette Act of 1975, which mandated health warnings on cigarette packets and cigarette advertisements (Corrao, 2000). This Act was passed in 1975 to provide certain restrictions related to the trade and commerce in, and production, supply and distribution of cigarettes. The Act required the manufacturers or persons trading in cigarettes to display a statutory warning that *'cigarette smoking is injurious to health'* in the same language used in the branding of the package and cartons of cigarettes and also a similar warning on advertisement of cigarettes. The purpose of this warning was mainly to inform citizens of the harmful effects of smoking so that the demand for cigarettes would be reduced.

Section 3 of the Act laid down restrictions relating to trade and commerce in tobacco making it obligatory for a person engaged in tobacco products trade to display the warning while the Section 4 describes the manner in which warning needed to be presented. Other sections of the Act addressed the confiscation of tobacco packages (Section 10) and liability to pay penalty in the event of not abiding by the provisions of the Act (Section 12).

The Cigarette Act, 1975, however, failed to accomplish much as it did not include in its purview non-cigarette tobacco products such as *beedis* and smokeless products. This Act was repealed with the passage of the new Act in 2003.

In the years following the Cigarette Act of 1975, there were a number of other single faceted national attempts at controlling tobacco use such as:

## Prevention and Control of Pollution Act, 1981

This Act includes smoking in the definition of air pollution.

## The Motor Vehicle Act, 1988

This Act makes it illegal to smoke or spit in a public vehicle.

## Cable Television Networks Amendment Act, 2000

This Act prohibits the transmission of tobacco, liquor and baby food commercials on cable television across the country.

## Legislative and Regulatory Action by State Governments

Though the Government of India was contemplating for comprehensive tobacco control legislation for quite sometime before 2003, some states moved ahead with state laws addressing specific components of that strategy (Table 3). Several states used the provisions of the Prevention of Food Adulteration Act to impose a ban on smokeless tobacco products. The Delhi government was the first to impose a ban on smoking in public places. Other states too have enacted bans on public place smoking.

*Table 3: State-level laws for tobacco control in India*

| State | Name of the act & the year of enactment | Features |
|---|---|---|
| Delhi | The Delhi Prohibition of Smoking and Nonsmokers' Health Protection Act, 1996. | Prohibition of smoking in public places; in the public service vehicles |
| Assam | The Assam Prohibition of Smoking and Nonsmokers' Health Protection Bill, 1999. | Same as Delhi |
| Meghalaya | The Meghalaya Prohibition of Smoking and Nonsmokers Health Protection Act, 1998. | Same as Delhi |
| Sikkim | The Sikkim Prohibition of Smoking and Nonsmokers' Health Protection Act, 1997. | Same as Delhi |
| Jammu & Kashmir | The Jammu & Kashmir Prohibition of Smoking and Nonsmokers' Health Protection in Public Service Vehicles bill, 1997. | Prohibition of smoking in public service vehicles; advertising of cigarettes, etc. Provision of penalties and ejection of violators from public service vehicles. |
| West Bengal | The West Bengal Prohibition of Smoking and Spitting and Protection of Health of Nonsmokers and Minors Bill, 2001. | |
| Goa | The Goa Prohibition of Smoking and Spitting Act, 1997. | |
| Himachal Pradesh | The Himachal Pradesh Prohibition of Smoking and Nonsmokers' Health Protection bill, 1997. | Same as Delhi |

### The Delhi Prohibition of Smoking and Nonsmokers Health Protection Act, 1996

This Act prohibits smoking in public places so that the nonsmokers are protected from environmental tobacco smoke (ETS). Salient features (Kishore J., 2005) of this Act are:

1. Selling cigarettes and other tobacco products to children under 18 years of age is illegal.
2. Storing, selling and distributing cigarettes, *beedis* or tobacco based products within 100 meters of schools, colleges and other educational institutions is illegal.
3. Smoking in public places and inside public transport is a punishable offence.
4. If anybody who smoke in public place or in public transport or does not display and exhibit board of "no smoking zone" shall be punished with fine of up to

Rs. 100/- and in case of second or subsequent offence, shall be punished with fine of up to Rs. 500/- and for the offence of advertising, selling cigarettes, *beedis* to a minor, or in the vicinity of educational institutions the fine shall be up to Rs. 500/- and in case of second or subsequent offence, shall be punished with up to Rs. 1000/- of fine or imprisonment up to three months or both.

Assam government followed Delhi and passed a similar Act in 1999. In July 2001, in the interest of public health, the sale of all brands of *paan masala* (containing tobacco) and chewing tobacco/*zarda/khaini* under any brand name, in the state of Andhra Pradesh was prohibited. In a similar order, in August 2002, *gutka* and *paan masalas* were banned for five years in the state of Maharashtra. Manufacture for sale, or store, *Gutka and paan masala* containing tobacco or not containing tobacco, by whatever name called, in the state of Goa was banned in January 2003. Similar ban was imposed in Bihar for five years in April 2003.

The tobacco industry segment, which manufactures and markets smokeless tobacco products in India, challenged some of these orders in the courts of law.

## The Cigarettes and Other Tobacco Products (Prohibition of Advertisement and Regulation of Trade and Commerce, Production, Supply and Distribution) Act, 2003

This Act is the result of more than a decade of consultation and has undergone many changes to assume its final form. The lawmakers started responding to the information about the dangers that tobacco posed to Indian society. It was considered expedient to enact a comprehensive law on tobacco in public interest and to protect the public health of country's citizens. With a view to achieve improvement of public health in general as enjoined by Article 47 of the Indian Constitution, Cigarettes and Other Tobacco Products (Prohibition of Advertisement and Regulation of Trade and Commerce, Production, Supply and Distribution) Act, 2003 came into being in the 54th year of the Republic of India after it was passed by both the Houses of the Indian Parliament (Rajya Sabha on 9th April, 2003 and Lok Sabha on 30th April, 2003). This Act, intended to protect public health, encompasses a wide array of evidence-based strategies to reduce tobacco consumption. For the purpose of this Act, the entire range of tobacco products is brought under the jurisdiction of the Central Government. Some of the key provisions and penalties to violators are listed in Table 4.

According to this Act, individual smokers are restrained from smoking in places where the law does not permit it. The rules under the Act further require owners, managers of public places, hotels and restaurants to display prohibitory signs. Manager or the owner of a hotel or restaurant is further responsible to ensure the segregation of smoking and non-smoking areas. Persons engaged in the production, supply, and distribution of tobacco products along with those having control over media and those likely to take part in advertisements are responsible for ensuring that the ban is upheld. No person is allowed to sell tobacco products to minors or within a range of 100 yards of educational institutions. The producer, supplier, distributor and seller are responsible for ensuring that the tobacco packages they trade carry the specific warnings. Inspectors of Food and Drug Administration, police officers not below the rank of sub-inspectors and any other officers authorized by the Centre and State Governments and the designated enforcement authorities under the law.

*Table 4: Key provisions and penalties of the Cigarettes and Other Tobacco Products Act, 2003**

| Provisions | Penalties |
|---|---|
| Prohibition of direct and indirect advertisement of tobacco products, with the exception of advertising at the point of sale and on tobacco packs. The rules under the law restrict point-of sale advertising in terms size, inclusion of a mandatory warning and disallowing the use of any pictures of the product itself.Ban on gifts, prizes, scholarships or sponsorship of sports or other cultural events using the trademark or brand name of tobacco products. | Advertisement is to be forfeited and disposed of. The first conviction is punishable with imprisonment of up to 2 years or a fine up to Rs. 1000 or both. Subsequent convictions are punishable with imprisonment of up to 5 years and a fine of up to Rs. 5000. |
| Prohibition of smoking in public places. | Offence would be made compoundable with a fine of up to Rs. 200. |
| Prohibition on sale of tobacco products to persons below the age of 18 years. Prohibition on the sale of tobacco within a radius of 100 yards of educational institutions. | Offence would be compoundable with summary trials and a fine of up to Rs. 200. |
| Legible and conspicuous health warnings including pictorial warnings (e.g. skull and cross-bones) on not less than one of the largest panels of the tobacco package with the text of the warning appearing in the same language(s) as the language(s) used on it. Indication of tar and nicotine contents of the tobacco products on the package along with the maximum permissible limits as prescribed by the rules under this Act. | Imprisonment up to 2 years or a fine of up to Rs. 5000 or both, for first conviction of a producer or manufacturer; subsequent convictions attract imprisonment of up to 5 years and with a fine of up to Rs.10,000.; imprisonment up to 1 year or a fine of up to Rs. 1000, or both, for the frst conviction of a seller or a distributor; imprisonment of up to 2 years or a fine of up to Rs. 3000 for subsequent convictions. |

***Source:*** *Report on Tobacco Control in India (2004) Government of India, Centres for Disease Control and Prevention, USA and World Health Organization.*
**see appendix*

Rules related to the implementation of the key provisions of the Act have been notified on 25th February, 2004 and came into effect from 1st May, 2004. The following provisions have been notified:

- Prohibition of smoking in public places
- Prohibition of advertisement of cigarettes and other tobacco products, and
- Prohibition of sale to minors.

  (see Rules in the appendix)

The Act is in effect for more than three years now it is yet to make its presence felt. In the country's capital city where it should be maximally effective seems to have done little to curb the menace of smoking among school children. Tobacco-product venders flourish just outside Delhi's school gates.

Effective implementation of the law calls for an informed community, empowered to assert the entitlements under the law, supplemented with a clear and simple mechanism for reporting violations. Some of the matters covered by the Act require technical expertise, such as deciding the permissible levels of tar and nicotine to be displayed on tobacco packs. There are other provisions such as smoking regulation that require extensive enforcement staff.

## Health Education and Mass Media Efforts

In the 1960s, when concept of 'prevention' was added to the health discourse, it referred to multi-pronged approach to disseminate warning about products and practices that health professionals considered potential health hazards along with educating the youth through school curricula. Therefore, the primary tool for tobacco control is comprehensive and active awareness of the population about the ill effects of tobacco on social, physical, financial and environmental aspects.

Both, the government and the Non-Governmental Organizations (NGOs) are engaged in educating the community. Research findings all over the world establish that it is necessary to reduce demand through educating masses about the health hazards, financial loss and adverse environmental effects related to tobacco use. These mass education efforts along with policy changes are targeted at reinforcing and changing the social norms towards no tobacco use. Public education is an integral part of the efforts to both prevent initiation of tobacco use and to encourage tobacco cessation. Consistent decline in tobacco use in United States and European countries could become possible only through education.

## Health Education in India

Intervention research on awareness related to tobacco avoidance and control has shown to positively alter tobacco use practices among the youth in India (Reddy *et al,* 2002). Interventions in the form of classroom curricula, posters, booklets, and debates at school level, and information for the families at home level, have shown positive results in India. Health education programme, which includes personal as well as mass media communication, is found to be quite effective. Communication inputs designed for these interventions were personal communications, films, folk dramas, radio programmes, cessation camps etc. In a study, these approaches could bring about cessation in 14% of the tobacco users (Aghi *et al,* 1992).

Health education efforts in India have been few but effective. These efforts have been effective mainly due to the paucity of information among the population on the inputs of tobacco use. However, efforts at the national level are required to counteract this menace, which can be largely curtailed through prevention and successful quitting as a result of health education.

### Government's Initiatives

Government of India has set up the Central Health Education Bureau (CHEB) and its state chapters called the State Health Education Bureaus. Around World No Tobacco Day on 31st May, every year the CHEB conducts a 4–6 weeks activity to disseminate awareness among general public. Similarly, the Directorate of Advertising and Visual Publicity (DAVP) and the Song and Drama Division under the Ministry of Information and Broadcasting are creating awareness among the masses on various public and social health issues.

Tobacco Control Awareness Education has traditionally received a low accord and there has been no systematic and concerted effort either by the central or the state agencies on the tobacco related issues. It is only recently, after setting up of the National Tobacco Control Cell, that awareness education through the print media and television has begun in a strategic manner.

In 1984, the National Cancer Control Programme was launched which included a component for educating the public about the dangers of tobacco to eliminate tobacco related cancers.

### National Tobacco Control (NTC) Cell

The National Tobacco Control Cell (NTC) established in February 2001, is supported by WHO's regional office in India and is located physically in the Ministry of Health at New Delhi. Its function is to provide impetus to the tobacco control efforts and to coordinate these activities at national level. The Cell's functions also include the development of strategic media plan to provide health education among the masses. The media plan of the NTC cell focuses specifically on protecting vulnerable segments such as the youth and passive smokers. The Tobacco Free Initiative (TFI) in WHO's India office is one of the largest programmes worldwide, clearly highlighting tobacco control to be a high priority for the country and WHO in India. The focus areas of work in the TFI are:

1. Planning and executing a comprehensive information, education and communication plan;
2. Capacity-building among NGOs working in the field of tobacco control.
3. Establishment and strengthening of tobacco cessation clinics; and
4. Undertaking research on policy issues related to tobacco.

### Television and Audio Advertising

NTC cell developed 13 anti-tobacco advertisements during 2002–2003. Anti-tobacco radio advertisements have also been developed and aired on various radio channels. An anti-tobacco mass media plan is also developed to reach the rural, semi-urban masses and the vulnerable audience — passive smokers and the urban youth.

### Production of Information, Education and Communication (IEC) Materials

The DAVP, in coordination of NTC cell designed and produced IEC materials related to tobacco control in all Indian languages, which include flip charts, brochures, bus panels, mobile exhibition kits and stickers.

### Organizing Health Melas

In these *melas* information is disseminated about various diseases including non-communicable diseases and those caused due to use of tobacco. These *melas* include mobile exhibitions on tobacco, displaying posters, handouts, audiovisual aids, projectors, movies, etc.

Initiatives taken by State Voluntary Health Associations, NGOs, Statewide Cancer Control Programmes and commemoration on World No Tobacco Day help in tobacco control programme.

## Litigation, Consumer Action and Judicial Verdict

The Indian judiciary has adopted an innovative approach to issues of public interest. A category of 'public interest litigation (PIL) was developed in 1970s, wherein any individual or organization could approach the court seeking its intervention on a matter of public interest. In such cases, it is not necessary for the plaintiff to be the directly affected party. Even a letter written to the apex court (a state High Court or the Supreme Court of India) by a citizen or a group of citizens can be treated as a petition, if the court decides that a matter of public interest is involved. This has been often referred to as '*epistolatory*' jurisprudence. The courts have, in many cases, even *suo moto* notice of newspaper reports on issues of public interest and issued notices to governments and even private parties. Such judicial activism has resulted in several landmark judgments in areas such as environmental pollution and provision of essential health care. These practices have had influence on tobacco-related litigation also. Issues related to tobacco control have featured prominently in the Indian courts of law and the judicial verdicts have had a major impact on government policies as well as tobacco trade practices.

### *Kerala High Court Verdict*

A PIL petition was filed before the High Court of Kerala by a woman who complained of problems caused by exposure to tobacco smoke from co-passengers during frequent travel by bus. This writ petition (No. 24160/1998) was first of its kind in India and was filed under Article 226 of the Constitution, contending that second-hand smoking violates the right to life that is guaranteed under Article 21 of the Constitution. The petition sought that appropriate measures be taken by the government to prosecute and punish persons guilty of smoking in public places as the same amounted to 'Public Nuisance', as defined under Section 268 of the Indian Penal Code.

In July 1999, the Court issued a path-breaking judgment that, for the first time in India, banned smoking in public places throughout the state of Kerala. The judgment stated that public health law to eliminate exposure to second-hand smoke is long overdue and the policy-makers pursue all the strategies that would help accomplish that goal including education, legislation, regulation, litigation and enforcement of the existing laws. The Court held that:

- Public smoking of tobacco is illegal, unconstitutional and violative of Article 21.
- Tobacco smoking in public places falls within the purview of the penal provisions.
- Print and the electronic media is directed to caution the public about the penal consequences of violation of ban on smoking in public places.

### *The Supreme Court of India Directive to Ban Smoking in Public Places Across India*

In November 2001, the Supreme Court of India stepped in to ban smoking in public places and directed the Centre and States to take necessary action to ensure implementation of the ban. This was in response to a PIL filed in the Supreme Court of India on 12th July, 1999 by Murali Deora, a former member of the Indian Parliament drawing attention to the infringement of the fundamental rights guaranteed under Articles 14, 19 and 21 of the Constitution of India and negation of the Directive Principles of State Policy articulated in Article 39(e) and Article 47 of the Constitution. The petition further contended that the current legislation had failed in achieving the objective, evident from the title of the Act itself (The Cigarette {Regulation of Production, Supply and Distribution} Act, 1975). It merely provided a mild specified warning that 'cigarette smoking is injurious to health, which is grossly inadequate in the light of the harmful effects of tobacco smoking. The petitioner contended that the Act had completely failed to regulate advertisements, promoting and glamourising cigarette smoking and thereby made no serious effort to stop the tobacco industry from shamelessly flaunting their products through every possible form of the media.

The petition sought that the business of tobacco manufacture be categorized as a noxious trade through legislation and compensation paid by tobacco companies, National Tobacco Policy be framed and prohibition of smoking in public places be imposed.

On 2nd November, 2001, in an interim order, the Supreme Court of India directed the central and the state governments to prohibit smoking in public places. The order stated that, *"it would be in the interest of the citizens to prohibit the smoking in public places till the statutory provision is made and implemented by legislative enactment. The persons not indulging in smoking cannot be compelled to or subjected to passive smoking on account of the acts of the smokers."*

This judgment reaffirmed the fundamental right of the public to protection against disease and the right to a healthy life and clean and wholesome environment, as provided in the Article 21 of the Constitution.

### *Ban on Tooth Pastes and Toothpowders Containing Tobacco*

The Government's order to prohibit the manufacture and sale of toothpastes/toothpowders containing tobacco was challenged in the Supreme Court by the tobacco industry. However, Supreme Court upheld the ban in the public interest.

Supreme Court has also said that the Central Government should bring law to ban gutka as it has lifted the ban imposed by various state governments on sale of gutka. This judgment does not, in any way, endorse the safety of *gutka* but merely emphasizes that the Central Government alone can issue orders imposing such a ban in matters where the primacy of power rests with it. It is, therefore, now a matter, which needs to be considered by the Central Government.

### *Class Action Suit for Damages*

Recently, the Consumer Education and Research Society (CERS) has initiated a Class Action suit for compensation on behalf of some patients with oral cancer, who developed the illness after being addicted to the chewing of *gutka*.

### *Civil Society's Initiatives*

Amidst the multi-nationals continuously promoting tobacco products and the governments in each country grappling with economic and political interests related to tobacco, the role of civil societies becomes pertinent as these groups advocate for regulating tobacco products, raising awareness among the masses, demanding regulation and litigating on other issues related to tobacco. Realizing the importance of civil society's contribution in the health sector, the World Health Organization has established a Civil Society Initiative (CSI) to achieve health goals in both developed and developing countries.

In 2001, nine national NGOs in India formed the Advocacy Forum for Tobacco Control (AFTC), which designed and implemented informative messages that clarified the benefits of having such a law in India to key Members of the Parliament. The Indian National Health Policy (NHP), 2002 recognized the significant contribution of NGOs and other civil society institutions in making the health services available to Indian people. To utilize their high motivational skills and maximize their contribution, the current NHP statement directs that 10% of the budget of all disease control programmes should be given exclusively to these institutions. NGOs in India have played a crucial role in creating a supportive environment for tobacco control.

## Policy Interventions

### *Taxation*

Some experts believe that taxation on cigarettes can curb the demand and can be helpful in decreasing consumption. The tobacco industry in India is subject to a range of taxes imposed by Central and State governments. According to an industry report, taxation on cigarette accounts for around 55% of the average price of the 20 cigarettes packet[4].

---

4 The Tobacco Industry, India: An economic analysis (2000), Economic Studies and Strategies Unit. Price Waterhouse, and Coopers : Canberra, Australia.

In 1998, US$1424 million worth excise duty was generated by tobacco products; nearly 82% of this came from the sale of cigarettes. These data highlight the minimal contribution of unorganized sector to excise revenue.

There are three reasons to raise tax on tobacco:

(i) To deter consumption

(ii) To correct for externalities such as healthcare cost.

(iii) To raise revenue

From economics point of view the law of demand is *ceteris paribus*, if the price of a commodity rises, the quantity demanded of the commodity will fall. Increasing taxation on tobacco products effectively lowers consumption in developing countries (Chaloupka, 2000). However, some studies say that tobacco would be an exception to this law by virtue of its addictive properties and that is the reason that the economic studies in this regard have reached unequivocal conclusions that higher prices are effective in reducing tobacco consumption, especially among the young and the poor (Joossens *et al,* 2000). The World Bank Report of 1999 concludes that the 10% increase in the price of tobacco products would reduce their use by 4% in the developed countries and by about 8% in the developing countries. While the demand for more expensive cigarettes is likely to fall with increased prices, this decrease in cigarette consumption could be offset by *beedis.* Consumers may not quit smoking as a result of higher prices but merely switch to *beedis,* the cheaper alternative. There is also a possibility of smuggling of tobacco products from neighbouring countries where taxes on these products are lower.

For various reasons, the tax rate on *beedis* and smokeless tobacco products are very low. To achieve greater control on tobacco use taxes on all types of tobacco products need to be increased as all have adverse health effects warranting taxation. (Sunley *et al,* 2000). There should be increased tax rates for *beedis* and chewing tobacco along with improvement in tax administration. The tax net has fallen almost exclusively on cigarette sector of the Indian tobacco industry. The *beedis* and chewing tobacco sector, which constitute larger consumption segments, have not been adequately taxed as they are mostly in the unorganized sector and are also the preferred products of poor who consume tobacco. Such a policy, however, ignores the reality that non-cigarette sectors will contribute to the largest burden of death and disability attributable to tobacco in India. It also does not take into account the fact that the price elasticity (the responsiveness of the quantity demanded by consumers to change in price) is higher among the poor and, therefore, the impact on consumption will be greater if the products consumed by the poor have a price increased through the tax mechanism.

The revenue generated from tobacco taxation needs to be spent on specific activities such as tobacco-related education, counter-advertising, and other tobacco control activities and research and environment.

## Closing All Advertising Avenues

One of the most important challenges to tobacco control is advertising. It has long been recognized that reducing or eliminating advertising of tobacco products is important for tobacco control. Many countries have taken steps to reduce tobacco advertising, including prohibition of advertising at the point of sale (Barnsley and Jacob, 2004). Recognizing the impact of tobacco advertising and promotional activities, the Framework Convention on Tobacco Control (FCTC) (Article, 13) has called upon member countries to undertake a comprehensive ban of all tobacco advertising, promotion and sponsorship to reduce the consumption of the tobacco products.

It is evident that advertising leads to increased tobacco consumption (Lovato, 2004) ban on advertising causes decline in prevalence of tobacco use. Most econometric studies have found that increased expenditure on tobacco advertising increases demand for cigarettes, while banning advertising leads to a reduction in tobacco consumption (Willemsen and Blij, 2004). In the United States alone, with just around 5% of the world's smokers, the tobacco industry spent more than $12.47 billion in 2002 (or more than $34 million every day) to promote their products (Hafez and Ling, 2005). In four countries where advertising bans have been introduced as a part of comprehensive tobacco control policy (Finland, France, New Zealand and Norway), a study has shown that per capita consumption of cigarettes dropped by between 14% and 37% after the implementation of the ban. Smoking prevalence among young people declined in the three of the four countries and remained stable in the fourth (Fielding and Chee, 2004). Although several countries have enacted laws prohibiting tobacco advertising on television, there are a large number of satellite channels that do not follow these laws. For instance, India, the world's largest film industry, has over 50 satellite TV channels, most of which advertise cigarettes and other tobacco products. Paid advertisements in favour to tobacco is one of the innovative methods used by tobacco companies to promote their products. Recently, a number of governments have banned all forms of tobacco advertising, while others are instituting tough restrictions, Finland, France, India, New Zealand, Italy, Portugal, Singapore and Thailand, among others, have banned all tobacco advertising, promotion and sponsorship (WHO, 2002).The Cigarettes and Other Tobacco Products Act, 2003, has banned direct and indirect advertising of all tobacco products. However, advertising has been permitted at the 'point of sale' of tobacco products. Venders and tobacco industry are not strictly observing the restrictions places on display boards at such sites. Further, there is the danger that the industry may rapidly increase the number and type of outlets where tobacco products are sold and festoon markets with display boards at supposed "points of sale". Therefore, the Act may not be adequately effective at controlling tobacco advertisements since it has ignored these avenues of advertising and promotion. It is, therefore, ideal if the Act is amended to extend the ban to such 'point of sale' advertising as well. Some developing countries like Thailand have recently passed legislation that may be effective in this area. The Thai experience provides insight into challenges that lie ahead for India.

## Protection of Vulnerable Groups: A Human Rights Approach

A recent report by Economic and Social Council (ECOSOC) of the United Nations states that 'Tobacco consumption is a major direct contributor to increasing non-communicable diseases and an associative contributor to communicable diseases such as tuberculosis. Poverty facilitates the spread of diseases and their treatment can impose a heavy financial burden on poor households. In developing countries, among poor families, the proportion of household expenditures used to purchase tobacco products can easily represent 10% of total household expenditures with lesser money left for basic items such as food, education and health. Studies also show that the poor consume the most toxic tobacco products e.g. unbranded *beedis* manufactured with poor quality control and sometimes laced with other narcotic drugs (Shah and Vaite, 2002). Tobacco consumption in males is inversely related to the level of education, with a higher prevalence among the illiterate and semiliterate (Reddy *et al,* 2000). Tobacco and poverty create a vicious circle, from which it is often difficult to escape. Tobacco tends to be consumed by those who are poorer. In turn, it contributes to poverty through loss of income, loss of productivity, disease and death. WHO's No Tobacco Day, 2004 theme 'Tobacco and Poverty' is in contrast to over-simplistic and widespread arguments that tobacco provides wealth to governments and growers.

In 2001, the National Human Rights Commission (NHRC) of India considered the issues related to tobacco control from the perspective of human rights and concluded that the following rights of an individual are violated due to lack of tobacco control mechanisms in India.

1. *Right to clean air*: A non-smoker is forced to inhale tobacco smoke in public places.
2. *Rights of children*: Born and unborn children are exposed to tobacco smoke. They are worst affected.
3. *Right to information*: Adequate information about the adverse health effects is generally not available to both smokers and non-smokers.
4. *Right to education*: All citizens have right to be educated about the tobacco products.
5. *Right to redressal*: Redressal mechanism to ill effects and injury due to tobacco should be adequately provided.
6. *Right to tobacco cessation programme*: Smokers have a right to have access to various cessation strategies.

The fundamental reciprocity between health and human rights is well established and need to put in place a proper regulatory framework to aid and nurture this synergy should be the guiding lights of policy-makers and analysts in this field. This is even truer of tobacco control than of many other policies related to public health.

## Tobacco Products Regulation, Testing and Laboratory Strengthening

The regulation of tobacco products is an important component of a comprehensive tobacco control strategy adopted by WHO Framework Convention on Tobacco Control (FCTC). Several countries have already enacted legislations incorporating provisions for tobacco product regulation. In India, Tobacco Products Act, 2003 calls for testing and disclosure of the tar and nicotine content of tobacco products. However, at present, laboratories providing facilities for testing tobacco products are grossly deficient in India.

The purpose of this regulation is to progressively reduce the level of harmful chemicals and alter their physical characteristics that influence the delivery of these chemicals. The purpose of regulation is to reduce initiation or maintenance of addiction, reduce uptake, reduce harm to active smokers and other tobacco users, eliminate toxic non-tobacco additives, facilitate quitting and protect non-smokers from environmental tobacco smoke (ETS).

WHO's Scientific Advisory Committee on Tobacco Product Regulation (SACtob) established in 2000 provides technical guidelines on matters related to tobacco product regulation. As such no cigarette is safe for human health. The erroneous impression created by the vested interests that 'low tar and low nicotine level' cigarettes are safe lead to altered consumption patterns that may have adverse health effects on population as well as individuals. Non-smokers, especially the youth, may be tempted to use tobacco products in the mistaken belief that they are safe. Based on the existing scientific evidence SACtob made the following conclusions and recommendations in 2002:

1. Tar, nicotine and carbon monoxide (CO) numerical ratings based on current ISO/FTC methods, and presented on cigarette packages and in advertising as single numerical values are misleading and should not be displayed.
2. All misleading health and exposure claims should be banned.
3. The ban should apply to packaging, brand names, advertising and other promotional activities.
4. Banned terms should include light, ultra-light, mild and low tar, and may be extended to other misleading terms. The ban should include not only misleading terms and claims but also names, trademarks, imagery and other means of conveying the impression that the product provides a health benefit.

Three articles of the FCTC address regulation of tobacco products in terms of their permitted content, testing methods, industry disclosure to government, consumer information and public disclosure. India needs to develop laboratory capacity for regulatory testing of tobacco products (both smoking and smokeless tobacco products). To monitor and discipline the tobacco industry, it is essential to develop a National Regulatory Authority with a clearly defined mandate and adequate resources.

## Politics and Economics of Tobacco Control

The tobacco lobby has argued that tobacco control measures can negatively impact the economy by creating massive employment loss.

## Smuggling and Effectiveness of Tax Policy

Smuggling activities also present a challenge to tobacco control policies in the region. It is now known that transnational tobacco companies do little to prevent, and may actually encourage such illegal activities. As the tobacco companies are continuously trying to dilute the laws for tobacco control, enforcement agencies, government, civil society organizations have to be vigilant about their tactics. Tax-led reduction in the demand for tobacco products has to contend with some escape routes that tobacco interests may avail of. Smuggled cigarettes from such countries may have lower prices on account of either no tax or lower tax rates or other factors pertaining to supply-side factors or as a result of deliberate policy by cigarette companies.

## Integration of Tobacco Control into Health and Developmental Programmes

Tobacco control programme needs to be comprehensive in nature incorporating the demand and supply reduction measures recommended by the FCTC and involving all the stakeholders. It should be integrated with existing delivery systems involving all concerned agencies. A comprehensive tobacco control for India should consist of:

1. Laws and Policies: A law is already in place in India (Cigarettes and Other Tobacco Products Act, 2003) and that should be adequately enforced. Law enforcers should be sensitized about its various provisions. It should be brought in conformity with the FCTC.
2. Fiscal Components: There should be a rational tax structure. *Beedis* and oral tobacco products should be taxed at sufficiently high rates. These taxes should ensure that the price rise takes inflation into account. The subsidies given to the industry should be discouraged and disincentives should be put in place, both for the industry and the consumer.
3. Educational Component: The mass media, which encompass radio, television, the print and electronic media can be used to educate people. Educational effort should be aimed at both preventing initiation as well encouraging users to quit. Harmful effects of tobacco use and the benefits of tobacco cessation should be conveyed to people. They should also be told about the methods of quitting available.
4. Advertising and Counter-advertising: All types of advertising, whether direct or surrogate should be effectively banned. To ensure successful implementation, it is essential that surrogate advertising be checked. Steps should be taken to check

cross-border advertising. There should be adequate counter-advertising, which de-glamourizes tobacco use.

5. Cessation Programmes: These programmes should address the needs of those who are already using tobacco products. Health professionals as well as tobacco users should be sensitized to the benefits of cessation.
6. Regulation of Products: Regulation should aim at progressively reduce the level of toxic chemicals and alter physical characteristics that influence the delivery of those chemicals. Laboratories should be developed for the testing of the tobacco products. These laboratories should not be owned, operated or influenced by the tobacco industry.
7. Supply-side Actions: Tobacco farmers should be informed about alternative crops, which are not harmful to human health. They should also be given government assistance during the transitional period. Smuggling should be prevented with the cooperation at the international level.

## Recommendations

To achieve the goal effectively, National Programme for Tobacco Control should be launched which should incorporate all essential components. Tobacco Cessation Programme should be integrated with the primary health care and all the patients contacting a primary care physician should be asked about their tobacco use status. Those desirous to quit should be promptly helped or should be referred to the specialized clinics. National Tobacco Control Programme should be integrated into developmental programmes such as poverty alleviation, rural development, women and child development and tribal welfare. These programmes can be used to spread the message about tobacco control. Tobacco control programme should use a setting approach. Defined settings such as schools, workplaces, homes and public places should be made smoke free. The role of primary health care services, and traditional health care providers, could play a decisive role in reaching *beedi* and smokeless tobacco users, informing them about the addictiveness and harm caused by tobacco use and by providing support for them to quit. Some adaptations of the usual approaches to cigarette users may be required.

WHO programme related to 'Healthy Schools', Healthy Workplaces' and 'Healthy Cities', are models wherein tobacco free norms are developed and observed in different settings. Students, parents, teachers and others should be made aware of, and involved in, tobacco control activities.

Tobacco demand is extremely high in India and is met by the poor farmers. A long-term perspective is needed that starts by investigating now in research aimed at identifying alternative high wage jobs for poor rural farmers. Tobacco diversification needs to be linked to rural development. Experiences from other countries such as Brazil, South Africa, Poland and Thailand, suggest that when there is political support for tobacco control from the leadership of a country, and it is supported by solid in-country research, and an open and transparent media, progress will happen (de Beer and Brigden, 2003). These ingredients are now in place in India. Continued and intensified action will bring the tobacco menace under control in the country.

## REFERENCES

Aghi MB; Gupta PC, Bhonsle RB and Murti PR (1992) Communication Strategies in Intervening In the Tobacco Habits of Rural Populations in India. In: Gupta PC; Hamner JE; Murti PR (eds). *Control of Tobacco-related Cancers and Other Diseases*. Proceedings of An International Symposium, 15–19 January, 1990. Oxford University Press: Mumbai, India.

Barnsley K and Jacob M (2004) Special Feature. Tobacco Advertising and Display of Tobacco Products at Point of Sale: Tasmania, Australia. Tobacco Control 2000; 9: 228–236. Available from URL:http://tc.bmjjournals.com/cgi/content/full/9/2/228 (on 17th October, 2004).

Brooks JE (1952) The Mighty Leaf: Tobacco through the Centuries. Little Brown and Company, Boston.

Chaloupka FJ; Hu T; Warner KE; Jacobs R and Yurekli A (2000) The Taxation of Tobacco Products. In: Jha P and Chaloupka FJ (eds) *Tobacco Control in Developing Countries*. Oxford University Press: Oxford. p. 237–272.

Corrao MA; Guindon GE; Sharma N, and Shokoohi DF (2000) *Tobacco Control Country Profiles*. American Cancer Society, Atlanta.

Fielding R and Chee YY (2004) Decline in Tobacco Brand Recognition and Ever-smoking Rates Among Young Children Following Restrictions on Tobacco Advertisements in Hong Kong. *Journal of Public Health*. Vol. 26 No. 1.

Hafez N and Ling PM (2005) How Philip Morris built Marlboro Into A Global Brand for Young Adults: Implications for International Tobacco Control, *Tobacco Control*, Vol. 14 No. 4.

Jha P; Paccaud F; and Nguyen S (2000) Strategic Priorities in Tobacco Control for Governments and International Agencies. In: Jha P; Chaloupka F (eds) *Tobacco Control in Developing Countries*. Oxford University Press: Oxford. p. 449–465.

John S (2001) Teething Problems of Tobacco Control in India. Association for Consumers Action on Safety and Health: Mumbai, India.

Joossens L; Chaloupka FJ; Merriman D and Yurekli A (2000) Issues in the Smuggling of Tobacco Products. In: Jha P and Chaloupka FJ (eds) *Tobacco Control in Developing Countries*. Oxford University Press: Oxford. p. 393–408.

Kabra K (1998) Some Neglected Aspects of the Economics of Tobacco. In: Abeden I (eds.) *Proceedings of the Conference on Economics of Tobacco Control: Towards an Optimal Policy Mix*. Applied Fiscal Research Centre, university of Cape Town: Cape Town.

Kenneth W (1998) The Economics of Tobacco and Health: An Overview. In: Abedian I;Vander Merwe R; Wilkins N and Jha P (eds) *The Economics of Tobacco Control: Towards An Optimal Policy Mix*. Applied Fiscal Research Centre. University of Cape Town: Cape Town South Africa.

Kishore J (2005) National Health Programs of India: National Policies and Legislations Related to Health. Century Publications: New Delhi.

Lovato C (2004) Impact of Tobacco Advertising and Promotion on Increasing Adolescent Smoking Behaviour. *Cochrane Database of Systematic Reviews.* Issue 3.

Morison SE (1994) *The Oxford History of American People.* Oxford University Press: New York.

Reddy KS; Arora M; Perry CL; Nair B; Kohli A; Lytle LA' (2002) Tobacco and Alcohol Use Outcomes of a School-based Intervention in New Delhi. *American Journal of Health Behaviour;* 26: 173–181.

Reddy KS; Prabhakaran D; Shah P; Shrivastava U; Prabhaker AK and Shah B (2000) Tobacco Consumption in North Indian Males is Inversely Related to Educational Level: Results of Three Cross-sectional Surveys. *World Conference on Tobacco or Health.*

Shah S and Vaite S (2002) Pavement Dwellers in Mumbai, India—Prioritizing Tobacco Over Basic Needs. In: *Tobacco and Poverty: Observations from India and Bangladesh.* PATH: Canada,63–72.

Sunley EM; Yurekli A and Chaloupka FJ (2000) The Design, Administration and Potential Revenue of Tobacco Excises. In: Jha P and Chaloupka FJ (eds) *Tobacco Control in Developing Countries.* Oxford University Press: Oxford. p 409–426.

Taha A and Ball K(1980) Smoking and Africa: The Coming Epidemic. *British Medical Journal.* 280 (2619): 991–993.

United Nations, E/2004/55. "Ad-hoc Inter-Agency Task Force on Tobacco Control, Report of the Secretary General." http://www.un.org/esa/coordination/ecosoc/Tobacco Rpt. 2004. pdf.

World Health Organization, The Tobacco Atlas (2002) http://www.who.int/tobacco/en/atlas31.pdf

Willemsen MC and Blij BD (2004) *Tobacco Advertising. Tobacco Control Fact-sheet.* Available from URL: http://factsheets.globlink.org/en/advertising.shtml (17th October 2004).

# APPENDIX I

# THE CIGARETTES (REGULATIONS OF PRODUCTION, SUPPLY AND DISTRIBUTION) ACT, 1975

No.49 of 1975 [16th August, 1975]

An Act to provide for certain restrictions in relation to trade and commerce in, and production, supply and distribution of, cigarettes and for matters connected therewith or incidental thereto.

Comment: This Act basically provides for statutory warning on the cigarette packets saying that it is injurious to health BE it enacted by Parliament in the Twenty-sixth Year of the Republic of India as follows:-

## 1. Short title, extent and commencement

(1) This Act may be called the Cigarettes (Regulation of Production, Supply and Distribution) Act, 1975.(2) It extends to the whole of India.(3) It shall come into force on such date as the Central Government may, by notification in the Official Gazette, appoint.

## 2. Definitions

In this Act, unless the context otherwise requires:

(a) "advertisement" includes any notice, circular and other document and also includes any visible representation made by means of any light, sound, smoke or gas;

(b) "cigarette" includes,(i) any roll of tobacco wrapped in paper or in any other substance not containing tobacco,(ii) any roll of tobacco wrapped in any substance containing tobacco, which, by reason of its appearance, the type of tobacco used in the filler, or its packing and labelling is likely to be offered to, or purchased by consumers as cigarette,but does not include beedi, cheroot and cigar;

(c) "distribution" includes distribution by way of sample.Whether free or otherwise;

(d) "export", with its grammatical variations and cognate expressions, means taking out of India to a place outside India;

(e) "foreign Language means a language which is neither an Indian language nor the English language;

(f) "import", with its grammatical variations and cognate expressions, means bringing into India from a place outside India;

(g) "Indian language" means a language specified in the English Schedule to the Constitution, and includes any dialect of such language;

(h) "label" means any written, marked, stamped, printed or graphic matter, affixed to, or appearing upon, any package;

(i) "package" include a box, carton, tin, or other container;

(j) "prescribed" means prescribed by rules made under this Act;

(k) "production", with its grammatical variations and cognate expressions, includes—

(i) packing, labelling, re-labelling, of containers,

(ii) re-packing from bulk packages to retail packages, and

(iii) the adoption of any other method to render the product marketable;

(l) "sale", with its grammatical variations and cognate expressions, means any transfer of property in goods by one person to another, whether for cash or on credit or by way of exchange and whether wholesale or retail and includes an agreement for sale, an offer for sale and exposure for sale;

(m) "specified warning", means the following warning namely, "Cigarette smoking is injurious to health."

**3. Restrictions on trade and commerce in, and production, supply and distribution of cigarettes**

(1) No person shall, directly or indirectly, produce supply or distribute cigarettes unless every package of cigarettes produced supplied or distributed by him bears thereon, or on its label, the specified warning.

(2) No person shall carry on trade or commerce in cigarettes unless every package of cigarettes distributed, sold or supplied by him bears thereon, on its label, the specified warning.

(3) No person shall import cigarettes for distribution or supply for a valuable consideration or for sale unless every package of cigarettes so imported by him bears thereon, or on its label, the specified warning.

(4) The specified warning shall on not less than one of the largest panels of the package in which cigarettes have been packed for distribution, sale or supply for a valuable consideration.

**4. Manner in which specified warning shall be made**

(1) The specified warning on a package of cigarette shall be-

(a) legible and prominent;

(b) conspicuous as to size and colour;

(c) in such style of lettering as to be boldly and clearly presented in distinct contrast to the other type, lettering or graphic material used on the package or its label and shall be printed, painted or inscribed on the package in a colour which contrasts conspicuously with the background of the package or its label.

(2) Every package containing cigarettes shall be so packed as to ensure that the specified warning appearing thereon, or on its label, is, before the package is opened, visible to the consumer.

**5. Restrictions on advertisements of cigarettes**

(1) No person shall advertise for the distribution, sale or supply of cigarettes, and no person shall take part in the publication of any such advertisement, unless the specified warning is included in such advertisement.

(2) Every specified warning included in an advertisement shall be conspicuous, legible and prominent.

(3) No person shall, whether directly or indirectly, import, for the purpose of carrying on any trade or commerce in cigarettes, any documents article or thing, containing any advertisement that violates the provisions contained in sub-section (1) or sub-section (2).

### 6. Language in which the specified warning shall be expressed

(1) Where the language used on a package containing cigarettes or on its label or in any advertisement relating to such package is

(a) English, the specified warning shall be expressed in the English language;

(b) any Indian language or languages, the specified warning shall be expressed in such Indian Language or languages;

(c) both English and one or more Indian Languages, the specified warning shall be expressed in English as well as in such Indian language or languages;

(d) partly English and partly any Indian language or languages, the specified warning shall be expressed in the English language as well as in such Indian language or languages;

(e) any foreign language, the specified warning shall be expressed in the English language;

(f) partly any foreign language and partly English or any Indian language or languages, the specified warning shall be expressed in the English language as well as in such Indian language or languages.

(2) No package of cigarettes or its label or any advertisement relating thereto shall contain any matter or statement, which is inconsistent with, or detracts from, the specified warning.

### 7. Size of letters

No warning shall be deemed to be in accordance with the provisions of this Act if the height of each letter used in such warning is less than three millimeters.

### 8. Power of entry and search

(1) Any police officer, not below the rank of a sub-inspector, may, if he has any reason to suspect that any provision of this Act has been, or is being, contravened, enter and search, at reasonable time, any factory, building, business premises or any other place where any trade or commerce in cigarettes is carried on or cigarettes are produced, supplied or distributed.

(2) The provisions of the Code of Criminal Procedure, 1973 (2 of 1974), shall apply to every search and seizure made under this Act.

**9. Power of seizure**

(1) If any police officer, not below the rank of a sub-inspector, has any reason to believe that, in respect of any package of cigarettes, the provisions of this Act have been, or are being, contravened, he may seize such package.

(2) No package of cigarettes seized under sub-section

(i) shall be retained by any officer for a period exceeding ninety days from the date of the seizure unless the approval of the District Judge, within the local limits of whose jurisdiction such seizure has been made, has been obtained for such retention.

## APPENDIX II

## CIGARETTES AND OTHER TOBACCO PRODUCTS *(PROHIBITION OF ADVERTISEMENT AND REGULATION OF TRADE AND COMMERCE, PRODUCTION, SUPPLY AND DISTRIBUTION)* ACT, 2003

A comprehensive law on tobacco in the public interest and to protect the public health; to prohibit the consumption of cigarettes and other tobacco products which are injurious to health with a view to achieving improvement of public health in general as enjoined by Article 47 of the Constitution; and to prohibit the advertisement of, and to provide for regulation of trade and commerce, production, supply and distribution of, cigarettes and other tobacco products and for matters connected therewith or incidental thereto: Enacted by Parliament in the Fifty-fourth Year of the Republic of India.

**Passed by the Houses of Parliament— Rajya Sabha on 9th April, 2003 & Lok Sabha on 30th April, 2003 (Act 32 of 2003)**

*Sections*

1. Short title extent and commencement.
2. Declaration as to expediency of control by the Union.
3. Definitions.
4. Prohibition of smoking in a public place.
5. Prohibition of advertisement of cigarettes and other tobacco products.
6. Prohibition on sale of cigarette or other tobacco products to a person below the age of eighteen years and in particular area.
7. Restrictions on trade and commerce in, and production, supply and distribution of cigarettes and other tobacco products.
8. Manner in which specified warning shall be made.
9. Language in which the specified warning shall be expressed.
10. Size of letters and figures.

***1. Short title, extent and commencement***

(1) This Act may be called the Cigarettes and Other Tobacco Products (Prohibition of Advertisement and Regulation of Trade and Commerce, Production, Supply and Distribution) Act, 2003.

(2) It extends to the whole of India.

(3) It shall come into force on such date as the Central Government may, by notification in the Official Gazette, appoint and different dates may be appointed for different provisions of this Act.

### 2. Declaration as to expediency of control by the Union

It is hereby declared that it is expedient in the public interest that the Union should take under its control the tobacco industry.

### 3. Definitions

In this Act, unless the context otherwise requires—

*(a)* "advertisement" includes any visible representation by way of notice, circular, label, wrapper or other document and also includes any announcement made orally or by any means of producing or transmitting light, sound, smoke or gas;

*(b)* "cigarette" includes—

(*i*) any roll of tobacco wrapped in paper or in any other substance not containing tobacco,

(*ii*) any roll of tobacco wrapped in any substance containing tobacco, which, by reason of its appearance, the type of tobacco used in the filter, or its packaging and labeling is likely to be offered to, or purchased by, consumers as cigarette, but does not include *beedi*, cheroot and cigar;

*(c)* "distribution" includes distribution by way of samples, whether free or otherwise;

*(d)* "export", with its grammatical variations and cognate expressions, means taking out of India to a place outside India;

*(e)* "foreign language" means a language which is neither an Indian language nor the English language;

*(f)* "import", with its grammatical variations and cognate expressions, means bringing into India from a place outside India;

*(g)* "Indian language" means a language specified in the Eighth Schedule of the Constitution, and includes any dialect of such language;

*(h)* "label" means any written, marked, stamped, printed or graphic matter, affixed to, or appearing upon, any package;

*(i)* "package" includes a wrapper, box, carton, tin or other container;

*(j)* "prescribed" means prescribed by rules made under this Act. "Production", with its grammatical variations and cognate expressions, includes the making of cigarettes, cigars, cheroots, *beedis*, cigarette tobacco, pipe tobacco, *hookah* tobacco, chewing tobacco, *pan-masala* or any chewing material having tobacco as one of its ingredients (by whatever name called) or snuff and shall include —

*(i)* packing, labeling or re-labeling, of containers;

*(ii)* re-packing from bulk packages to retail packages; and

*(iii)* the adoption of any other method to render the tobacco product marketable;

*(k)* "public place" means any place to which the public have access, whether as of right or not, and includes auditorium, hospital buildings, railway waiting room, amusement centres, restaurants, public offices, court buildings, educational institutions, libraries, public conveyances and the like which are visited by general public but does not include any open space;

*(l)* "sale", with its grammatical variations and cognate expressions, means any transfer of property in goods by one person to another, whether for cash or on credit, or by way of exchange, and whether wholesale or retail, and includes an agreement for sale, and offer for sale and exposure for sale;

*(m)* "smoking", means smoking of tobacco in any form whether in the form of cigarette, cigar, *beedis* or otherwise with the aid of a pipe, wrapper or any other instrument;

*(n)* "specified warning" means such warnings against the use of cigarettes or other tobacco products to be printed, painted or inscribed on packages of cigarettes or other tobacco products in such form and manner as may be prescribed by rules made under this Act;

*(o)* "tobacco products" means the products specified in the Schedule.

### *4. Prohibition of smoking in a public place*

No person shall smoke in any public place:

Provided that in a hotel having thirty rooms or a restaurant having seating capacity of thirty persons or more and in the airports, a separate provision for smoking area or space may be made.

### *5. Prohibition of advertisement of cigarettes and other tobacco products*

*(i)* No person engaged in, or purported to be engaged in the production, supply or distribution of cigarettes or any other tobacco products shall advertise and no person having control over a medium shall cause to be advertised cigarettes or any other tobacco products through that medium and no person shall take part in any advertisement which directly or indirectly suggests or promotes the use or consumption of cigarettes or any other tobacco products.

*(ii)* No person, for any direct or indirect pecuniary benefit, shall —

(*a*) display, cause to display, or permit or authorize to display any advertisement of cigarettes or any other tobacco product; or

(*b*) sell or cause to sell, or permit or authorize to sell a film or video tape containing advertisement of cigarettes or any other tobacco product; or

(*c*) distribute, cause to distribute, or permit or authorize to distribute to the public any leaflet, hand-bill or document which is or which contains an advertisement of cigarettes or any other tobacco product; or (*d*) erect, exhibit, fix or retain upon or over any land, building, wall, hoarding, frame, post or structure or upon or in any vehicle or shall display in any manner whatsoever in any place, any advertisement of cigarettes or any other tobacco product:

***Provided that this sub-section shall not apply in relation to —***

(*a*) an advertisement of cigarettes or any other tobacco product in or on a package containing cigarettes or any other tobacco product;

(*b*) advertisement of cigarettes or any other tobacco product which is displayed at the entrance or inside a warehouse or a shop where cigarettes and any other tobacco products are offered for distribution or sale.

(*iii*) No person, shall, under a contract or otherwise promote or agree to promote the use or consumption of —

(*a*) cigarettes or any other tobacco product; or

(*b*) any trademark or brand name of cigarettes or any other tobacco product in exchange for a sponsorship, gift, prize or scholarship given or agreed to be given by another person.

### *6. Prohibition on sale of cigarette or other tobacco products to a person below the age of eighteen years and in particular area*

No person shall sell, offer for sale, or permit sale of, cigarette or any other tobacco product —

(*a*) to any person who is under eighteen years of age, and

(*b*) in an area within a radius of one hundred yards of any educational institution.

### *7. Restrictions on trade and commerce in, and production, supply and distribution of cigarettes and other tobacco products*

(*i*) No person shall, directly or indirectly, produce, supply or distribute cigarettes or any other tobacco products unless every package of cigarettes or any other tobacco products produced, supplied or distributed by him bears thereon, or on its label, the specified warning including a pictorial depiction of skull and cross bones and such other warning as may be prescribed.

(*ii*) No person shall carry on trade or commerce in cigarettes or any other tobacco product unless every package of cigarettes or any other tobacco product sold, supplied or distributed by him bears thereon, or on its label, the specified warning.

(*iii*) No person shall import cigarettes or any other tobacco products for distribution or supply for a valuable consideration or for sale in India unless every package of cigarettes or any other tobacco products so imported by him bears thereon, or on its label, the specified warning.

(*iv*) The specified warning shall appear on not less than one of the largest panels of the package in which cigarettes or any other tobacco products have been packed for distribution, sale or supply for a valuable consideration.

*(v)* No person shall, directly or indirectly, produce, supply or distribute cigarettes or any other tobacco products unless every package of cigarettes or any other tobacco products produced, supplied or distributed by him indicates thereon, or on its label, the nicotine and tar contents on each cigarette or as the case may be on other tobacco products along with the maximum permissible limits thereof: Provided that the nicotine and tar contents shall not exceed the maximum permissible quantity thereof as may be prescribed by rules made under this Act.

## *8. Manner in which specified warning shall be made*

*(i)* The specified warning on a package of cigarettes or any other tobacco products shall be —

(a) legible and prominent;

(b) conspicuous as to size and colour;

(c) in such style or type of lettering as to be boldly and clearly presented in distinct contrast to any other type, lettering or graphic material used on the package or its label and shall be printed, painted or inscribed on the package in a colour which contrasts conspicuously with the background of the package or its labels.

*(ii)* The manner in which a specified warning shall be printed, painted or inscribed on a package of cigarettes or any other tobacco products shall be such as may be specified in the rules made under this Act.

*(iii)* Every package containing cigarettes or any other tobacco products shall be so packed as to ensure that the specified warning appearing thereon, or on its label, is, before the package is opened, visible to the consumer.

## *9. Language in which the specified warning shall be expressed*

*(i)* Where the language used on a package containing cigarettes and any other tobacco products or on its label is —

*(a)* English, the specified warning shall be expressed in the English language;

*(b)* any Indian language or languages, the specified warning shall be expressed in such Indian language or languages;

*(c)* both English and one or more Indian languages, the specified warning shall be expressed in the English language as well as in such Indian language or languages;

*(d)* partly English and partly any Indian language or languages, the specified warning shall be expressed in the English language as well as in such Indian language or languages;

*(e)* any foreign language, the specified warning shall be expressed in the English language; contents.

(*f*) partly any foreign language and partly English or any Indian language or languages, the specified warning shall be expressed in the English language as well as in such Indian language or languages.

(*ii*) No package of cigarettes or any other tobacco products or its label shall contain any matter or statement, which is inconsistent with, or detracts from, the specified warning.

### 10. Size of letters and figures

No specified warning or indication of nicotine and tar contents in cigarettes and any other tobacco products shall be deemed to be in accordance with the provisions of this Act if the height of each letter or figure, or both used on such warning and indication is less than the height as may be prescribed by rules made under this Act.

### 11. Testing laboratory for nicotine and tar contents

For purposes of testing the nicotine and tar contents in cigarettes and any other tobacco products the Central Government shall by notification in the Official Gazette grant recognition to such testing laboratory as that Government may deem necessary.

### 12. Power of entry and search

(*i*) Any police officer, not below the rank of a sub-inspector or any officer of State Food or Drug Administration or any other officer, holding the equivalent rank being not below the rank of Sub-Inspector of Police, authorized by the Central Government or by the State Government may, if he has any reason to suspect that any provision of this Act has been, or is being, contravened, enter and search in the manner prescribed, at any reasonable time, any factory, building, business premises or any other place —

(*a*) where any trade or commerce in cigarettes or any other tobacco products is carried on or cigarettes or any other tobacco products are produced, supplied or distributed; or

(*b*) where any advertisement of the cigarettes or any other tobacco products has been or is being made.

(*ii*) The provisions of the Code of Criminal Procedure, 1973, shall apply to every search and seizure made under this Act.

### 13. Power to seize

(*i*) If any police officer, not below the rank of a sub-inspector or any officer of State Food or Drug Administration or any other officer, holding the equivalent rank being not below the rank of Sub-Inspector of Police, authorised by the Central Government or by the State Government, has any reason to believe that—

(a) in respect of any package of cigarettes or any other tobacco products, or (*b*) in respect of any advertisement of cigarettes or any other tobacco products, the provisions of this Act have been, or are being, contravened, he may seize such package or advertisement material in the manner prescribed.

*(ii)* No package of cigarettes or any other tobacco products or advertisement material seized under clause (*a*) of sub-section (*1*) shall be retained by the officer who seized the package or advertisement material for a period exceeding ninety days from the date of the seizure unless the approval of the District Judge, within the local limits of whose jurisdiction such seizure was made, has been obtained for such retention.

### 14. Confiscation of package

Any package of cigarettes or any other tobacco products or any advertisement material of cigarettes or any other tobacco products, in respect of which any provision of this Act has been or is being contravened, shall be liable to be confiscated; Provided that, where it is established to the satisfaction of the court adjudging the confiscation that the person in whose possession, power or control any such package of cigarettes or any other tobacco products is found is not responsible for the contravention of the provisions of this Act, the Court may, instead of making an order for the confiscation of such package, make such other order authorized by this Act against the person guilty of the breach of the provisions of this Act as it may think fit.

### 15. Power to give option to pay costs in lieu of confiscation

*(i)* Whenever any confiscation of any package of cigarettes or any other tobacco products is authorized by this Act, the court adjudging it may, subject to such conditions as may be specified in the order adjudging the confiscation, give to the owner thereof an option to pay, in lieu of confiscation, costs which shall be equal to the value of the goods confiscated.

*(ii)* On payment of the costs ordered by the court, the seized packages shall be returned to the person from whom they were seized on condition that such person shall, before making any distribution, sale or supply of such packages of cigarettes or other tobacco products, get the specified warning and indication of nicotine and tar contents incorporated on each such package.

### 16. Confiscation not to interfere with other punishments

No confiscation made, costs ordered to be paid under this Act shall prevent the infliction of any punishment to which the person affected thereby is liable under the provisions of this Act or under any other law.

### 17. Adjudication

Any confiscation of cigarettes or any other tobacco products may be adjudged or costs may be ordered to be paid —

(*a*) without any limit, by the principal civil court of original jurisdiction within the local limits of whose jurisdiction such confiscation has been made, costs have been ordered to be paid,

(*b*) subject to such limits as may be specified by the Central Government in this behalf, by such other court, not below a civil court having pecuniary jurisdiction exceeding rupees five thousand, as the Central Government may, by notification in the Official Gazette, authorize in this behalf.

### 18. *Giving opportunity to the owner of seized packages*

(*i*) No order adjudging confiscation or directing payment of costs shall be made unless the owner or person in possession of the package of cigarettes or any other tobacco products has been given a notice in writing informing him of the grounds on which it is proposed to confiscate such package, and giving him a reasonable opportunity of making a representation in writing, within such reasonable time as may be specified in the notice, against the confiscation mentioned therein, and, if he so desires, of being heard personally or through a representative in the matter: Provided that, where no such notice is given within a period of ninety days from the date of the seizure of the package of cigarettes or of any other tobacco products, such package shall be returned, after the expiry of that period, to the owner or the person from whose possession it was seized.

(*ii*) Save as otherwise provided in sub-section (*1*), the provisions of the Code of Civil Procedure, 1908, shall, as far as may be, apply to every proceeding referred to in sub-section (*1*).

### 19. *Appeal*

(*i*) Any person, aggrieved by any decision of the court adjudging a confiscation, ordering the payment of costs, may prefer an appeal to the court to which an appeal lies from the decision of such court.

(*ii*) The appellate court may, after giving to the appellant an opportunity of being heard, pass such order as it thinks fit confirming, modifying or reversing the decision or order appealed against or may send back the case with such directions as it may think fit for a fresh decision or adjudication, as the case may be, after taking additional evidence, if necessary; provided that an order enhancing any fine in lieu of confiscation or confiscating of goods of greater value shall not be made under this section unless the appellant has had an opportunity of making a representation and, if he so desires, of being heard in person or through a representative in his defense.

(*iii*) No further appeal shall lie against the order of the court of appeal.

## 20. Punishment for failure to give specified warning and nicotine and tar contents

*(i)* Any person who produces or manufactures cigarettes or tobacco products, which do not contain, either on the package or on their label, the specified warning and the nicotine and tar contents, shall in the case of first conviction be punishable with imprisonment for a term which may extend to two years, or with fine which may extend to five thousand rupees, or with both, and for the second or subsequent conviction, with imprisonment for a term which may extend to five years and with fine which may extend to ten thousand rupees.

*(ii)* Any person who sells or distributes cigarettes or tobacco products which do not contain either on the package or on their label, the specified warning and the nicotine and tar contents shall in the case of first conviction be punishable with imprisonment for a term, which may extend to one year, or with fine which may extend to one thousand rupees, or with both, and, for the second or subsequent conviction, with imprisonment for a term which may extend to two years and with fine which may extend to three thousand rupees.

## 21. Punishment for smoking in certain places

*(i)* Whoever contravenes the provisions of section 4 shall be punishable with fine which may extend to two hundred rupees.

*(ii)* An offence under this section shall be compoundable and shall be tried summarily in accordance with the procedure provided for summary trials in the Code of Criminal Procedure, 1973.

## 22. Punishment for advertisement of cigarettes and tobacco products

Whoever contravenes the provision of section 5 shall, on conviction, be punishable—

*(a)* in the case of first conviction, with imprisonment for a term which may extend to two years or with fine which may extend to one thousand rupees or with both, and

*(b)* in the case of second or subsequent conviction with imprisonment for a term which may extend to five years and with fine which may extend to five thousand rupees.

## 23. Forfeiture of advertisement and advertisement material

Where any person has been convicted under this Act for the contravention of the provision of section 5, the advertisement and the advertisement material for cigarettes and other tobacco products may be forfeited to the Government and such advertisement and advertisement material shall be disposed of in such manner as may be prescribed by rules made under this Act.

### 24. Punishment for sale of cigarettes or any other tobacco product in certain places or to persons below the age of eighteen years

*(i)* Any person who contravenes the provisions of section 6 shall be guilty of an offence under this Act and shall be punishable with fine, which may extend to two hundred rupees.

*(ii)* All offences under this section shall be compoundable and shall be tried summarily in accordance with the procedure provided for summary trials in the Code of Criminal Procedure, 1973.

### 25. Prevention, detention and place of trial of offences under Sections 4 and 6

*(i)* Notwithstanding anything contained in any other law for the time being in force, the Central Government or the State Government may, by notification in the Official Gazette, authorize one or more persons who shall be competent to act under this Act: Provided that the person so authorized may, if he has reasonable ground for believing that any person has committed an offence under section 4 or section 6, may detain such person unless the accused person furnishes his name and address, and otherwise satisfies the officer detaining him that he will duly answer any summons or other proceedings which may be taken against him.

*(ii)* Any person detained under sub-section (*1*) shall forthwith be taken before a Magistrate to be dealt with according to law.

*(iii)* Any person committing an offence under section 4 or section 6 shall be triable for such offence in any place in which he may be or which the State Government may notify in this behalf, as well as in any other place in which he is liable to be tried under any law for the time being in force.

*(iv)* Every notification issued under sub-sections (*1*) and (*3*) shall be published in the Official Gazette, and a copy thereof shall be exhibited for information to the public in some conspicuous place or places as the State Government may direct.

*(v)* Every person authorized under sub-section (*1*) shall be deemed to be a public servant within the meaning of section 21 of the Indian Penal Code.

### 26. Offences by companies

*(i)* Where an offence under this Act has been committed by a company, every person who, at the time the offence was committed, was in charge of, and was responsible to, the company for the conduct of the business of the company, as well as the company, shall be deemed to be guilty of the offence and shall be liable to be proceeded against and punished accordingly: Provided that nothing contained in this sub-section shall render any such person liable to any punishment, if he proves that the offence was committed without his knowledge or that he had exercised all due diligence to prevent the commission of such offence.

*(ii)* Notwithstanding anything contained in sub-section (*1*), where any offence under this Act has been committed by a company and it is proved that the offence has been committed with the consent or connivance of, or is attributable to any neglect on the part of, any director, manager, secretary or other officer of the company, such director, manager, secretary or other officer shall be proceeded against and punished accordingly. *Explanation* —For the purposes of this section —

(*a*) "company" means a body corporate and includes a firm or other association of individuals; and

(*b*) "director", in relation to a firm, means a partner in the firm.

### 27. Offences to be bailable

Notwithstanding anything contained in the Code of Criminal Procedure, 1973, an offence punishable under this Act shall be bailable.

### 28. Composition of offences

*(i)* Any offence committed under section 4 or section 6 may either before or after the institution of the prosecution be compounded by such officer authorised by Central Government or State Government and for an amount which may not exceed two hundred rupees.

*(ii)* Where an offence has been compounded under sub-section (*1*), the offender, if in custody, shall be discharged and no further proceedings shall be taken against him in respect of such offence.

### 29. Protection of action taken in good faith

No suit, prosecution or other legal proceeding shall lie against the Central Government or any State Government or any officer of the Central Government or any State Government for anything which is in good faith done or intended to be done under this Act.

### 30. Power to add any tobacco products in the Schedule

The Central Government, after giving by notification in the Official Gazette, not less than three months' notice of its intention so to do, may, by like notification, add any other tobacco product in respect of which it is of opinion that advertisements are to be prohibited and its production, supply and distribution is required to be regulated under this Act, and thereupon the Schedule shall in its application to such products be deemed to be amended accordingly.

### 31. Power of Central Government to make rules

*(i)* The Central Government may, by notification in the Official Gazette, make rules to carry out the provisions of this Act.

*(ii)* Without prejudice to the generality of the foregoing power, such rules may provide for all or any of the following matters, namely:—

*(a)* specify the form and manner in which warning shall be given in respect of cigarettes or other tobacco products under clause (*o*) of section 3;

*(b)* specify the maximum permissible nicotine and tar contents in cigarettes or other tobacco products under the proviso to sub-section (*5*) of section 7;

*(c)* specify the manner in which the specified warning shall be inscribed on each package of cigarettes or other tobacco products or its label under sub-section (*2*) of section 8;

*(d)* specify the height of the letter or figure or both to be used in specified warning or to indicate the nicotine and tar contents in cigarettes or other tobacco products under section 10;

*(e)* provide for the manner in which entry into and search of any premises is to be conducted and the manner in which the seizure of any package of cigarettes or other tobacco products shall be made and the manner in which seizure list shall be prepared and delivered to the person from whose custody any package of cigarettes or other tobacco products has been seized;

*(f)* provide for any other matter which is required to be, or may be, prescribed.

*(iii)* Every rule made under this Act and every notification made under section 30 shall be laid, as soon as may be after it is made, before each House of Parliament, while it is in session, for a total period of thirty days which may be comprised in one session or in two or more successive sessions, and if, before the expiry of the session immediately following the session or the successive sessions aforesaid, both Houses agree in making any modification in the rule or notification or both Houses agree that the rule or notification should not be made, the rule or notification shall thereafter have effect only in such modified form or be of no effect, as the case may be; so, however, that any such modification or annulment shall be without prejudice to the validity of anything previously done under that rule or notification.

### *32. Act not to apply to cigarettes or other tobacco products which are exported*

Nothing contained in this Act shall apply to any cigarette or other tobacco products or package of cigarettes or other tobacco products which is exported:

Provided that nothing in this section shall be deemed to authorize the export of any package of cigarettes or other tobacco products, not containing the specified warning and indication of nicotine and tar contents to any country if the law in force in that country requires that the same or similar warning and nicotine and tar contents shall be specified on each package of cigarettes or other tobacco products. *Explanation*— For the purpose of this section, any cigarette or other tobacco products or package of cigarettes or other tobacco products shall be deemed to be exported before the commencement of this Act, if the necessary steps for export have already been taken notwithstanding that the actual export has not taken place.

**33. Repeal and savings**

*(i)* The Cigarettes (Regulation of Production, Supply and Distribution) Act, 1975, is hereby repealed.

*(ii)* Notwithstanding such repeal, anything done or any action taken under the provisions of the aforesaid Act, shall, in so far as such thing or action is not inconsistent with the provisions of this Act, be deemed to have been done or taken under the provisions of this Act as if the said provisions were in force when such thing was done or such action was taken and shall continue in force accordingly until superseded by anything done or any action taken under this Act.

## The Schedule

**[*See* section 3(*p*)]**

1. Cigarettes
2. Cigars
3. Cheroots
4. *Beedis*
5. Cigarette tobacco, pipe tobacco and *hookah* tobacco
6. Chewing tobacco
7. Snuff
8. *Pan-masala* or any chewing material having tobacco as one of its ingredients (by whatever name called).
9. *Gutka*
10. Tooth powder containing tobacco.

## APPENDIX III

## MINISTRY OF HEALTH AND FAMILY WELFARE NOTIFICATIONS

**(Department of Health)**

***Notification***

New Delhi, the 25th February, 2004

**S.O. 238(E).** —In exercise of the power conferred by Sub-section (3) of Section 1 of the cigarettes and other Tobacco products (Prohibition of Advertisement and Regulation of Trade and Commerce, Production, Supply and Distribution) Act, 2003 (34) the Central Government hereby appoints 1st day of May, 2004 as the date on which the provisions of section 1,2,3,4,5,6(a), 12(1)(b), 12(2), 13(1)(b) 13(2), 14,16,19,21,22,23,24,25,26,27,28,29,30 and 31 of the said Act shall come into force [F.No.P-16011/2/2003-PH]

Bhavani Thyagarahjan, Jt. Secy. Ministry of Health and Family Welfare (Department of Health).

***Notification***

New Delhi, the 25th February, 2004

Cigarettes and other Tobacco Products (Prohibition of Advertisement and Regulation of Trade and Commerce, Production, Supply and Distribution) Rules, 2004 G.S.R. 137. — In Exercise of the power conferred by section 31 of the Cigarettes and other Tobacco Products (Prohibition of Advertisement and Regulation of Trade and Commerce, Production, Supply and Distribution) Act, 2003 (34 of 2003), the Central Government hereby makes the following rules, namely: -

1. **Short title and commencement** — (1) These rules may be called the Cigarettes and other Tobacco Products (Prohibition of Advertisement and Regulation of Trade and Commerce, Production, Supply and Distribution) Rules, 2004 (2) They shall come into force on the 1st day of May, 2004.
2. **Definitions** — In these rules, unless the context otherwise requires,—
   (a) "Act" means the Cigarettes and other Tobacco Products (Prohibition of Advertisement and Regulation of Trade and Commerce, Production, Supply and Distribution Act, 2003
   (b) "section" means a section of the Act
   (c) "open space" mentioned in Section 3(1) of the Act shall not include any places visited by the public such as open auditorium, stadium, railway station, bus stop and such other places; and
   (d) words and expressions used herein and not defined in these rules but defined in the Act, shall have the meaning, respectively, assigned to them in the Act.
3. **Prohibition of smoking in a public place** —
   (a) The owner or the manager or in charge of the affairs of a public place shall cause to be displayed prominently a board, of a minimum size of sixty centimeter by thirty centimetre in the Indian languages(s) as applicable, at least one at the entrance of the public place and one at conspicuous place(s) inside, containing the warning "No Smoking Area - Smoking here is an offence
   (b) The owner or the manager or in charge of the affair of a hotel having thirty rooms or restaurants having seating capacity of thirty persons or more and the manager of the airport shall ensure that —
      (i) The smoking and non-smoking areas are physically segregated;
      (ii) The smoking area shall be located in such manner that the public is not required to pass through it in order to reach the non-smoking area; and
      (iii) Each area shall contain boards indicating thereon "Smoking Area/Non-Smoking area."

**4. Prohibition of advertisement of cigarette and other tobacco products—**

(a) The size of the board used for advertisement for cigarettes and any other tobacco products displayed at the entrance or inside a warehouse or a shop where cigarettes and any other such tobacco products are offered for distribution or sale shall not exceed ninety centimeter by sixty centimeter and number of such boards shall not exceed two.

(b) Each such board shall contain in the Indian language as applicable, one of the following warning occupying twenty-five percent of top area of the board, namely: -

(i) Tobacco causes cancer, or

(ii) Tobacco kills

(c) The board referred to in sub-rule (2) shall contain only the brand name or picture of the tobacco products and no other promotional message and picture.

**5. Prohibition of sale to minors**

(a) The owner or the manager or the in-charge of the affairs of a place where cigarettes and other tobacco products are sold shall display a board of minimum size of sixty centimeter by thirty centimeter at conspicuous place(s) containing the warning "Sales of tobacco products to a person under the age of eighteen years is a punishable offence", in Indian language(s) applicable.

(b) The onus of proof that the buyer of the tobacco products is not a minor lies with the seller of the tobacco products. The seller, in case of doubt, may request tobacco purchaser to provide appropriate evidence of having reached eighteen years of age.

[F. No. P-16011/2/2003-PH]

Bhavani Thyagarahjan, Joint. Secretary Prohibition on sale of Cigarettes and other Tobacco Products around Educational Institutions Rules, 2004.

**Ministry of Health and Family Welfare**
(Department of Health)

***Notification***

New Delhi, the 1st September, 2004

G.S.R.561(E). In exercise of the powers conferred by Section 31 read with Section 6 of the Cigarettes and other Tobacco Products (Prohibition of Advertisement and Regulation of Trade and Commerce, Production, Supply and Distribution) Act, 2003 (No.34 of 2003), the Central Government hereby makes the following rules, namely:-

***1. Short Title, Extent and Commencement***

(a) These rules may be called the Prohibition on Sale of Cigarettes and Other Tobacco Products around Educational Institutions Rules, 2004.

(b) They shall extend to the whole of India.

(c) They shall come into force on the 1st day of December, 2004.

**2. Definitions**

In these rules, unless the context otherwise requires

(a) Act means the Cigarettes and other Tobacco Products (Prohibition of Advertisement and Regulation of Trade and Commerce, Production, Supply and Distribution) Act, 2003;

(b) Educational institution means places/centers where educational instructions are imparted according to the specific norms and include schools, colleges and institutions of higher learning established or recognized by an appropriate authority;

(c) Section means a section of the Act; and

(d) Words and expressions used herein and not defined in these rules but defined in the Act, shall have the meanings, respectively, assigned to them in the Act.

***3. Prohibition of Sale of Cigarettes and other Tobacco Products Around***

*Educational Institutions*

(a) Display of Board: The owner or manager or any person in-charge of affairs of the educational institution shall display and exhibit a board at a conspicuous place(s) outside the premises, prominently stating that sale of cigarettes and other tobacco products in an area within a radius of one hundred yards of the educational institution is strictly prohibited and that it is an offence punishable with the fine which may extend to two hundred rupees.

(b) Measurement of Distance: Distance of one hundred yards shall be measured radially starting from the outer limit of boundary wall, fence or as the case may be, of the educational institution.

(F.No.P-16011/2/2003-PH)

Bhavani Thyagarahjan, Joint Secretary.

## APPENDIX IV

**SUPREME COURT ORDERS IN MURLI S. DEORA Vs. UNION OF INDIA CASE IN THE SUPREME COURT OF INDIA CIVIL ORIGINAL JURISDICTION WRIT PETITION (CIVIL) No. 316 OF 1999 Murli S. Deora ... Petitioner Versus Union of India and Others ... Respondents**

## ORDER

Heard the learned counsel for the parties.

Fundamental right guaranteed under Article 21 of Constitution of India, inter alia, provides that none shall be deprived of his life without due process of law. Then — why a non-smoker should be afflicted by various diseases including lung cancer or of heart, only because he is required to go to public places? Is it not indirectly depriving of his life without any process of law? The answer is obviously - 'yes'. Undisputedly, smoking is injurious to health and may affect the health of smokers but there is no reason that health of passive smokers should also be injuriously affected. In any case, there is no reason to compel non-smokers to be helpless victims of air pollution. The statement of objects and reason of (The) Cigarettes (Regulation of Production, Supply and Distribution Act, 1975, inter alia, provides, "Smoking of cigarettes is a harmful habit and, in course of time, can lead to grave health hazards. Researches carried out in various parts of the world have confirmed that there is a relationship between smoking of cigarettes and lung cancer, chronic bronchitis; certain diseases of the heart and arteries; cancer of bladder, prostrate, mouth pharynx and oesophagus; peptic ulcer etc., are also reported to be among the ill-effects of cigarette smoking." Similarly, the statement of objects and reasons of The Cigarettes and Other Tobacco Products (Prohibition of Advertisement and Regulation of Trade and Commerce, Production, Supply and Distribution) Bill, 2001, provides, "Tobacco is universally regarded as one of the major public health hazards and is responsible directly or indirectly for an estimated eight lakh deaths annually in the country. It has also been found that treatment of tobacco related diseases and the loss of productivity caused therein cost the country almost Rs.13,500/- crores annually, which more than offsets all the benefits accruing in the form of revenue and employment generated by tobacco industry." In this view of the matter, when this petition under Article 32 of the Constitution of India came for orders on 31st August, 2001, we have passed order for implementing 1975 Act. At that time of hearing, learned Attorney General as well as counsel for the parties submitted that considering harmful effect of smoking, smoking in public places is required to be prohibited. On this submission, we sought response of the Central Government. As no affidavit was filed during the stipulated time by the Central Government, on 28th September, 2001, we were required to adjourn the matter. Today also, when the matter came up for hearing, no response is filed on behalf of the Central Government. However, learned Attorney General with all emphasis at his command submitted that appropriate order banning smoking in public places be passed. Learned counsel for the petitioner also submitted to the aforesaid effect. Counsel appearing for other respondents also supported the same. In the petition, it is pointed out that tobacco smoke contains harmful contents including nicotine, tar, potential carcinogens, carbon monoxide, irritants, asphyxiates and smoke particles which are the cause of many diseases including the cancer. It is alleged that three million people die every year as a result of illness related to the use of tobacco products of which one million people belong to developing countries like India. The World Health Organization is stated to have estimated that tobacco related deaths can rise to a whopping seven million per year. According to this organization, in the last half century in the developing countries alone smoking has killed more than sixty million people. Tobacco smoking also adds to the air pollution. Besides cancer, tobacco smoking is responsible for various other fatal diseases to the mankind. It is further submitted that statutory provisions are being made for prohibiting smoking in public places and the Bill introduced in the Parliament is pending consideration before a Select Committee. The State of Rajasthan has claimed to have passed Act No.14 of 2000 to provide for prohibition of smoking in place of public work or use and in public service vehicles for that State. It is stated that in Delhi also there is prohibition of smoking in public places. Learned Attorney General for India submits and all the counsel appearing for the other parties agree that considering the adverse effect of smoking in public places, it would be in the interests of the citizens to prohibit the smoking in public places till the statutory provision is made and implemented by the legislative enactment. The persons not indulging in smoking cannot be compelled to or subjected to passive smoking on account of acts of the smokers. Realizing the gravity of the situation and considering the adverse effect of smoking on smokers and passive smokers, we direct and prohibit smoking in public places and issue directions to the Union of India, State Governments as well as the Union Territories to take effective steps to ensure prohibiting smoking in public places, namely:

1. Auditoriums
2. Hospital buildings
3. Health institutions
4. Educational institutions
5. Libraries
6. Court buildings
7. Public office
8. Public conveyances, including railways.

Learned Attorney General for India assured the court that Union of India shall take necessary effective steps to give wide publicity to this order by electronic as well as print media to make the general public aware of this order of prohibition of smoking. We further direct the Registrar General to intimate the State Governments/Union Territories as well as the Commissioners of Police as mentioned in our orders dated 31st August, 2001 and 28th September, 2001 of this Court with directions for submission of their compliance report in this Court within five weeks from today. Union of India shall also file its response at the earliest. List after six weeks..........

(M.B. Shah)

New Delhi,

November 2, 2001. (R.P. Sethi)

Cigarettes and Other Tobacco Products (Prohibition of Advertisement and Regulation of Trade and Commerce, Production, Supply and Distribution) Act, 2003.

CHAPTER 12

# Tobacco Use: 2020 and Beyond

*"There will be 1 billion deaths from tobacco in the 21st century unless strong and sustained action is taken now."*

— Richard Peto and Alan Lopez, 2002

With the dawn of new millennium, in the first decade of the new century, one tends to think how the future is like to be. On the basis of the current trends, one is inspired to speculate the likely comforts and the threats the future may possibly offer. These speculations, both at individual level and the national and global level provide a direction for further action and taking necessary steps wherever needed. Indian scholars, policy-makers, media persons and others like anywhere in the world made such speculations about the future India by identifying the forces that are likely to shape the country. In none of these forecasts was the threat of tobacco ever identified as a clear and present danger that would grow to endanger India's developmental efforts in the twenty-first century. Yet, that is the reality we have to contend with, as we envision the future. Tobacco control, therefore, becomes imperative for urgent multi-sectoral action, as we resolve to remove the threats and enhance the opportunities for India's unimpeded development.

Tobacco is truly a global problem presented by the European navigators and the explorers in an epoch propitious toward receiving it as a panacea to the world. It provided countless options for experimentation to be used in different ways, however, its smoking as cigarette culminated in most widely prevalent form all over the globe. No wonder cigarette is most widely studied due to this reason only. Cigarette is the most common preventable cause of morbidity and mortality. In India and other Asian countries smokeless tobacco in the form of chewing is also quite common which is sold in attractive packing. Tobacco is a form of marketed malady and its use has become engineered addiction promoted by tobacco companies. The multinational tobacco industry operating at the global level promotes and profits from the deadly tobacco trade. Such a global threat is bound to have far reaching consequences if appropriate measures are not adopted to counter the threat with a global thrust.

### *Number of tobacco users will increase in developing countries*

According to the Economic and Social Council (ECOSOC) of United Nations Report 2002,[1] there will be 1% annual decline in the prevalence of tobacco use world-wide. In developed countries an increasing awareness of damaging health effects of smoking together with the anti-smoking measures, banning of advertising and increased taxation, have had a strong negative effect on consumption of tobacco products. Therefore, tobacco demand in developing countries is decreasing and will reach about 2.05 million tons in 2010. Consumption of tobacco in these countries was 10% in 1998 when consumption was 2.23 million tons. Slower population increase and growth in income are also the contributory factors.

In the developing countries, tobacco consumption is expected to rise to 5.09 million tons by 2010 as against 4.2 million tons in 1998 at the annual growth rate of 1.7% during this period. Maximum increase in demand is expected to occur in China. The share of China in total world tobacco demand is likely to remain around 37% in 2010.

However, the absolute number of persons smoking tobacco and the amount of tobacco smoked will increase in the developing countries such as India because of the following reasons:

(i) The population size will increase in these countries at a rate higher than the rate of decline in the prevalence of tobacco use. Therefore, the absolute number of people will increase.

(ii) There will be a progressive rise in per capita income levels in the developing countries. It will provide more disposable money to be spent on tobacco consumption. A steady shift in the production sites of tobacco to developing country locations will decrease the local cost of tobacco products. Purchasing power of people will increase and there will be more tobacco smokers.

(iii) Tobacco companies, after decline of tobacco consumption in the developed countries, are diverting their energy to the developing countries as their potential costumers. Aggressive attempts by the multinational tobacco companies to expand their sales in the developing countries in order to compensate for declined sale in the developed world, will be an additional reason that the prevalence of tobacco use will increase in the developing countries.

Table 1 depicts the prevalence of smoking in 2002 and the estimated number of smokers in the years 2020 and 2050 at reduced and constant prevalence rates.

---

[1] United Nations Economic and Social Council. Report of the Secretary-General of the Ad Hoc Inter-Agency Task Force on Tobacco Control, E/2002/44, New York, 2002.

*Table 1: Current and projected estimates of the number of smokers by country category and year (2000, 2020 and 2050) for alternate scenarios of reduced and constant prevalence rates.*

| *Country category (by level of development)* | *Number of smokers (millions) at reduced prevalence (-1% per year)* | | | *Number of smokers (millions) at constant prevalence.* | |
|---|---|---|---|---|---|
| | 2000 | 2020 | 2050 | 2020 | 2050 |
| Developed | 196.5 | 177.0 | 134.7 | 216.4 | 222.6 |
| Developing | 977.4 | 1055.2 | 1093.4 | 1290.1 | 1807.2 |
| Economies in transition | 108.0 | 90.1 | 60.4 | 110.2 | 99.8 |
| Total World | 1282.5 | 1385.1 | 1341.8 | 1693.5 | 2217.9 |

**Source:** *ECOSOC Report, 2002.*

The population in India is likely to grow by about 300 million between 2000 and 2020. Most of the increase in the number of people will be in the age group of 15 to 59 years. This is the most vulnerable age group to acquire and continue tobacco use. Even if the tobacco use falls globally by 1% as per estimates of ECOSOC modeling, there is likely to be a net annual increase in the absolute number of persons consuming tobacco in India. By 2050, this will translate into a large burden of deaths and disability arising from tobacco-related diseases. If the tobacco control programme does not yield the desired results and the prevalence of tobacco use remains the same or the decline is less than the projected 1% per year, the situation would be even more grim. With the fall in the domestic price of the tobacco products, the situation will further worsen.

Because of decline in tobacco consumption in the developed countries, India's ability to export tobacco to the world market is diminishing. The tobacco markets in the developing countries are being increasingly captured by transnational tobacco companies, which operate from developed countries. In such a case, the surplus of tobacco produced in India will aggressively seek an increase in the internal market, in one form or the other. It is not surprising that the large-scale increase in the manufacture and sale of oral tobacco products in India coincided with the fall of India's tobacco exports to countries belonging to the erstwhile Soviet bloc. Tobacco production continues unabated and as tobacco exports decline, India would experience the worst situation of increasing number of people using tobacco and falling victim to its deadly effects over the next half century. India will fall victim of its own agricultural success in tobacco. The situation demands the implementation of vigorous demand-reduction measures.

Between 80,000 and 99,000 children and adolescents in the world take to smoking everyday who get lured by the glare and glamour of tobacco advertising and tobacco marketing that sells a deadly product as the taste of fashion and freedom[2]. Presented in attractive packets depicting some celebrities using them, the tobacco products are sold to young people who easily identify with these celebrities and get hooked to use of these tobacco products.

According to National Organization for Tobacco Eradication (NOTE) about 6,000 teenagers start using tobacco products in India every day[3]. Advertisement, peer pressure, availability and the curiosity to experiment are the main reasons for initiation. It is estimated that out of 100 teenagers smoking today, 50 will eventually die of tobacco related diseases in times to come. Two-third of country's smoking population begin at an early age and by the time they realize the risk, they become addicted to it.

As per estimates there are about 1.3 billion tobacco users worldwide of which approximately one billion men and more than 250 million women consume almost 6 trillion sticks of cigarettes (and *beedis)* annually or 15 billion sticks every day. If the current trends continue, it is expected that by 2025, the number of tobacco users will be 1.6 billion[3].

## Tobacco Mortality

Worldwide, 1.3 billion people smoke and, unless urgent action is taken, 650 million of them will die prematurely due to tobacco use in the next 30–50 years. Half of these deaths will occur in productive middle age thus robbing the dying individuals of 20 to 25 years of life. Tobacco is estimated to have caused 3 million deaths a year in early 1990s, one in six deaths in late 1990s[4] and death toll is steadily increasing and it is currently responsible for the deaths of one in 10 adults worldwide (about five million deaths each year). If current smoking patterns continue, by 2020, tobacco will cause one out of three deaths and some ten million deaths each year by 2025[5]. 70% of these deaths will be in the developing countries alone. By 2030, tobacco is expected to be the single biggest cause of death worldwide, accounting for more than 10 million deaths each year – more than total of deaths from malaria, maternal and major childhood conditions, and tuberculosis combined[6].

Worldwide, the only two major causes of death whose effects are now increasing rapidly are HIV and tobacco. If current tobacco use patterns persist, there will be one billion deaths

---

2 WHO Press Release (2000) European Union Directive Banning Tobacco Advertising Overturned: WHO urged concerted response.

3 India Vision 2020; New Delhi: Planning Commission, Government of India, 2002. Available from URL:**http://planning** commission.nic.in/plans/planrel/;l_vsn2020,pdf

4 Curbing the epidemic – Governments and the Economics of Tobacco Control, World Bank, 1999.

5 Tobacco-free Initiative, World Health Organization, 2004.

6 The World Health Report 1999, World Health Organization, Geneva.

from tobacco during 21st century, compared with 100 million during the whole 20th century[7]. 450 million of these one billion deaths will occur in the first 50 years (Peto and Lopez 2001). It is estimated that currently 5 million deaths or 8.8 percent of all deaths are caused by tobacco related morbidity every year globally of which about 1 million deaths occur in China alone[8]. Most of the tobacco attributed deaths worldwide in 1990s have occurred in developed countries to the tune of 2 million annually and around 1 million per year in the developing countries (3 million tobacco related deaths globally)[9]. However, the situation is changing rapidly now.

There are two main reasons for this large scale increase in tobacco deaths. First, the world population in middle and old age will increase. Second, the proportion of deaths in middle and old age that is caused by tobacco will increase over the next few decades, due to the delayed effects of the large increase in cigarette smoking among young adults over the past few decades (Peto *et al.,* 1999). Among cigarette smokers, the risk of death from tobacco in middle or old age is really substantial (about 1 in 2) only for those who start smoking in early adult life (Doll *et al.,* 1994). Hence, when there is a large upsurge in cigarette smoking among the young adults in a particular country, this will produce a large upsurge in tobacco deaths half a century later. The number of deaths from tobacco at the dawn of 21st century is strongly influenced by the number of young adults who took up smoking around 1950 while the number of young adults who are taking up smoking now will strongly influence the number of deaths due to tobacco around the year 2050 and beyond.

Among persons of both genders, the proportion of all deaths attributed to smoking increased overtime. However, the increase is relatively greater in women, resulting in narrowing of gender gap. The main increase in cigarette use by young adults took place during the first half of twentieth century for men in developed countries, but it took place during the second half of the century for the women in developed countries and for men in developing countries (WHO, 1997). For men in developed countries the epidemic of tobacco deaths may already be about as large as it will ever be, with tobacco now responsible for about one-third of all male deaths in middle age (Peto *et al.,* 1994). For women in most developed countries, however, the epidemic still has far to go – indeed in many European countries such as France or Spain the main increase in female tobacco deaths is only just beginning, although in the United States the proportion of death in the middle age that is due to tobacco is now almost as great in women as in men (Peto *et al.,* 1994). Taking both sexes together, US cigarette consumption per adult was 1, 4 and 10 per day in 1910, 1930 and 1950, after which it remained relatively constant for some decades. As a delayed result of this pre-1950 increase in cigarette consumption, the proportion of all US deaths at ages 35–69 attributed to tobacco rose from 12% in 1950 to 33% in 1990.

---

7 World Health Organization. Tobacco or Health? First Global Status Report, Geneva, Switzerland; 1996.

8 Tobacco: Global Trends, ASH (UK) Briefing July, 2001.

9 World Health Organization, An International Treaty of Tobacco Control, 2003.

In the age groups 35–69 years, the proportion of all deaths due to smoking among women increase from 2% in 1955 to 13% in 1995, while among men it increased from 20% to 36%. One in eight female deaths (13%) between the ages of 35 and 69 in developed countries in 1995 was due to smoking, and for men and women combined, each smoker who died in this age group lost significant numbers of life expectancy due to smoking (WHO, 1996). Since the women of the developing countries are the target as the potential customers for the tobacco companies the number of women smokers in the developing countries is likely to increase and hence an increased number of tobacco-related deaths in women in these countries will take place 30–50 years later.

There are wide variations between regions and, in particular, in the prevalence of smoking among women in different regions. In Eastern Europe and Central Asia, 59% of men and 26% of women smoked in 1995, which was more than any other region. In East Asia and the Pacific, where the prevalence of male smokers is equally high, at 59%, just 4% of women were smokers. This gap between men and women smokers is an opportunity, but one that must be grabbed quickly to prevent the epidemic of tobacco deaths in women as being seen in men today. Tobacco related diseases are on the rise among women, particularly younger women. This is not only because more and more women are starting to use tobacco products but also due to the fact that millions are exposed to second hand smoking on daily basis. Second hand smoking is an important women's issue (it is dealt with in a different chapter) and needs to be dealt with seriously. Women everywhere are exposed to second hand smoking and suffer serious health consequences because of it. In the Asian region, where significant numbers of men are smokers, millions of women and children suffer from second hand smoking.

In China, male cigarette consumption averaged 1, 4 and 10 per day in 1952, 1971 and 1992, and the proportion of Chinese male deaths at ages 35–69 attributed to tobacco was measured to be 12% in 1990 and is projected to be 33% in 2030 (Liu *et al.,* 1998 and Niu *et al.,* 1998). Two-thirds of the young men become persistent smokers, and about half of those who do so will eventually be killed by the habit: so, about one-third of all the young men in China will eventually be killed by tobacco, if current smoking patterns continue. About 30% of the world's cigarettes are consumed in China which suffers more than 1 million tobacco deaths every year. This figure is likely to at least double by 2025.

Tobacco threat relates to a rise in the absolute number of tobacco users in India as well as to the proportion of deaths attributable to tobacco. The World Health Organization (WHO) estimates that the proportion of deaths that result from tobacco-related diseases will rise in India, from 1.4 % of all deaths in 1990 to 13.3% of all deaths in 2020 (WHO 2003).

Worldwide, there are now around 5 million deaths a year caused by tobacco but this number reflects smoking patterns several decades ago, and worldwide cigarette smoking has increased substantially over the last fifty years (WHO, 1997). On current smoking patterns, about 30% of the young adults become persistent smokers and relatively few give up. The main diseases by which smoking kills people are substantially different in America (where vascular diseases and lung cancer predominate) (Peto *et al.*, 1994), in China (where chronic obstructive pulmonary disease predominates) (Liu *et al.*, 1998) and in India (where almost half the world's tuberculosis deaths take place, and the ability of smoking to increase the death from TB may well be of particular importance) (Gajalakshmi and Peto, 1999 and Gupta and Mehta, 2000).

There are already 1.3 billion smokers worldwide now, and by 2030 another billion young adults will have started to smoke making tobacco deaths to be around 10 million a year. It will rise somewhat further in the later decades. So, tobacco will cause about 150 million deaths in the first quarter of the 21st century and 300 million in the second quarter. Predictions for the third and, particularly, the fourth quarter of the 21st century are inevitably somewhat speculative, but if over the next few decades about a quarter or a third of the young adults become persistent smokers and about half of them are eventually killed due to tobacco, then about 15% of the adult mortality in the second half of the century will be due to tobacco, implying 600–900 million tobacco deaths in 2050–2099 (Peto and Lopez, 2000).

The number of tobacco deaths before 2050 cannot be greatly reduced unless a substantial proportion of the adults who have already been smoking for some time give it up. For, a decrease over a next decade or two in the proportion of children who become smokers will not have its main effects on mortality unless the third quarter of the century. If many of the adults who now smoke were to give up over the next decade or two, halving global cigarette consumption per adult by the year 2020, then this would prevent about one-third of the tobacco deaths in 2020 and would almost halve tobacco deaths in the second quarter of the century. Such changes would avoid about 20 or 30 million tobacco deaths in the first quarter of the century and would avoid about 150 million in the second quarter. This dream can only be fulfilled if some effective tobacco-cessation measures are adopted.

If, by progressive reduction over the next decade or two in the global uptake rate of smoking by young people, the proportion of young adults who become smokers were to be halved by 2020, then this would avoid hundreds of millions of deaths from tobacco after 2050. It would, however, avoid almost none of the 150 million deaths from tobacco in the first quarter of the century, and would probably avoid 10 or 20 million of the 300 million deaths from tobacco in the second quarter of the century.

## The Future of the Global Tobacco Treaty Negotiations

The tobacco business is fundamentally a global enterprise. The sale of raw leaf and the manufactured tobacco products, the smuggling of cigarettes to evade taxes, and the effects of print and television advertising all cross national borders. The consequences of this enterprise are staggering – by the year 2025, an estimated 10 million people will die annually from tobacco-related diseases, 70% of them from the developing countries.

To respond to this global public health crisis, in 1995 the World Health Assembly of the WHO explored the feasibility of an International Treaty on Tobacco Control and create a global mechanism to counter the political influence of the tobacco industry. In May 1999, WHO's Framework Convention on Tobacco Control (FCTC) provided the basic tool for the countries to enact comprehensive tobacco control legislation and take on the powerful tobacco industry. The treaty commits nations to ban all tobacco advertising, promotion, and sponsorship (with an exception of constitutional constraints) and to require large warning labels covering at least 30% of the display area of the cigarette pack.

The Framework Convention on Tobacco Control (FCTC) was adopted by its 192 member states calling for an international attempt to regulate tobacco use; a record breaking 50 countries out of 192 pledged financial and political support. In adopting and signing the treaty, the WHO's member states have expressed their firm commitment to tackle the public health challenges posed by tobacco and have resolved to address issues such as price and tax measures, cross-border smuggling, tobacco advertising and promotion, and people's right to clean indoor air.

The Treaty became international law on 27th February, 2005 on completion of 40 ratifications which was the minimum requirement for the FCTC to enter into force. On 26th May, 2006, of the 168 signatories of FCTC, 128 countries have ratified it.

As stated in the Preamble of the treaty, the objective of the FCTC is "to protect present and future generations from the devastating health, social, environmental and economic consequences of tobacco consumption and exposure to tobacco smoke." The preamble also recognizes the need for countries to give priority to their right to protect public health. The FCTC requires all parties to undertake a comprehensive ban on tobacco advertising, promotion and sponsorship within five years of ratifying the treaty. FCTC's crucial role in fighting tobacco menace is bound to provide desirable results in times to come.

## Future of Tobacco Industry

Anti-tobacco activists generally speculate and argue that in a gigantic Armageddon of US super-litigation, tobacco industry has no future and it will witness shrinkage in times to come due to vast expenditure on lawsuits. Others feel that the industry is likely to survive even the most severe litigation assaults. Even the worst judgments will leave the tobacco industry intact. But suppose the courts did deliver that knockout or the companies could not raise prices because foreign tobacco companies not involved in the litigation entered the market. This means the companies have to find the money from shareholders rather than customers. Even if litigation could take down Philip Morris, it would be *shareholders* that lost everything. But the most valuable entity owned by the shareholders is the Philip Morris (PM) business and its global brand Marlboro with a market value of US$82 billion. They would have to sell the tobacco business as a going concern complete with the existing factories, distribution channels, management, and brands. The pension funds, mutuals, and individuals that currently own PM shares would take the hit. The company would go on, though with different owners.

Litigation will continue to have many benefits and rich rewards, not least as a rolling "truth machine" and a reason for the companies to overhaul their business practices. However, it cannot stop the sale of a product that people want or need to buy, nor can it eliminate the inherent value in a big business run as a growing concern able to meet the demand.

Diversification in completely new businesses will not prove to be a commercial reality for the main companies involved because there is no advantage to non-tobacco business to be merged with tobacco[10]. The problem with the diversification is that the benefits flow one way. Pure tobacco stocks are volatile and prone to regulatory or litigation risks. For a tobacco business, a merger with a food or financial services operation helps to dampen the fluctuations in the overall stock price. The problem is that it is hard to see any advantages to a viable food or financial services business in being merged with tobacco. Not only is there the volatility of the tobacco part of the business and the risk that all the assets will be seized to pay for tobacco litigation claims, but also boycotts, management distraction, shareholder actions and so on.

Diversification only really works where there is a synergistic advantage in which the parts of the conglomerate benefit from being part of the whole. Some of the tobacco brands could be valuable to other businesses, but the problem for the tobacco companies is that the governments are clamping down on tobacco advertising and rightly suspect that so-called brand diversification is mainly an attempt to circumvent tobacco advertising restrictions[11].

Regulators will assert proper jurisdiction over tobacco and force the companies to make products that are less harmful by setting emissions limits and product standards – for example, to reduce or remove carbon monoxide, carcinogenic nitrosamines, or many other toxins in tobacco smoke. Over time the delivery of nicotine through tobacco will evolve from combustion, through heating and oral use, and eventually to extracts and purified distillates.

Before describing a possible future for tobacco, it is necessary to name some unlikely culprits behind the epidemic of tobacco related disease. It is believed the pharmaceutical regulators are responsible for thousands and maybe millions of unnecessary tobacco related deaths. It is a shocking truth, but perverse regulation of the market for nicotine has granted an unregulated monopoly to the worst, most deadly suppliers of the tobacco industry.

---

10 WHO Press Release No.27, 30th March, 2001.

11 Tob Control 2000; **9**:237-238 ( Summer ).

Nicotine the psychoactive chemical is likely to become recognized as the real "product". The tobacco companies will face competition from new forms of nicotine delivery unconnected with tobacco and will have to respond by using the power of their brands to move into this market. It is speculated that nicotine will continue to be widely used in society and many will be addicted, but the risk to users will be reduced; atleast the option to reduce risk will be available. Concern about "addiction" rather than "disease" will become the defining reason not to use nicotine. Concern about "addiction followed by disease" will become the dominant reason not to smoke tobacco.

There has to be a clear distinction between the use of the drug nicotine and the harm caused by its manner of delivery. This is a crucial distinction. Health promotion efforts have implicitly tried to tackle the harm and the underlying drug use simultaneously. This approach has had some success with some groups in some societies. The problem is the remaining people who continue to take nicotine by smoking tobacco. For them, it is possible to tackle the harm caused by the manner of delivery independently of the drug syndrome. This is not to say that nicotine dependence should not be tackled, but "drug problems" are social phenomena and should be tackled by addressing the underlying socioeconomic and cultural causes, backed up with treatment for dependence.

The impetus for change will come from steady regulatory pressure on the harm caused by nicotine delivery through tobacco smoke. We already know there are many patents and techniques for reducing toxins in tobacco smoke for example, to remove nitrosamines, carbon monoxide, phenols, hydrogen cyanide, and many more. This would be the start of a long process of "purifying" nicotine delivery. Smokers take the nicotine they need from smoke, but they inhale the toxins that come with the nicotine. By reducing the concentration of toxins in the smoke *relative to nicotine* the smoke will become genuinely less hazardous unlike so-called low tar cigarettes. Continuous regulatory pressure would force innovation in tobacco product design that would suggest an evolution from burning to heating tobacco, and then perhaps into products which are sucked or chewed, or the active ingredients extracted and repackaged.

In parallel, it is necessary to open the nicotine market to competitors of Big Tobacco. That means changing the approach of some very entrenched conservative pharmaceutical regulators who have never had to face their de facto complicity in protecting and nurturing tobacco interests. One of the toughest questions with new nicotine products is the extent to which established tobacco control policies, such as taxation, advertising restrictions, and health promotion campaigns should be applied. These products are highly desirable alternatives to smoking tobacco, but they are not safe and are addictive. To compete with tobacco they would have to be marketed, as lifestyle products rather than medicines. At the moment, the regulatory approach is "reckless extreme caution" in the shape of a total ban on competitive nicotine products that offers the entire market to tobacco.

## Tobacco and the Millennium Development Goals (MDGs)

The Millennium Development Goals (MDGs) concretely defines 8 goals which the international community promised to achieve by 2015. The improvement of public health, which is central to the achievement of most of the MDGs, is directly threatened by the increase in tobacco consumption in the following ways:

1. **Eradication of extreme poverty and hunger:** Tobacco use contributes substantially to malnutrition, disability and other major causes of poverty. In Bangladesh, over 10.5 million malnourished people can have an adequate diet if money spent on tobacco is spent on food instead, saving the lives of 350 children under age 5 each day. Among lower income households in Egypt, more than 10% of household expenditures go to cigarettes or other forms of tobacco.

2. **Achievement of universal primary education:** Money spent by poor households on tobacco is money that cannot be spent on education, depriving people of educational opportunities that could help them lift out of poverty. Currently the poorest households in Bangladesh spend almost 10 times as much on tobacco as they do on education. The labour-intensive nature of tobacco production means that in many tobacco-producing countries, children work in the tobacco fields rather than attend school.

3. **Promotion of gender equality and empowerment of women:** The number of women who smoke is expected to nearly triple over the next generation to more than 500 million. The vast majourity of this increase will occur in low-and-middle income countries, where tobacco companies are focusing slick advertising campaigns that portray smoking as part of women's freedom, emancipation and empowerment. The rise in smoking rates among women poses a significant threat to advances in the economic and health status of women.

4. **Reduction in child mortality:** Children born to women who smoked during pregnancy have lower birth-weight than those born to non-smoking women. Exposure to tobacco in utero is a major cause of spontaneous abortion, still-birth and neo-natal mortality, and is a likely cause of sudden infant death syndrome (SIDS).

5. **Improvement in maternal health:** Women who smoke are at much higher risk of cardiovascular disease, chronic obstructive pulmonary disease, as well as lung cancer, oral cancer and cervical cancer. Smoking during pregnancy seriously compromises maternal health and is a major cause of complications in pregnancy, premature births, stillbirths and low birth weight delivery. It is also associated with long-term developmental and behavioural problems among children of smokers.

6. **Combating HIV/AIDS, malaria and other diseases:** Smokers with the HIV virus develop full-blown AIDS twice as quickly as nonsmokers[12]. Tobacco use also

---

[12] US Department of Health and Human Services, "Tips for Teens: The Truth about AIDS." http://www.health.org/govpub/PHD725/

promotes the onset and outcome of tuberculosis, a disease that mainly affects the poor. In India, a recent study shows that half of the all male TB deaths can be attributed to tobacco[13].

7. **Ensuring Environmental sustainability:** About 200,000 hectares of forest are cut down every year around the world to make way for tobacco farming and wood to cure tobacco[14]. Tobacco growing requires large amounts of harmful pesticides and fertilizers. Cigarette manufacturing also creates an enormous amount of solid waste.
8. **Developing a global partnership for development:** Governments, international agencies, NGOs, donors and others need to work together to ensure that tobacco control gets the funding and political attention it deserves. The entry into force of the Framework Convention on Tobacco Control (FCTC) should provide new impetus for strengthening these global partnerships and spurring others to get involved in both funding and capacity building.

Enhanced support by the international donors for tobacco control efforts in low and middle income countries could possibly reverse this tragedy, while helping to achieve the ambitious Millennium Development Goals (MDGs) that the international community has agreed upon. Joint effort by the concerned can save the world from this marketed tragedy of a communicated disease.

**At National Level**

There are several ways in which menace of tobacco can be countered and diminished, if there is a political will and collective societal commitment to strengthen tobacco control in India. This can be accomplished with following steps to be taken:

1. **Taxes on all tobacco products are raised:** In 2002, the excise tax revenue from tobacco was around Rs 5600 crores (Rs 56 billion), which was derived mostly from taxes on cigarettes constituting only 14% of India's tobacco market. *Beedis* and oral tobacco products were virtually untouched. If these sectors are also included under the ambit of taxation a large sum of revenue can be generated. Even if a total ban were to be imposed on manufacture and sale of oral tobacco products, the taxation of smoked tobacco products (cigarettes and *beedis*) alone could produce an additional revenue of Rs 6000 crores (Rs 60 billion) through a combination of excise tax parity and an earmarked cess.

---

13 Gajalakshmi V *et al.*, "Smoking and Mortality from Tuberculosis and Other Diseases in India: Retrospective study of 43000 adult male deaths and 35000 controls." The Lancet 2003; 362 (9391):1243-1244. http://www.pranjnopaya.org/pdf/indiapdf

14 World Health Organization, Tobacco and Poverty: A Vicious Cycle (2004). http://www.who.int/tobacco/resources/publications/wntd/2004/en/index.htm

2. **Additional revenue generated is spent on social sector initiatives:** The money generated is utilized for the welfare of the poor and effective tobacco control programmes. Since poor are the predominant tobacco consumers in India, it is sometimes argued that increased tax burden on tobacco products would adversely affect the poor. Apart from the fact that increased tobacco taxes would raise tobacco product prices and thereby, reduce consumption of these harmful products (especially by the poor who are more price-sensitive), the best way to counter the argument is to spend a large fraction of tobacco tax revenue on social sector programmes especially intended to benefit the poor. Investment in education and alleviating poverty will address the main social determinants of tobacco use and help vulnerable groups to escape the curse of tobacco addiction. Rest of the money could be utilized in strengthening tobacco-cessation programmes. The creation of such a large fund for tobacco control will also enable the Central Government to provide adequate resources to the states for undertaking effective tobacco control programmes.

3. **Ban is imposed on oral tobacco products:** Because of various political and economic reasons it may not be possible to impose ban on all tobacco products in the country, however, ban on oral tobacco products could be a feasible option. Though these products are relatively new in the Indian market they are rapidly victimizing people to their addiction especially the women and children who are otherwise deterred from smoking by social taboo but can chew tobacco without such inhibitions. Low priced and easy to carry pouches of smokeless tobacco products are easily accessible to children. Moreover, ban on smoking in public places does not extend to smokeless tobacco products and can be freely used anywhere and everywhere. High rates of oral cancer are likely to result at younger ages from such addictions becoming established in children and young adults. India has the highest prevalence of oral cancers in the world and a ban on oral tobacco products would be a relevant step in the direction of tobacco control programme. Very few countries manufacture oral tobacco products and none on the scale that India does. Countries such as Australia have banned the manufacture and importation of oral tobacco products and have effectively prevented their entry through smuggling. Ban on these products in India can raise the possibility of smuggling from other countries which has to be effectively dealt with. While the whole world is struggling with the mistake of having permitting smoked tobacco products to become established as legal commodities before their harm was adequately recognized, India can at least take steps to eliminate the most recent entrant into the market, on the grounds of manifest and potential threat to health.

4. **Enforcement of existing laws and regulations is strengthened:** The comprehensive and powerful Anti-tobacco Act of 2003 which is in conformity with the Framework Convention on Tobacco Control (FCTC) needs to be effectively implemented. Law enforcing agencies, both at central and state level should be

strengthened quantitatively as well as qualitatively. This would mean involvement in periodic training, establishment of easy reporting and early response systems to deal with violations, coordination mechanisms for concerted efforts by different enforcement agencies and monitoring methods for evaluating success and failures. Community mobilization by creating awareness is equally important in effective implementation of the law.

5. **Coordinating mechanisms at central and state levels are established:** Tobacco control programme involves multi-sectoral actions at multiple levels. This requires efficient planning, effective coordination and close monitoring. A national coordinating body needs to be constituted.

6. **People are mobilized through mass education and community empowerment:** Community participation and public support is essential for effective implementation in a society. It is essential, therefore, to increase the knowledge, motivation and skills of the people through mass education, and to create strong community-level coalitions to combat tobacco through government-supported civil society action. Media can play an effective role in this effort.

7. **Tobacco-cessation programme is promoted:** If we really wish to reduce tobacco-related burden by 2020, it is absolutely essential to promote tobacco cessation effectively and extensively, as most of the burden of death and disease due to tobacco over the next two decades would arise from current consumers of tobacco. Success in tobacco-cessation would yield early benefits in terms of reduced cardiovascular death rates, as the risk of heart disease is substantially reduced (close to normal) by stopping smoking for three years. The cancer risk is lowered more slowly. Counseling services for tobacco-cessation need to be made available at primary health care level. Research needs to identify cessation techniques which are especially appropriate for oral tobacco users and young persons, since most of the available global cessation research has focused on adult smoking.

8. **Import of tobacco products is restricted in the country:** India can effectively restrict the entry of tobacco products from other countries by setting stringent regulatory standards for domestic tobacco products, which the foreign tobacco products have to match. Even if some of the foreign manufacturers comply with these regulations, their uniform application to both foreign and domestic tobacco products will ensure a strong and effective regulatory environment which will, in turn influence domestic consumption.

9. **Land under tobacco cultivation is progressively reduced:** When there is lesser consumption of tobacco, there will be lesser demand and hence reduced production of tobacco over time. However, the aggressive attempts of the tobacco industry to fully utilize the domestic production of tobacco to produce a variety of tobacco products as well as interventions by the government to provide distress subsidies to tobacco farmers may delay such a market response. It will be in the

interest of tobacco control if the supply of tobacco is also reduced, alongside effective measures to reduce the demand. The land under tobacco cultivation may be progressively reduced, by encouraging farmers to switch to alternative crops. It is essential that steps are also taken to ensure that this reduction in domestic supply is not compensated by entry of tobacco from other countries. This can be done through a strong regulatory regime and well-designed import restrictions which will not attract the censure of World Trade Organization (WTO).

Future predictions are by their nature speculative but some things are certain: the tobacco epidemic, with its attendant health and economic burden, is both increasing and also shifting from developed to developing nations; and more women are smoking.

The industry is consolidating, and also shifting from the West to developing regions, where there may be less government control and public debate about the role of transnational tobacco companies.

The future looks bleak; the global tobacco epidemic is worse today than it was 50 years ago. And it will be even worse in another 50 years unless an extraordinary effort is made now. Several countries have already shown that smoking rates can be reduced. These successes can be reproduced by any responsible nation, but only through immediate, determined, and sustained governmental and community action. The future epidemic depends on understanding of the issue, and policies, politics and actions taken today.

### *What Needs to be Done*

It is the responsibility of the Government to initiate legislative and administrative measures to control tobacco menace at the national level which requires multi-sectoral action by several different government agencies. The Union Government of India should undertake following measures:

1. A co-ordination committee to develop, implement and monitor a National Programme for Tobacco Control (NPTC) should be constituted to integrate demand-reduction and supply-reduction strategies.
2. National Regulatory Authority for regulating the constituents and emissions of tobacco products should be established.
3. An independent National Laboratory for testing of tobacco products free from the influence of tobacco industry should be established.
4. The existing laws to control tobacco should be effectively implemented and new laws be enacted to curb cross-border advertising. To reduce tobacco consumption through price mechanisms, a progressively increasing tax policy should be adopted for all tobacco products.
5. Tobacco industry and tobacco farming should be discouraged by discontinuing direct and indirect subsidies and financial incentives.

6. Government should establish partnership with civil society organizations and the private sector for advancing the implementation of the NPTC.
7. Government should levy an earmarked tobacco cess, whose revenue would be utilized for strengthening health programmes in the country.
8. A National Coordinating Body with all stakeholders to be its members (except tobacco industry) to guard and monitor the implementation of NPTC needs to be established.
9. The NTPC should be integrated with other national health programmes.
10. A nationwide surveillance system for monitoring the patterns of tobacco products, consumption among different population groups and trends in major tobacco-related diseases, along with systems for monitoring the determinants of tobacco consumption should be established.

## REFERENCES

Doll R, Peto R, Wheatley K. Gray R. and Sutherland I.: Mortality in Relation to Smoking: 40 Years Observations on Male British Doctors. *British Medical Journal*; 309:901–911, 1994.

Gajalakshmi C.K. and Peto R.: Retrospective Study of 48,000 Deaths in Chennai (Madras) , India. In: *Proceedings of the XV Asian Pacific Cancer Conference*, Chennai, 1999.

Gupta P.C. and Mehta HC: A Cohort Study of all Cause Mortality Among Tobacco Users in Mumbai, India. *International Journal of Public Health*, 2000.

Liu B.Q., Peto R. Chen ZM. Boreham J. Wu YPLi J.Y., Campbell T.C. and Chen J.S.: Emerging tobacco hazards in China: 1. Retrospective Proportional Mortality Study of one Million Deaths. *British Medical Journal*; 317:1411–1422, 1998.

Niu S.R.; Yang G.H.; Chen Z.M.; Wang J.L.; Wang G.H.; He X.Z.; Schoepff H.;Boreham J.; Pan H.C. and Peto R. Emerging Tobacco Hazards in China: 2. Early Mortality Results from a Prospective Study. *British Medical Journal;* 317:1423–1424, 1998.

Peto R.; Chen Z.M. and Boreham J.: Tobacco – The Growing Epidemic. *Nature Medicine*; 5:15–17, 1999.

Pet R. and Lopez A.D.: The Future Worldwide Health Effects of Current Smoking Patterns. In: Global Health in 21st Century (eds) Everette Koop by Jossey-Bass, New York, 2000.

Peto R. Lopez A.D.: Future Worldwide Health Effects of Current Smoking Patterns. In: Koop CD; Schwarz MR eds. *Critical Issues in Global Health*. Jossey-Bass, New York, 2001.

Peto R. Lopez A.D. Boreham J. Thun M. and Heath C. Jr: Mortality from Smoking in Developed Countries 1950–2000: *Indirect Estimates from National Statistics*. Oxford University Press, 1994.

World Health Organization: A Global Status Report. World Health Organization, Geneva, 1997.

# INDEX

## A



## B



## C

## O



## P



## Q



## R

## S



## T

## U



## V



## W



## Y



## Z